PSYCHIATRIC/ MENTAL HEALTH NURSING

Second Edition

PSYCHIATRIC/ MENTAL HEALTH NURSING

Contemporary Readings

Barbara A. Backer, M.S., M.A., R.N.
Patricia M. Dubbert, PH.D., R.N.
Elaine J. P. Eisenman, M.S., R.N.

Wadsworth Health Sciences Division
Monterey, California

Sponsoring Editor: *Aline Faben*
Production Editor: *Constance D. Brown*
Manuscript Editor: *Jaqueline Isabell*
Permissions Editor: *Mary Kay Hancharick*
Interior and Cover Design: *Lois Stanfield*
Typesetting: *Instant Type, Monterey, California*
Printing and Binding: *Malloy Lithographing, Inc., Ann Arbor, Michigan*

Wadsworth Health Sciences Division
A Division of Wadsworth, Inc.

Printed in the United States of America

10 9 8 7 6 5 4 3 2

Library of Congress Cataloging in Publication Data

Main entry under title:

Psychiatric/mental health nursing.

   Articles reprinted from various sources.
   Includes bibliographies.
   1. Psychiatric nursing—Addresses, essays, lectures.
I. Backer, Barbara A.   II. Dubbert, Patricia M.
III. Eisenman, Elaine J. P.   [DNLM: 1. Psychiatric Nursing—collected
works. WY 160 P97205]
RC440.P739 1985   610.73'68   84-29937
ISBN 0-534-04644-4

Foreword

IN THE PAST THIRTY years we have seen the field of psychiatric nursing develop from its almost unlettered unfancy into a highly sophisticated entity. That psychiatric nursing has come a long way in these three decades is well exemplified in this excellent anthology whose contents, for the most part, are derived from nursing literature and describe nursing practice. The progress made by psychiatric nurses in this period has changed the image of the psychiatric nurse from one who worked with psychiatric patients as custodian and carer for physical ills to that of a therapist—intervening on the basis of psychosocial and physiological assessments.

Rather than repeat what is readily available in other books, the editors have focused on the "how to" of psychiatric nursing. In selecting papers which apply theoretical concepts to actual clinical situations the editors have deliberately focused on the set of observations necessary before the nurse can put theory into action. To this end they have included an excellent section on the gathering of data—the first step in the solution of any problem, including problems in relationships. In this section, as in the others, the selection of articles is both comprehensive and finite and suggests that the book's contents will stimulate one's thinking to answer such questions as—who is the patient, what does the nurse need to know, and what is the scope of the nurse's practice. These themes are present throughout the book as a variety of modes of intervention are discussed by each author.

The articles in this book should provide a needed resource for nursing students and practitioners. They will also serve to provide information to other professionals about the nature of psychiatric nursing.

Claire M. Fagin, Ph.D., R.N.

Preface

THIS BOOK IS FOR all nurses who encounter problem behaviors in their clients. Although the focus is on clients who are labelled psychiatric patients, one does not have to be on a psychiatric unit to encounter patients who are manipulative, abused, depressed, alcoholic, or hallucinating. And nurses who work in all kinds of settings need supportive supervision and stress management skills. As in the first edition, our primary goal has been to build a collection of articles that illustrates the many exciting facets of contemporary psychiatric/mental health nursing. In doing this, we selected articles that are relevant for a wide audience—not just psychiatric nurses and students in psychiatric nursing courses or graduate programs. The articles in this book were chosen because they provide scientifically based, practical suggestions, which nurses can use in managing a variety of problem behaviors, and because they provoke readers to think about important issues in working with problem behavior clients. The resulting book is a unique collection of papers that serve as an important resource for graduate nurses who want new ideas for improving their practice and for students making the transition from classroom theory to client interaction.

The second edition includes sixteen new articles by authors of various theoretical persuasion, drawn from many different journals, and seven original contributions for areas that we believe are important, but which were not covered adequately in any single published paper we reviewed. Seven of the journal articles reprinted in the first edition were retained "by popular demand" of educators who had used the text for their courses. The papers vary greatly in style and documentation. Some may not appear at first glance to be contemporary (for example, those published more than 10 years ago). However, some of these papers are classics in psychiatric nursing, and others, although published a number of years ago, still rank among the best for discussing the specific content area. In general, the recent papers are more likely to contain references to research supporting the authors' opinions or suggestions. This trend reflects increasing expectations for scientifically based professional nursing practice. Where such documentation is missing, our readers will find a wealth of opportunities for clinical research or may be encouraged to write updated review articles on that topic.

In this second edition, Unit One includes articles about the nature of psychiatric nursing, including new articles about its historical development, and about the support systems and personal coping skills nurses need to go on giving quality care day after day. Unit Two is devoted to assessment techniques and issues. Units Three and Four, the largest portion of the book, are made up of articles on the management of specific problems encountered in the care of patients; Unit Three focuses on the individual, Unit Four on groups and families. Finally, Unit Five provides a series of thought provoking articles about important unresolved problems and controversial issues in psychiatric/mental health practice, including the possibility of changing the social systems of hospitals.

Barbara A. Backer

Patricia M. Dubbert

Elaine J. P. Eisenman

Contents

Contents

PSYCHIATRIC/ MENTAL HEALTH NURSING

Part One

PSYCHIATRIC/ MENTAL HEALTH NURSING

I t has been said that health-care providers in the area of mental health/illness must learn to live with ambiguity and uncertainty, since this area of practice does not fall as readily and neatly into the cause and effect, treatment and care modalities as other health-care specialties. Practitioners working for the first time in a clinical psychiatric setting may wonder what it is they are supposed to do with and for clients. Initially, the role of the nurse may seem vague and undefined, and role overlap with other members of the interdisciplinary health-care team may evoke feelings of conflict and consternation. Beginning practitioners may ask themselves: "How can I possibly just talk to clients all day?" "What if I don't understand what the client is saying?" "How do I cope with my own feelings of uncertainty, stress, and worry in this setting?"

The first two articles in this unit are written by two leaders in psychiatric/mental health nursing, Claire Fagin and Hildegard Peplau. Although initially published in 1967, Fagin's article continues to offer definitive content regarding the role of the psychiatric nurse. Peplau's article remains timely in its presentation of differentiating psychiatric nursing practice according to educational preparation. The remaining articles discuss various aspects of psychiatric/mental health nursing, including nurse-client collaboration, clinical supervision, and stress management.

Fagin describes the unique role of the nurse in psychiatry and how this role differs from that of therapists in other disciplines. The professional nurse needs to be aware of herself, her feelings, and the expectations of others. An essentially interpersonal philosophy of psychotherapeutic nursing emphasizes the nursing role as one in which the nurse helps the client establish more comfortable interpersonal relationships. The methodology of implementing this role is discussed.

In Peplau's article the distinction is made between the roles of the nurse who has basic nursing education and works in psychiatry and the psychiatric nurse who has specialist or graduate training. Peplau summarizes explanatory theories and concepts of mental illness based on intrapersonal, interpersonal, and systems models in table format. She points out that what nurses may do in any given setting is based not only on the competencies of the nurses but also on the prevailing definition of mental illness in that setting. Definition of interdisciplinary roles, cost of certain types of care, and number of staff available to provide care are also factors that may influence nursing roles.

The significance of collaborative relationships between nurses and clients is the topic of Bayer and Brandner's article. In their description of peer practice in nursing, the authors point out how the nurse and the client work together in the problem-solving process, discovering the client's healthy strengths as well as looking at behavioral responses the client has "chosen" to preserve his or her human system. The nurse and client then look at the client's available choices and solutions. A primary focus in the peer practice of nursing is supporting the health and strengths of the client.

Who provides caring for the caregiver? Benfer discusses the idea that clinical supervision can be utilized as a support system for the caregiver. Mental health professionals may experience many stresses and strains in working with emotionally disturbed clients. How do these caregivers cope with stress and their emotional responses to clients? Benfer suggests that, in order to provide care, the caregiver must experience being cared for. She proposes that clinical supervision, which helps us investigate our own interactions and behaviors with our clients as well as to recognize our own strengths and potential for growth, can be a positive support system.

Nickle-Gallagher utilizes mental health technologies along with Orem's self-care deficit theory of nursing to help clients achieve, maintain, or regain capabilities for managing their own health related self-care. She describes her practice of mental health nursing in a rehabilitation center by presenting her work with one particular client. She clearly makes the point that it was her unique and special education as a mental health nurse that enabled her to provide the individualized care that this client required.

Although some stress is inevitable in most careers, Scott reports that excessive occupational stress is one of the most frequently cited reasons for leaving the field of nursing. Because an event becomes a stressor in relation to our interpretation of that event, we are sometimes responsible for our own stress. Scott provides some guidelines for early identification of stress, such as pinpointing high-risk situations on the job. In nursing, these stressors may include inadequate staffing, client emergencies, and problems in interpersonal relationships. Coping strategies for management of stress, such as relaxation exercises and assertive behavior, are presented. Scott suggests that student nurses may want to look at their current stress levels and coping strategies, since these patterns may very well carry over into their graduate nursing roles.

Chapter One

PSYCHOTHERAPEUTIC NURSING

Claire M. Fagin

PSYCHOTHERAPEUTIC NURSING CONSISTS OF those acts, those interventions through which nurses help patients use new or healthy patterns in consistent and continuous ways. To do this the nurse moves on three avenues of approach: through the milieu, that is, through manipulating the organization of the social system in the patient setting; through her one-to-one relationship with the patient; and through her interactions with groups of patients.

The nurse may work in all these ways simultaneously or in one way exclusively. For example, she may have a one-to-one interview with a patient in a structured setting where she is aware of the social system which affects the patient but is not a part of it. Or the one-to-one relationship may occur within the context of a milieu—home, hospital, or institution of any kind—which the nurse may attempt to change.

The place of treatment need not be the hospital. It could be the home, the community center, the storefront. And within this frame of reference, it is not only the patient who is deemed sick; his family also, as a social system, is seen as functioning in a pathologic way. There is, in other words, an integration constructed within this family unit which serves to elicit and continue disturbing behavior on the part of the patient.

The nurse's intervention with groups of patients also has a specific configuration. Even though she may work with groups of patients in the same structured way as other therapists, she also works with groups of patients and plans intervention with groups on the ward or in the home where the setting is far less structured. It is in these less structured areas that our theoretic frame of reference regarding nursing therapy is not well

From "Psychotherapeutic Nursing," by Claire M. Fagin. Copyright © 1967, American Journal of Nursing Company. Reproduced with permission from *American Journal of Nursing*, February, Vol. 67, No. 2, pp. 298-304.

developed. In the more structured aspects of individual and group interviews, nurses can borrow and adapt from the approaches of other professional workers. However, in our manipulations of the more typical nursing roles, we are less scientific even though we have much pragmatic evidence. But, this has neither been shared nor researched.

For example, seven dimensions of nursing practice may be identified:

Time Spent With Patients.   Nursing personnel live with their patients within the hospital for an entire tour of duty. If we think of the concept of anxiety, it is obvious that one cannot live with anxiety for extended periods—neither patients for their twenty-four-hour day nor nurses for their eight. Nursing personnel must, therefore, be able to intervene in anxiety-producing situations wherever these occur—in the hospital, in the home, or in the clinic.

The Spatial Area.   Nursing personnel have to be able to participate effectively in areas as varied as bedroom, bath, dining room, living room, or recreation area. This is in sharp contrast to the psychiatrist or social worker, whose spatial area generally is structured.

Variety of Patients.   The nurse must relate simultaneously with many individuals who have varying degrees of health and illness with multiple and possibly conflicting needs.

Care for the Whole Patient.   The nurse's ability in relation to patients' physical as well as emotional care needs can be extremely useful in her psychotherapeutic efforts. It can also pose a problem, however, of too great intimacy for the patient and a lack of clarity of role for the nurse. Again, this is in sharp contrast to the psychiatrist or the social worker whose roles tend to remain more or less constant.

Rapid Adjustments.   Throughout her working day, the nurse moves frequently from relating to individual patients to relating to groups of patients. Her effectiveness is determined by her ability to make rapid adjustments to these changes in situations and to creatively utilize and influence the interactions. In other words, the movement from individual therapy to group therapy and vice versa should not be seen as an interference with the relationships but as a learning experience in the daily life of the patients.

Care for Patients as a Group.   Frequently nurses are involved with groups of patients. Group interactions are inherently complex, especially in terms of the meaning of relationships and communications between nurse and patients, patient and patients, and nurse and family.

On-the-Spot Decision Making.   The nurse has to make moment-to-moment decisions, compromises, improvisations, and take risks for prolonged periods of time.

Although each nurse may add to this list on the basis of her own experience, considering these seven dimensions has been useful in thinking through nursing roles and relationships.[1]

To achieve therapeutic effectiveness, the first step the nurse must take is to look at the preconceptions she brings to the situation. What is of particular concern is her concept of illness which, overtly and covertly, influences her philosophy of nursing and her approach to therapy. The nurse must understand the meaning of illness in our society and, more particularly, the meaning of mental illness.

Action for Mental Health.   The report of the Joint Commission on Mental Illness and Health noted sharply that attitudes about mental illness were obstacles to therapeutic efforts. They found an underlying attitude of rejection and disapproval of mental illness and the mentally ill which frequently engendered more rather than less estrangement of the sick person (1). The patient, too, holds these attitudes and, therefore, he tends to reject himself for some of the same reasons that others do: fear of his acts, his destructive impulses, his anger, and his helplessness. Lack of awareness of our own feelings about mental illness and the mentally ill covertly influences our behavior. This is true, of course, of preconceptions in general.

By way of illustration, let's take the preconception some people have of nurses. Occasionally, it is said that nurses are authoritarian and cold hearted. The nurse who is not authoritarian may provoke anxiety in patients who think this. Such a patient comes to the nurse expecting that she will give him answers and tell him what to do. If, instead, the nurse is warm and spontaneous and tries to make decisions *with* the patient instead of *for* the patient, his preconceptions may clash with reality. But if this nurse also notes the cues to the patient's anxiety and tries to understand and clarify with the patient what is going on, there is possibility for growth.

The nurse's concepts and attitudes also are relevant. For example, the nurse working with a specific cultural group needs to examine her preconceptions about this group, test them with reality, and then attempt changes if her findings so dictate.

The recognition and subsequent alteration of one's preconceptions are essential modes of behavior in any area in which the nurse finds herself. And unless she is clear on the degree to which her preconceptions are accurate and on how they influence her thinking, she cannot begin to

---

[1]This list is based on but not identical with that developed through collaborative efforts with Gwen Tudor Will and Agnes Middleton.

be therapeutically effective in any relationship: one-to-one, group, or milieu. Morris Schwartz points out:

> There has been increasing acceptance of the idea that non-organic mental illness is not a disease entity lodged within the patient. Rather, it is seen as a pattern of difficulty that the person manifests in relating to himself and others. This pattern of difficulty is seen not only as a product of what a patient "is" but of what he does and what others think about him and do to, and with, him. This line of thinking further maintains that, if the patient's difficulties are to be alleviated—his thinking and behavior changed—not only must the patient do something about himself but personnel who are part of his daily social environment must develop attitudes and behavior toward him that best fit his needs and are most appropriate for his current and changing condition.(2)

This concept leads to the view that is within the behavior, within the interpersonal relations which develop between staff and patient, that the patient can learn and grow and, therefore, get well. Such a concept can determine a philosophy of psychotherapeutic nursing that is essentially interpersonal. It is, for example, no longer believed that a therapeutic hour each day, alone, helps the patient get well but, rather, that one or many persons in many situations with the patient can bring about therapeutic results. Patients, and their families as well, are seen as active participants in treatment.

Quite simply, one might say that a patient comes into contact with psychiatric personnel because he is having difficulty in living; specifically, difficulty in living with other people. One of the purposes of nursing intervention, then, is to provide experiences in living which will enable the patient to establish relationships that are less anxiety provoking and more comfortable, making possible other less threatening, less forbidding relationships.

METHODOLOGY

The obvious question is, "How does the nurse do this?" First of all she *observes* and *collects data*. Part of this data is theory: information about personality development, interpersonal interaction, the concept of anxiety, and how social systems operate (3). She acquires this knowledge from the literature and from her own observations and research.

In addition to theory, the data include specific observations about the patient: his verbal and nonverbal communications; that is, his words, actions, expressions, and gestures. The extent to which the patient uses gestures rather than verbal communication, for example, will indicate something about the level of personality development at which he is operating.

In addition to these observations, the nurse needs to look at her own words, actions, and gestures and, even more important, at her thoughts and feelings for the clues they give. Thoughts and feelings of patients are not always obvious yet they often are the first clues that something is amiss with patients, the group, or the social setting. They may, on the other hand, tell us that things are going well and that the situation is comfortable.

Harry Stack Sullivan said that two overall goals in interpersonal relations were satisfaction and security (4). These two broad categories are helpful in grouping patients' needs. Satisfaction, for example, is produced when needs that are primarily biologic are met; security when needs that are primarily interpersonal are fulfilled. Both of these categories are of concern in nursing since a patient's problems often are entwined with frustrations in both biologic and interpersonal areas. A patient on a special diet who is always hungry may feel a lack of physiologic satisfaction but, since food plays a significant role in our interpersonal context from birth to death, he also may have his need for security breached. Or a man seriously mutilated in an accident may be more troubled by the change in his self-image than with his severe pain.

Needs which have to do with maintenance of the self, that is, who we are and what we are, are included in the category of security needs. For example, such needs as the feeling of respect for oneself, for approval, prestige, love, friendship, recognition, power, and so forth, obviously deal with personal security. When these needs are unmet or, in other words, when there is a threat to the self-esteem, a feeling of anxiety may be experienced. All of us are familiar, in one degree or another, with the discomfort of anxiety, as well as with the desire to avoid such discomfort. The wish to avoid anxiety gives rise to patterns of behavior that will meet needs or, at least, preserve the self with a minimum of discomfort.

Anxiety is essentially an emergency emotion that warns the individual that something is likely to interfere with the self-concept. This emotion can be generated interpersonally by co-workers, patients, family, or others in the situation, or it may be generated by something in the present situation which unconsciously reminds the individual of a painful experience in the past.

People have different ways of seeking relief from the feeling of helplessness that arises with anxiety. Some persons may become more dependent and submissive, clearly demonstrating the helplessness that they feel. Others may respond with defiance or stubbornness, or they may become demanding. Each response that a person makes is apt to bring a response from others which may reinforce the way the person feels or alter it.

8

Most people have experienced anxiety from being with a very anxious person. But this reaction often is not realized until a later time. This process—one person's anxiety being communicated to another person—may become circular if there is no awareness of the anxiety and no understanding of it. Self-observation, therefore, is crucial in being therapeutic.

The second function is to *make inferences* from the data gathered. Here the nurse looks at the data and tries to relate her own observations of the situation to the theory and also to past situations she and others have observed. She makes an attempt to decode and infer meaning from the communications, and to look at the whole: herself and the patient, the nonverbal and the verbal communications, and at the theory.

Third, the nurse *structures her interventions according to her inferences.* These three—collecting data, making inferences, and structuring nursing interventions—may occur on a rapid moment-to-moment basis or over a long period of time. The nurse working with a patient thinks about what is happening and plans her interventions accordingly. But she also thinks about the relationships of today's activities with those of the week before and the weeks to follow; she thinks of the continuous process, the themes that emerge, the unique patterns, the recurring patterns.

Fourth, she also *evaluates.* The correctness or incorrectness of particular interventions or of inferences she draws about the patient's responses, the feeling tone of the group, progress, regression, obvious or subtle changes, or even no change are looked at in this process. Evaluation is a separate function, yet it also is a part of the nurse's other therapeutic functions.

The nurse cannot practice psychotherapeutic nursing unless she is able to take these four steps independently as well as interdependently. Unless she can use her own intellectual abilities, she will function only in rote fashion and not consistently and continuously in terms of the specific situation in which she is interacting with the patient.

For example, if the principle is accepted that behavior is reciprocal—that is, what we do with patients influences their responses—the nurse can alter her behavior on the basis of what she knows about the situation. But this may elicit any of a variety of responses from the patient since no set response to a particular behavior can be predicted. In determining a correct and useful response to make to the patient, the nurse uses the skills with which understanding is built—observing, listening, studying, decoding, inferring, acting, and evaluating. Patients' needs, however, are often expressed in obscure and confusing ways, and any conflict between the nurses' and the patients' interpretation of what is being communicated must be resolved if there is to be understanding of the problems the patients are facing.

So far this paper has focused on the ideas which are relevant to the three avenues of approach in psychotherapeutic nursing intervention—the one-to-one relationship, group relationships, and the milieu. The remainder of the paper will identify some specific techniques that can be used in each of these three areas.

INDIVIDUAL THERAPY

A useful beginning in individual, or one-to-one therapy is to look at how the patient might see the nurse. Every patient will have ideas about the nurse and her job because of the cultural stereotype. But each nurse needs to examine this stereotype for herself. If the patient has had pleasant experiences with nurses, he might see the nurse as someone who cares for or helps people, who goes out of her way to do something for someone. This concept of doing something for someone may be of positive value with patients who are dependent, yet unable to express their dependency in a way that will get them constructive help. Such a patient may find it difficult to seek help or to express his needs for help. The nurse, on the other hand, can go to the patient. Some writers describe this approach to patients as positive aggression (5). That is, the nurse goes after the patient and meets the patient on his own terms. The one-to-one relationship, thus, may be started in an unstructured way and continued on an appointment basis when both nurse and patient so choose. The nurse by virtue of role is in a position to seek out the patient and to see him in a variety of places rather than waiting for him to come to her.

Another aspect of nursing that is essential with many patients is the nurse's ease in physical caring and doing for others. In this instance, the mother-surrogate role, spelled out by Peplau, has particular relevance (6). In tending the patient physically, the nurse demonstrates how much she cares, but the anxiety and disapproval which the patient's mother may have conveyed to him in her caring is absent. Caring activities are vehicles for deepening the relationship; the nurse may find it is when she is giving physical care that the patient will discuss his real concerns. But the patient who has difficulty in what he views as intimacy with another person will have increased anxiety if the nurse is not clear about the differences between her professional and her social roles, and about her own needs. The nurse may have a need to be liked and accepted by patients. The clearer she is on how this need affects her behavior the more useful she will be. By consciously manipulating her own behavior she can help the patient find himself through the acceptance, learnings, and subsequent satisfactions of their relationship.

When the nurse is helping a patient express and resolve his dependency needs, it is essential that she be alert to minute changes in his responses. She addresses herself to the healthy aspects of the patient. As she watches, listens, and infers meaning, she is able to sense when he has made some movement which she then uses in helping him to gradually assume more responsibility for himself and lessen his need to continue his mentally ill behavior. If the nurse does not notice the change in behavior, she will continue to deal with the patient as if it had not occurred, and thus make it more difficult for him to sustain the improvement. A small change in behavior may be a big step for the patient, and if the nurse fails to sense it, the patient may become greatly discouraged.

The very subtle cues which may come from the patient, particularly in terms of any movement toward a higher level of functioning, are extremely important. Even a small amount of understanding will reinforce his healthy behavior and help him feel that he is not completely "crazy." Understanding the patient's communication makes the whole process of illness more rational and brings about a sharing experience which for the patient may be a unique event. Each experience of this kind gives him hope that other experiences like this can happen to him, that he isn't so different from others, that he can be understood.

One difficult aspect of the one-to-one relationship is the silent listening and observing that is necessary. This skill is not easy to acquire because the nurse often feels unsuccessful if she hasn't been able to get the patient to talk to her. But if she recognizes the importance of the nonverbal cues and develops her ability to observe them, she will uncover signs she previously would have ignored.

One essential aspect of therapy is reflection on the meaning of what the nurse sees or hears, reflection that encourages the patient to expand on it further. The nurse who jumps in to say something, or says the first thing that comes to her mind, will shut off the patient's flow of self-expression. If she can sustain her own tension and anxiety and respond thoughtfully to the patient's comments, she will often learn more about the patient's particular modes of behavior. She may find out what he is looking for in other people; themes or consistencies may become obvious; knowledge may be obtained, for example, about a phase of his development. Is he operating for the most part at an infantile level? If so, what might be done to help him move to the next level of development?

The one-to-one relationship allows the nurse to structure her interventions to include experiences geared toward helping the patient accomplish a particular developmental task. But, one-to-one therapy is not always feasible nor always desirable. Some patients respond better to group therapy, and for some nurses group work is their métier.

WORKING WITH GROUPS

Obviously, the important aspect in groups is the reaction of personalities on one another. There is stimulation and contagion of emotion from one patient to another, and correlation of one person's problems with those of others—of help particularly to those patients who find it hard to verbalize their difficulties.

Another value of a group experience for a patient may be a realization that his problems are not unique. This realization tends to dispel his guilt and sometimes even lessens the weight of his problem. In the group, the individual obtains support not only from the therapist but from other patients as well. A problem the nurse needs to keep aware of is that of competition among patients for attention from the therapist and for status in the group.

Sensitivity to the needs and tensions in the group is very important. A common error is to focus more on individual rather than on group interaction. Another is to fail to recognize the unofficial patient leader and channel his leadership into healthy rather than destructive patterns.

A therapist working with groups learns to verbalize the underlying feelings of the group only when they are near the surface and only when many group members share them. In other words, the feelings should be easily perceived. In general, probing questions are ruled out, both in individual and in group therapy. Patients will discuss the topics of importance to them when they are ready to do so. The responsibility to make choices and to institute change belongs to them.

Group therapy draws only part of its methodology, dynamics, and techniques from psychiatry; sources of knowledge about the particular ways in which groups operate, cultural and class values and configurations, and concepts of role come from sociology, social psychology, and anthropology. Such ideas as role complementarity and role set have relevance in individual therapy, but these ideas are even more significant in situations where there are multiple "others" to assume roles in relation to particular problem situations.

Although group interviews deal predominately with current problems—following the patient's leads—the therapist develops a sensitivity to group themes, individual incongruities, topics around which the group clusters, silences, and the direction which patients are taking. She notes whether silences occur around specific topics or whether there are situational changes. Continued silence by some patients may mean that they are too embarrassed or too ashamed for the group discussion. Their usual patterns of withdrawal might be reinforced by the discussion. Sensitivity to this behavior would lead the nurse to help plan subsequent individual approaches.

This paper, focusing on psychotherapeutic function, is not meant to imply any view of the nurse as omnipotent. Although she may work independently, there are, of course, times when she collaborates with members of other disciplines. However, when and how she collaborates is a subject for another paper.

THE MILIEU

In the third avenue of approach—the milieu—the nurse has the authority as well as the responsibility for creative action. Many authors believe that the milieu is the most important treatment modality for psychiatric patients. In the first place, psychiatric patients often are not able to express themselves in a traditional interview, and often are not able to talk easily about many aspects of their lives. Second, improvements in the milieu reach a greater number of patients than do other therapies. Third, and probably most important, the patient lives in a situation 24 hours a day, 7 days a week; the benefits of a few scheduled therapy hours often can be undone, or at least not capitalized upon, by the social setting.

In examining and creating a therapeutic milieu, a philosophy of psychotherapeutic nursing must first be developed and then implemented in the situation. For example, admission routines are a good place to start. Frequently, the way a patient is treated on admission reinforces his negative feelings about himself and about hospitals. The procedure often is depersonalized, the patient's belongings are removed, and few explanations are given. Good practice would be to see that he has everything he needs, and to introduce him, regardless of his behavior, to patients and personnel he is going to live with in his immediate area.

For example, a graduate student told about seeing, on her first day on a psychiatric ward, a tall, thin, well-groomed young man pacing the long hall. Occasionally, he would pause, look into the living room, but would never enter. The student introduced herself to him; he told her his name was Bob. Presently, another patient joined them, remarked upon her Boston accent, and spent a few moments in conversation. Soon Bob resumed his pacing. At lunchtime, the student asked one of the nurses to tell her about Bob. The nurse replied, "Who knows him? He has been here for three weeks but doesn't say very much and just seems to wander about the ward. He's a chronic schizophrenic."

Three days later, when the student returned to the ward, she was told that Bob was becoming catatonic, had been posturing, was not able to swallow, and consequently had not eaten. He had been given sodium amytal and had been sleeping most of the afternoon. Following this report she saw him lying on the bed, unshaven and unkempt. She brought him a tray for supper and when she awakened him to eat, she noticed that he appeared dazed, frightened, and had tremors. In order to alleviate some of his fears, she forewarned him about all of her actions and told him that she would help him eat and remain with him. To her surprise, he ate all the food on the tray, but did not speak. Following supper, he stood up. The student asked him if he would like to walk in the hall; he responded by turning toward the door. He was unsteady, so she offered to hold his arm. They walked into the hall and the first words he said were, "Have you been to Boston lately?" Obviously, he remembered her.

She spent most of the evening pacing the hall with him. His verbalization was autistic for the most part. At one point, he told her he was frightened and he took her hand in his as they paced. An undergraduate nursing student relieved her for dinner and coffee break. Bob went to bed at 10:00 p.m. after the graduate student had told him she would return in two days. The night staff discussed Bob and his feelings of depersonalization as evidenced by some of his activities. When the student returned two days later, she found that Bob had been eating and that members of the staff, especially the nursing students, were taking turns pacing with him in the hall. When the graduate student began walking with Bob again, he was walking with a shuffling gait but shortly changed to a normal gait. At times, he was confused, but he told her about his brothers and sisters, and some of his interests. He was initiating conversation, not merely responding to the nurse's questions.

The staff nurse assigned to the patient was amazed at the change in his behavior and said, "His medication must finally be working." But the student said she thought the interpersonal attention he had been receiving might well be related to the change, pointing out that at the beginning of the week he was alone most of the time and no one had seemed to know anything about him (7).

This example illustrates a patient's awareness of events at times when he does not seem to know what is going on, the overlapping nature of the one-to-one and milieu approaches, and the contagious effect of one person's behavior on another. In this case, it was the nursing student who picked up the behavior of the graduate student. Sometimes, a nurse's behavior will be reflected by patients on the unit who, when they see how a patient is treated, may also begin to behave toward the patient in similar ways. In fact, patients, like other people, are influenced as much by the nurse's behavior as by what she says.

In implementing a psychotherapeutic philosophy, another area to examine is that of communications. Are there opportunities for staff and patients to meet formally and informally? And for personnel to share information, both verbal and written? Is the ward routine so arranged that nurses can devote time to listening to patients and to each other? Does the setting allow for exploiting life issues? For example, is it possible for interviews to be held when necessary and when indicated rather than only at prescribed hours during the day?

The direction of communication and the way decisions are made is another index of the philosophy of care. If the patient is to benefit from the milieu, he must participate in it so that his behavior actually influences what is going on. The same principle holds for the optimum functioning of all levels of nursing personnel. Personnel who are involved in decision making have an investment in the policies they have helped to frame.

Program, policies, and routines should insure that the patient is protected from traumatic handling by any personnel associated with the unit. In addition, there must be gratification divorced from consideration of whether the patient deserves it or not. Patients need gratification as part of their treatment; they don't win it on the basis of good behavior. Tolerance of symptoms and leeway for regression is necessary within the treatment environment, but protective interference by the staff at the moment when it is necessary to protect the patient from his own guilt, anxiety, or depression, or to protect other patients, is also a part of effective milieu therapy.

A patient may not be able to handle a permissive environment, especially at the beginning of hospitalization. Acceptance of him, his problems, and his symptoms may make him anxious. In this instance, patients and personnel need to recognize the difference between acceptance of symptoms and indifference or permissive enjoyment of problem behavior. Accepting a patient does not mean approval of everything he does. Approval of negative feelings may, in fact, be a hindrance rather than a help. The patient group, itself, will indicate over and over to individual patients the concept of permissiveness and acceptance that really exists. And the patient will sense this from the nurse's responses to him and from what he observes of her acceptance of other patients.

A treatment milieu also has rules or limits—rules for social and for physical behavior that are really necessary, rules that are clearly understood and carefully observed. First of all, dangerous, aggressive behavior against self and others obviously cannot be permitted. Some forms of obscene language and some forms of acting out also may be too seductive under certain circumstances. Judiciously planned, rules, limits, or routines will help to increase a patient's sense of security.

Routines should be part of the design, however, rather than a challenge to patients to behave in ways which would then call out reward, punishment, acceptance, or rejection on the part of the personnel. Whatever the rules, let them be few, explicit, and understood by staff as well as by patients. Nothing is more attractive to patients than testing limits, especially with new staff.

Creative manipulation of the milieu is an exciting aspect of psychotherapeutic nursing. It suggests an infinite variety of work roles with personnel and patients, and poses a fruitful arena for nursing research.

SUMMARY

The role of the nurse as a therapeutic agent has been identified, using three overlapping avenues of approach — the one-to-one relationship, the group relationship, and the milieu. The philosophic frame of reference has been that the patient has become ill as a result of the experience he has had in living. His illness then can be influenced, interrupted, or altered by what other people do, to and with him. Behind a patient's rejecting behavior is potential for warmth and responsive behavior. This potential can be reached through persistence in offering the patient a responsive and respectful relationship.

References

1. Joint Commission on Mental Illness and Health. *Action for Mental Health,* Final report. New York, Basic Books, 1971.

2. Schwartz, M. S. and Shockley, Emmy L., *Nurse and the Mental Patient.* Science Editions, John Wiley and Sons, New York, 1966, (Paperback) Introduction.

3. Fagin, Claire M. *Study for Desirable Functions and Qualifications for Psychiatric Nurses.* New York, National League for Nursing, 1953. (Mimeographed)

4. Sullivan, H. S. *Conceptions of Modern Psychiatry.* Washington, D.C., William Alanson White Psychiatric Foundation, 1947, p. 6.

5. Bruce, Sylvia J. Adolescence, delinquent and distressed. *Nurs. Outlook* 8:499-501, Sept. 1960.

6. Peplau, Hildegard E. Principles of psychiatric nursing. In *American Handbook of Psychiatry,* ed. by Silvano Arieti, New York, Basic Books, 1959, Vol. 2, pp. 1840-1856.

7. Davidites, Rose Marie. (Unpublished paper)

Chapter Two

PSYCHIATRIC NURSING: ROLE OF NURSES AND PSYCHIATRIC NURSES

Hildegard Peplau

THE PSYCHIATRIC NURSE'S ROLE is today in an "identity crisis." The crisis is being resolved, in different ways and at different speeds, in various countries. The emerging role of psychiatric nurses in the various countries is in relation to the developments in mental health as a field and to the social sciences as another source of explanatory theory relevant to mental health.

It may be most useful to think of *nurses* who practice in psychiatric settings and *psychiatric nurses*, who also work in such facilities. Nurses have only *basic* nursing education, of which a part includes knowledge and supervised practice related to psychiatric work. Psychiatric nurses have specialized *post-basic* nursing education and therefore have more knowledge and competence for their work.

The *role of nurses* in psychiatric settings of all types is the same generalized one as in other types of health care institutions, but adapted to the special considerations of psychiatric patients. This role includes assessment of nursing needs of patients, developing nursing care plans, implementing such plans through direct nursing care or through other nursing personnel, evaluating the results of nursing care and coordinating the care of other health professionals. The nurse also helps to create and maintain an environment in the service unit that is beneficial for patients. Through visitors

From "Psychiatric Nursing: Role of Nurses and Psychiatric Nurses," by Hildegard Peplau, *International Nursing Review*, 1978, Vol. 25. Reprinted by permission.

and other programme plans the nurse stimulates continuing relationships between patients and their family members and community contacts. In addition, of course, nurses carry out medical orders. The knowledge base which the nurse uses to guide these nursing practices is whatever is included in the basic nursing curriculum. Additionally, inservice and continuing education opportunities should be available so that the knowledge base will be gradually up-dated and expanded.

The *role of psychiatric nurses* also depends upon the length of post-basic nursing education, the scope and depth of knowledge included in it and the clinical modalities for which supervised clinical practice is provided. There is great variation in what psychiatric nurses are able to do, for their competence is largely dependent on the foregoing factors. It is not a matter of intelligence. There are just as many intelligent nurses as there are intelligent persons in all other health professions. It is a matter of educational opportunity to develop that intelligence into competence for practice in psychiatric nursing.

What nurses or psychiatric nurses do—or learn to do—in any given country has much to do with prevailing definitions of the phenomena called "mental illness" and of definitions of the nature of the corrective professional work that is needed to put patients in the direction of "mental health." It is a characteristic of all professional work—that of physicians, nurses, lawyers, dentists, etc.—that the starting point for deciding the practices, and therefore the role, must be an understanding of the problems, difficulties, needs, or phenomena, which the practices or role to be used are intended to fix, correct, change or improve in some way. As shown in Table 1, the conceptions and theoretical explanations of "mental illness" are changing. Only three major trends are shown. There are, of course, many "schools of thought" about what is mental illness. Some of them are blends of these three trends; others are elaborations of one piece of one trend. In any given hospital or mental health centre it is possible to find most, if not all, of the prevailing schools of psychiatric thought. Each physician on a hospital staff may represent and adhere to a different psychiatric theory to explain the phenomena called "mental illness."

The dilemma of nurses and psychiatric nurses is clear. No basic or post-basic nursing programme can teach all possible theories used by psychiatrists in their work. There isn't that much time! Should one theoretical framework be taught to nurses? If so, which one and on the basis of what criteria should it be selected? Or, should nurses take an eclectic approach—learning a little bit about as many different theoretical orientations as possible but not gaining any depth in one of them? In the latter case, what would be the nursing practices, for these, like medical practices, flow from the theories that are used.

A consideration of some characteristics of patients living in hospitals is in order. Some of the usual things that nurses do in general hospitals are bathing, feeding, toileting patients, attending to mouth and skin care or positioning or changing dressings or other kinds of bodily care. In psychi-

TABLE 1

Changing Conceptions and Theories Explanatory of Mental Illness

Intra Personal	Inter Personal	Systems
Within-person phenomena	Between-persons phenomena	Within social systems phenomena
Medical model: -Psychoanalysis—intrapsychic; -Biochemical—disturbed body function; -Genetic—inherited traits; -Behaviour modification—extinguish problem behaviour by rewarding acceptable behaviour.	Dyadic interaction model: -Psychotherapy—therapist a model for changing client's problematic pattern integrations with sick-making and sick-maintaining others; -Therapeutic modalities—individual and group; -Dyadic therapy—patient and significant other person.	Social interaction model: -Family therapy—therapist promotes change in family network of patterns, linkages, and strategies of family; -Milieu therapy—an environment that provides various mechanisms for change of behaviour in groups.
Mental illness is a disease of a person; the "patient" is "sick."	"Mental illness" is a disturbance in a relationship with two or more people; the relationship is problematic.	The "identified patient" is merely the signaller of a disturbed system in a "closed family"; the family is disturbed.
The "cause" of mental illness lies in the patient's past, in his genetic inheritance, and/or in bodily dysfunction—neurological, biochemical, etc.	The "generic roots" of mental illness lie in past relationships but the "purpose" of present behaviour, which replicates and perpetuates past relationships, determines the continuation of the behaviour.	One member of a family is assigned or takes (for some purpose) the role of signaller of on-going family system disturbances; that member is "labelled" mentally ill.

TABLE 1 *(continued)*

Changing Conceptions and Theories Explanatory of Mental Illness

Intra Personal	Inter Personal	Systems
Within-person phenomena	Between-persons phenomena	Within social systems phenomena
Spectator observation is used: -The patient's symptoms are studied. -A diagnosis of the type of "mental illness" is made. -Treatment is ordered for the patient: Drugs, EST, behaviour modification, activity schedules, etc.; -Acute disturbance and acting-out are seen as signs of illness and are often "treated" with drugs, restraint, seclusion, etc.	Participant observation is used: -Interactions between patient/patients, patient/staff member and patient/visitor are studied so all become aware of them. -Diagnosis of problematic pattern-integrations of patient with others is studied. -Diagnosis of "type" of "mental illness" is done when required for official records. -Drugs are used to reduce severe anxiety. -Acute disturbance is treated as panic and acting-out is a basis for discussion of purpose and pattern-integration.	Sociological observation is used: -The entire family and its network of patterns and strategies are studied so all family members become aware of them. -Options for revised or new patterns or strategies are openly considered. -No diagnosis is indicated. -Separate sessions with parents, children, or one member may be held but not to discuss absent members.
-The professionals *do not* observe or study their behaviour in interaction with the patient's behaviour.	-Professionals observe and study their participation in interaction with patients.	-The "treatment" experience is open and aims to open up a closed family. -The professional is an educative agent

-Family are "informants." -Care: Doing things *to* or *for* the patient.	-Family data are taken in front of patient. -Care: doing things *with* the patient.	for system change and detached from the family system.
The concern is about symptoms, entities and their amelioration. The sick person is seen as "different" from others.	The concern is for processes, mainly interpersonal and intellectual processes. The person's behaviour is seen as different in degree not in kind—an exaggerated expression of ordinary human processes.	The concern is about systems, networks and ways in which they are maintained. The patterns of behaviour of family members are seen as needful and purposeful, based on past experience often being replicated, but open to awareness and change.
The tendency is to hospitalize the "mentally ill," to remove from family (often to exclude family) and to protect the community. -The family tends to "close ranks" and enlarge distance from the "sick" person. "Chronicity" in patients is explained as evidence of genetic defect, failure of the organism to respond to drugs, EST, etc., or failure of the patient as a person.	The tendency is to maintain in the community, using out-patient care and short-term hospitalization when absolutely necessary. -Family members may be invited to dyadic or individual therapy. They are participants in care of patient. Chronicity in hospitalized patients is explained as "institutional pathology," failure of the therapist to infer patterns and apply successful interventions, lack of explanatory theory, or insufficient time.	The work with families is done on an out-patient basis—in the home when possible; the tendency is *not* to hospitalize or treat individually the "identified patient."
-The institutional tendency is toward routines and custody and occurs as a consequence of staff failure to observe staff participation in evoking patient disturbances and in perpetuating psychopathology,	Out-patient care prevents institutionalization and its effects and allows the patient opportunities for contacts in which to try out new behaviours that may result from therapy.	

TABLE 1 (continued)

Changing Conceptions and Theories Explanatory of Mental Illness

Intra Personal	Inter Personal	Systems
Within-person phenomena	Between-persons phenomena	Within social systems phenomena
unwittingly. -Institutions tend to become "closed systems."		
Theories used: Descriptive psychiatry, genetics, bio-chemistry, biology, psychoanalysis, conditioning theories (behaviour modification), psychology.	Theories used: Interpersonal psychiatry, social science—especially socio-psychological interaction theories, communication theory, behavioural theory.	Theories used: General systems theory, social science—especially socio-psychological interaction theories, family theory, communication theory, matrix theory, behavioural science theory.

atric hospitals patients do these activities for themselves and only a minimal surveillance of them by nurses may be needed. Patients' beds need to be made, but patients also do this. Furthermore, if a patient has had a mother who was compulsively orderly and demanded precision in bedmaking, any rebellion of that patient about bed-making in the hospital may be a healthy, independent stance, in which event the nurse would be well advised not to make an issue of bed-making. But that would, of course, depend on whether refusal of the bed-making was taken as a sign of health or of illness, which would depend upon the theoretical framework being used, by physician and nurse, to explain the patient's behaviour.

Nurses pass out medications. It is common in psychiatric hospitals to medicate patients, often quite heavily. Nurses can, of course, observe and report drug effects. But the effects to be observed are also related to the theoretical aim in giving them. The aim may be to take the edge off severe and recurring anxiety of the patient, thereby enabling nurse/patient talks of a substantial, beneficial kind, or the aim of the medication may be to "tranquillize," to produce in the patient the effect of quiet that may stimulate thought undisturbed by talk.

Nurses also often schedule patients for activities, on and off a hospital unit, providing surveillance of adherence to such schedules. Nurses may also arrange and participate in ward activities: ward government meetings, birthday parties for patients, coffee-break sessions when patients have completed "cleaning duties," if these are required of them in a unit. The "activities of daily living" in a hospital unit are often considered to be the nurses' concern. These include such activities as hours of arising in the morning, nap times if permitted, sleep hours— deciding these matters and providing surveillance of these activities.

The critical question is whether the nurse is to carry out these activities within an intrapersonal framework—being a detached observer and mother-surrogate—or whether an interpersonal framework will guide the nurse, as a participant observer, alert to verbal tactics and considering them from a standpoint of nonreplication of "sick-making others" in the previous interpersonal environment of the patient. No one can monitor or direct the nurse/patient verbal exchanges at all times. Only the nurse who has a theoretical knowledge of communication theory, and who can recall and use it during nurse/patient verbal exchanges, can be held responsible for the short and long-term effects of such exchanges.

The work of nurses in psychiatric settings can be defined in different ways: (a) as manager of the routines of life on a unit with kindness, but only a modicum of unselected theory; or (b) as a change agent who uses substantial theory to guide nurse-interactions with patients with the aim of evoking substantial change in patient behaviour. Two generalizations in psychiatric literature are instructive. One is the generalization that panic in patients is staff-induced, most specifically when there are covert, undiscussed, staff disagreements as to what care should be or how it is to be carried out. The other is the idea of illness-maintenance by staff, which is, of course, unwitting. The latter idea generated from study of "the other twenty-three hours"; i.e., after a patient's fifty-minute hour of therapy with a physician. If these two generalizations are taken seriously, as they should be, then nurses, in order to be more fully knowledgeable and responsible in their work, need substantial post-basic nursing education in theories that aid them to see qualities of illness-maintenance in their daily work, and aid them to change their own participant behaviour so as to become agents for new and more self-evolving behaviour in patients (Table 2).

The definition of the nature of "mental illness" is in effect the definition of the work which the patient is to do in order to change himself into a more fully-functioning person. The role of physician and nurse and other mental health workers flows out of the definition of the patient's work (Table 3). The question of who will define the patient's work is another matter; whether it be defined in very general terms, as in Table 3, or in terms more specifically related to the particular patient.

In some community mental health centres in the United States the professional staff is organized into "focus teams." Each team includes physicians, nurses, social workers and psychologists but not according to a particular ratio. Each team serves a defined population in a geographical area of the region served by the mental health centre as a whole. Initially each team spends some time seeking a consensus on its views of mental illness. When a patient first comes to the centre the receptionist calls whichever team member who has that hour free to do the "intake," the initial history. At its next "team meeting," usually held every other day, the team reviews the intake, decides more specifically what work of the patient may be required, and assigns one team member to arrange appointments through the receptionist and to proceed with the work. The criteria for assignment include who has the necessary competence and who has time free to take on another patient. The work might be brief counselling, individual psychotherapy of somewhat longer duration, participation in group therapy, family therapy, referral to a "sheltered workshop" and the like. Very nearly all team members are competent to do the various forms of therapy, including the psychiatric nurses and general nurses who are members of the team. The work of each team member is subject to periodic data review by one other team member; when a case is to be closed a team review and decision is made.

It is easy to see that there is a great deal of planned role overlap. All professionals provide psychotherapy although some may prefer group therapy, some individual therapy, and some prefer family therapy. Some teams also include graduate students in nursing (master's programme in psychiatric nursing) as well as psychiatric residents and psychology and social work students. They are supervised in their clinical work by faculty in their respective programmes but the final team review before discharge also occurs.

TABLE 2
Some Illness-Maintaining Behaviours of Nurses with In-Patients

1. The nurse using a patient (who was similarly exploited at home) to do errands for her (bring coffee, clean office, carry messages).

2. The nurse burdening the patient with tales of her exciting social life—putting the patient in the position of "audience" and at the same time having little interest, if any, in his concerns; to cheer him up by "one-upping" him!

3. The nurse making "pets" of a few patients and thereby reinforcing previous "pet" status for those patients and reinforcing "unfavourable comparison" for other patients. Giving gifts to some but not all patients.

4. Arbitrating sibling-like disputes among two patients so that one loses and one wins, as in sibling disputes at home.

5. Responding to dependency bids in ways that confirm and reconfirm the patient's self-view: "I am helpless, dependent," etc.

There are also some separate roles. Diagnosis and prescription of medication is a physician role. Study of a home is a social work or psychiatric nurse function. Follow-up care after discharge is most often a nursing function due to medication that may be involved. Psychological testing is a psychology role. Fees that are charged to patients are the same for all psychotherapists but are adjusted according to the economic status of the patient.

The aim of the mental health centres is to provide "talking" therapy for all patients, to do that early and only for as long as needed.

The concern in the development of community mental health centres has been with early and effective treatment to prevent hospital admissions and to stop the continuing backlog of patients in public mental hospitals. Another aim has been to keep families and communities involved—to see "mental illness" as a problem of a family which it must help to solve. The family is a part of the problem and of its solution.

There are similar developments with respect to mental retardation and psycho-geriatrics. Special homes are of course available for patients who have for years been in such institutions, but the trend is toward home-care and community-based supportive services. Nurses are often the

TABLE 2 *(continued)*
Some Illness-Maintaining Behaviours of Nurses with In-Patients.

6. Responding to patient bids for derogation or punishment by giving it, thereby confirming and reconfirming these patient self-views.

7. Permitting, inviting and responding to "tale bearing" in which one patient "tattles" on another, thereby reinforcing the patient's "informer role" which further isolates the patient from constructive interaction with other patients as peers.

8. Allowing or permitting "coalitions across generations"; i.e., participating in nurse/patient discussion to the detriment of some other staff member. This replicates the patient's previous pattern of "pitting one against another" which may have effectively disunited mother and father, who are then reunited in concern for the now "identified patient."

9. Entering into pseudo-chum relationships with patients.

10. Non-useful channelling of anxiety into over-medication, seclusion, EST, or work rather than into investigation of circumstances that evoked the anxiety in a given situation.

11. Using various problematic verbal inputs such as "mixed messages," "double-binds," etc.

primary care persons who visit homes, arrange for services needed, and contact physicians when there is a medical problem. In institutional care, nurses, of course, are needed for direct, bedside care of the severely handicapped (idiots, hydrocephalics, etc.) and for the medically ill psychogeriatric patient (CVA's, Parkinson's, etc.). With regard to the less severely retarded who are institutionalized, the "training" is seen as the function of special teachers, while nurses use "activities of daily living" and group modalities other than therapy (behaviour modification; remotivation groups) to stimulate the human development and social behaviour of the retardate. Similarly, in psycho-geriatrics, nurses are studying the aging process and developing nursing interventions which prevent or slow up institutionalization and which tend to ensure human functioning at the highest level possible for each patient.

In public mental hospitals the tendency is to place the most compe-

TABLE 3

Different Definitions of Mental Illness and Therefore of the Work of the Patient and the Role of the Nurse

Definition	Work of the Patient	Role of the Nurse
Socially unacceptable behaviour of the patient has previously been "rewarded"; he has unfortunately been "conditioned" to behave in these ways.	Submit to treatment using behaviour modification (reconditioning) techniques.	Surveillance of patient following treatment plan. Pass out rewards. General nursing routine care.
Unacceptable behaviour is the result of genetic inheritance.	Submit to whatever ameliorative treatment of symptoms is ordered.	Surveillance and custody. Reporting. General nursing routine care.
Unacceptable behaviour is due to a biochemical imbalance.	Submit to tests and prescribed treatment drugs to rectify the imbalance.	Surveillance. Reporting. Pass medications: tranquillizers, stimulants, lithium, hormones, etc. Observe effects. General nursing routine care.
Unacceptable behaviour is due to	Submit to prescribed treatment	Surveillance. Reporting.

TABLE 3 (continued)

Different Definitions of Mental Illness and Therefore of the Work of the Patient and the Role of the Nurse

Definition	Work of the Patient	Role of the Nurse
some unknown but adverse brain activity.	(electro-stimulation, electro-shock, lobotomy, etc.).	Pre- and post-treatment "preparation." General nursing (and surgical nursing) care.
Unacceptable behaviour reflects problems in living with people and lack in intellectual and interpersonal competencies to understand and solve those problems.	Participate in psychotherapy sessions and in ad hoc talking sessions with the available professionals, so as to investigate, understand and resolve those problems and in the process gaining new intellectual and interpersonal competencies on an experiential/educative basis.	Use all "activities of daily living" as a basis for observation, discussion and intervention in ways that enhance the patient's intellectual and interpersonal competencies to change his own behaviour. Also general nursing care. Using "situational counselling" to aid patients involved in disputes, violence, other grossly unacceptable behaviour, to investigate the problem inherent in the acting-out situation. Referral for other professional

28

services, i.e. clergy, and coordination and follow-up on discharge.

The unacceptable behaviour is due to "lack of insight" into intrapsychic causes.	Seek psychoanalysis for those who can afford it.

tent psychiatric nurses in admission wards or with newly admitted patients. Such nurses provide counselling, individual and group psychotherapy, and "specialing" for patients in panic. In "chronic wards" the effort is toward resocialization, with nurses most often being the programme planners.

An attempt has been made in Table 4 to show an array of possible activities connected with the role of the nurse and psychiatric nurse in ious kinds of psychiatric/mental health settings. What nurses and psychiatric nurses will actually do in any given setting depends upon:

TABLE 4

Summary: Role of Nurses and Psychiatric Nurses

Nurses (basic nursing education only)	Psychiatric nurses (post-basic nursing education)
Assess patient needs.	*All activities listed under "nurse," plus:*
Develop nursing care plans.	Intake (history taking).
Implement nursing care plan: -Carry out direct care; -Assign and supervise nursing personnel.	Sociological observation of homes.
Evaluate effects of nursing care.	Member of mental health team: -Counselling; -Individual psychotherapy; -Group psychotherapy;
Create and maintain an environment in service unit of benefit to patients.	-Family therapy; -Supervisory review of clinical data (own and other);
Stimulate patient relationships with family: -Dyadic patient/visitor conferences with nurse.	-Discharge planning with team; -Follow-up and evaluation of patient outcomes; -File case reports.
Carry out medical orders: -Pass prescribed medications; -Monitor medication effects; -Carry out physical procedures.	"Special" patients in panic.
	Model for constructive intervention in "ward disturbances."
Surveillance of bathing, mouth care, toileting, bed-making, food intake, sleep.	Experiential teaching of nurses.
General nursing routines, especially for severely retarded and medically ill psycho-geriatric patients.	Writing professional nursing papers. *In hospital*
Prepare for and/or participate in special treatments: behaviour	Work with newly admitted patients as above.
	Work with acutely disturbed patients, especially re panic.

30

1. the competence brought to the work as a consequence of basic or post-basic nursing education;

2. the definition of mental illness and therefore of the work of "mentally ill" patients, that prevails in a given setting;

3. the extent of consensus around the question of whether each profession should or should not have only discrete, unique, circumscribed roles or whether there can be overlap (as, for example, in talking with patients which all profes-

---

TABLE 4. *(continued)*

Summary: Role of Nurses and Psychiatric Nurses

Nurses (basic nursing education only)	Psychiatric nurses (post-basic nursing education)
modification, electroshock, lobotomy.	Work with autistic and otherwise acutely disturbed children.
Referrals to other professions—clergy, social work, etc.	Work with acting out and otherwise acutely disturbed adolescents.
Coordination of patient care of other professionals.	
Schedule patient activities (off the unit): -Surveillance of adherence to schedule.	Serve as a resource and consultant to nurses.
Arrange and participate in unit "activities of daily living": -Ward government; -Various modalities of group activity; -Remotivation and resocialization groups; -Work groups; -Patient parties.	Present patient data at staff meetings.
	Arrange supervisory review of clinical data with equally or more experienced professional colleague.
Make follow-up home visits after discharge.	
Talking with patients: -Situational counselling; -Disrupt illness maintenance.	
Attend in-service education sessions and ward staff meetings.	
Attend outside continuing education meetings.	

sions do) and if so, to what extent (i.e., only counselling, counselling and the various psychotherapies);

4. the cost of certain kinds of care (e.g. psychotherapy), the difference in status and salary levels (e.g. physicians, nurses, etc.) and the numbers of persons needed and available to provide certain kinds of care may also be countervailing or influential factors.

References

De Schouwer, P. and Bart, A.: The Role of Nursing Personnel within the Psychiatric and Mental Health Team—as seen by a Medical Administrator. WHO Working Group, Saarbrücken. 10–13 March 1975 (mimeographed).

Staunton, A. and Schwartz, M.: Mental Hospitals (Basic Books, New York, 1954).

Chapter Three

NURSE/PATIENT PEER PRACTICE

Mary Bayer and Patty Brandner

AS CONSUMERS BECOME MORE concerned about the high cost and inconvenience of illness, more knowledgeable about medical and health care, and insistent on making decisions on their own health care, they are seeking new answers to such basic human problems and new ways to meet their health needs.

Meanwhile, the health system hierarchy is struggling to maintain authority over the consumer. We believe that nursing should withdraw from this effort and join forces with consumers to achieve a more enhancing health care system.

Before the client can feel a true partnership with nursing, however, a major change must occur: nurses must not only acknowledge clients' rights to have intelligence, but also encourage them to use it! That is one of the fundamentals of what we call peer practice in nursing. The patient here is a peer; one abandons the old stance of the doctor as "father," the nurse as "mother," and the patient/client as "child."

We believe an alternate attitude begins with the nurse's concept of her- or himself as a unique, never duplicated-in-the-past-present-future member of the human species; the holistic approach is applied to the nurse as well as to the client. The ongoing task of the nurse is to understand how her own human system functions and to be responsible for its integrity. With this awareness, she does not have to be afraid of becoming "emotionally involved" with clients nor of using them to gratify her personal needs.

Further, the nurse values her own time and that of others; she does

From "Nurse/Patient Peer Practice," by Mary Bayer and Patty Brandner. Copyright © 1977, American Journal of Nursing Company. Reproduced with permission from *American Journal of Nursing*, January, Vol. 77, No. 1, pp. 86–90.

not waste it. She recognizes that cooperation in peer relationships uses life energy more productively than do the competitive ways that characterize our present health care system. Maintaining authority and/or servility requires energy. That energy can be used more efficaciously to promote health for the relatively short time life offers each human being.

From this basic respect for life comes the recognition that each person has "health," which includes the ability to solve the problems of living; that each person is in control of her or his life-behavior; that each has a background of personal interactions, socialization, and education that he uses to make behavior choices. Survival in our society requires a complex of skills for problem-solving; nurses recognize those skills as a component of "health" and, working in a peer relationship with the clients, "diagnose" the clients' strengths, their "healthy" behaviors.

As the nurse and the client discover the healthy strengths together—the nurse bringing her special knowledge to the process and the client contributing his own uniqueness and survival ability—the two can pool choices for further health enhancement. The nurse can offer choices only from her experience and knowledge; the client can accept or reject those choices only as they fit his own health needs. At all times during the interaction, the client's intellect is engaged in the problem-solving process.

We outline problem-solving steps this way to each client:

1. Identifying *one* problem

2. Discovering and listing the choices for a solution

3. Exploring the consequences of each choice

4. Making the choice

When nurse and client pool choices, the client has a greater variety from which to choose. When professional colleagues also are invited to offer their suggestions, the client has a still greater chance to make health-supportive decisions.

To help the client to a clearer understanding of peer nursing practice, we explain how the human system operates. We describe how the four major facets of each human being—physical, emotional, social, and intellectual—are integrated into a unique system and the primary need is to maintain the system's integrity.

That primary function is often masked because every culture assigns roles to its members according to age, sex, race, educational, and economic levels, and the like. Nonetheless, the human system continues struggling, either awarely or unawarely, to maintain a balance among its component facets to survive.

We recognize that, because every client has existed within his own system for as long as he has lived, he is the "resident expert" on himself. Not only does that client know more about himself than does any other person, but he also knows how he has integrated his own human system to survive until now. In today's health care system, this vital information is seldom elicited.

In the peer practice of nursing, the nurse's role is to help clarify the manner in which each client responds to assaults on his unique human system. Then, working as peers and using a problem-solving approach, the two can identify and evaluate the choices available. Once all of the possible choices are laid out and probable consequences of each are determined, the client chooses the solution which appears to be the most self-enhancing.

Bringing the client's intellect as well as emotions into the therapeutic interaction provides the base for his future successful problem-solving. The nurse supports the client's past problem-solving (by which, after all, he has survived to that moment) and recognizes that professional help has been sought because the individual's usual pattern of problem-solving is not appropriate for the current situation.

While the nurse is responding to the system or problem, she also strengthens the client's healthy behaviors and facets by calling attention to them. Most clients are responding to one or more assaults to their systems, and the nurse's role is to help the client deal with the effects of the assault and to serve as a consultant while the client attempts to reintegrate his human system. As consultants, we find that it is helpful to share examples of ways in which various facets can respond to assaults.

ASSAULTS ON THE SYSTEM

We note that no matter on which facet or facets an assault occurs, the categories of choices remain virtually the same. Some of the choices may appear bizarre in view of the seemingly insignificant assault but, because of the complexity of each human system, a choice that is possible for one person may be totally inappropriate for another. For example, in Maine where the winters are long and severe, often a body is found in the spring with a suicide note beside it saying, "I just couldn't take one more snow storm this year." To someone in Florida, that might seem an insane response to a spring snow storm. But the people of Maine understand.

Physical Assaults.   An assault to the physical facet might be a cut finger. The primary response is physical: bleeding. A secondary response follows quickly, one that seems to be integrative, representing simultaneous responses from the other facets. At the physical level there may be continued bleeding, perhaps an increase in pulse and respirations. Emotionally there may be anger, disgust, fear. The intellect may register pain and begin evaluating the severity of the injury. At the same time the social facet may be concerned over spilling blood onto a friend's new rug.

Once these responses are integrated, the individual automatically begins problem-solving either with past patterns of response or by use of the intellect. The choices for dealing with the cut finger might include ignoring it, helping oneself, turning to another for assistance—or possibly getting drunk, popping a pill, or even committing suicide. In the case of a cut finger, most persons probably consider that the best choice would be to cleanse the wound and apply a bandage; some might rush off to the family doctor.

Emotional Assaults.   As mental health nurse-therapists, we have been testing our peer nursing theory as we interact with so-called "emotionally disturbed" clients. We discuss the physical, emotional, social, and intellectual responses with each client as part of our nursing intervention. We express the view that each person is responding in the most enhancing ways of which he is aware at that time. We perceive this as individual behavior to preserve the integrity of the human system. We don't label clients "sick"; we talk about "protective skills" or "behavior choices" rather than about "defense mechanisms." We point out immediately that we want to discuss the "good things about you" for assessment of healths and strengths with which we, client and nurse, can work.

During the first interaction, we identify behavior responses as "choices" by which the client tries to preserve his human system. Reviewing the problem-solving process, we identify additional choices: "going crazy," "getting sick," drinking, running away, ignoring, attempting suicide, and so on. Many of these choices are ones that the client may have made in the past.

Many of our clients have been in traditional therapy before reaching us and have believed their "craziness" to be outside their control. They feel frightened and desperate, directed by forces outside themselves. They express surprise, recognition, and relief when they hear that we consider their behavior of their own choosing and that there are other choices they can make. With hope, often eagerness, clients examine solutions for health that the therapist can offer, but which only the clients can know will be enhancing in their situations.

With our clients we explore the responses of the human system to assaults on the emotional component. Take a verbal insult as an example. The primary response is emotional, usually in the form of hurt feelings or embarrassment. The secondary response involves all facets: flushed face, increased pulse; anger at the assailant and/or self; and asking self "why" or remembering previous insults: "be nice," "don't show anger," "what will my friends think."

The problem-solving choices are many: running away, ignoring (by stuffing the feelings back down), confronting and clarifying, getting drunk, taking drugs, fighting back, and so on. Individuals limited in response patterns and ability to conceptualize consequences realistically will often respond with the same choice regardless of the severity of the assault. Those who are aware of a wide range of choices, as well as the probable consequences of each, will usually choose a solution appropriate to the situation, with little energy lost in the selection process.

Intellectual Assaults.   Hospitalized persons, because of their vulnerability, are particularly susceptible to intellectual assault, which often occurs when staff members talk about him in jargon he cannot understand. The covert message to the patient is "There, there, darling. You relax and *we'll* decide what is to be done."

The primary response of the assaulted intellect is often "I'm too stupid to understand." The secondary responses appear simultaneously throughout the system: flushed face and tensed muscles; anger, fear, frustration, shame; "It isn't right to question a doctor's judgment"; "They know better than I do."

Again, the same choices are available, but where a person is at the mercy of others (as hospitalized patients can feel), the choices often take more subtle forms: stuffing feelings back down, regressing to a more dependent state (described in nursing notes as "cooperative" "no complaints") or displacing the feelings onto "safer" people than those who have charge of the individual's health situation.

Social Assaults.   Persons who would rather look after themselves, but who are forced to seek outside help, frequently perceive social assaults. When a patient enters the system on his own two feet and then is requested to replace street clothes with a hospital gown and hop into bed immediately, he may consider this an assault. The primary response takes place within the *social* facet: "I must look ridiculous in this get-up" or "People don't go to bed when they feel OK." The secondary, integrated responses might be blushing, tensed muscles; embarrassment, frustration, apprehension, anger; "Better cover up my bare legs"; "What would my friend think of me now?"; "I must be sicker than I thought" or memory of previous hospitalizations.

Although patients have been known to gather up their clothes and take them off at this point, most will internalize their feelings by verbalizing their anxiety in a joking way (so as not to risk disapproval from the staff) or by ventilating to friends and family.

In each case, a primary response occurs at the facet under assault; followed by secondary responses at all facets. The intellect integrates the various responses and either awarely or unawarely proceeds into a problem-solving sequence in order to restore equilibrium to the system. We help clients to become aware of this process and together engage intellects to examine choices and consequences.

As consequences of behavior choices are explored, the nurse discusses with the client the concept that past choices were made because a limited range may have been seen at the time or the individual chose the least threatening, therefore the most protective, of those choices seemingly available. The nurse encourages the client to accept past choices, even those with self-destructive consequences, as "protective skills" by which the individual kept alive until a wider range of choices was available and more self and social understanding had been gained.

UNDERSTANDING THE CONSEQUENCES

When persons realize that past choices were made from a need to protect their survival in a hostile, unchangeable environment; that these choices are considered "skills" since the human system did survive; and that behavior is in the control of the individual, then feelings of guilt, self-blame, shame, frustration, and fear can be relinquished. The knowledge that each human system is in control of its own behavior frees the individual from self-defeating energy use.

Then, working in a peer relationship, the client and therapist each contribute from their unique human systems, and the probable consequences of each choice can be predicted. For example, running away can offer temporary relief, but often involves facing the problem again at a later date, possibly in another form. Stuffing feelings back down may work at the moment, but usually results in displacement of anger onto others or in eventual depression or psychosomatic illness. Potentially self-destructive choices such as getting drunk, taking drugs, getting physically and/or mentally ill are often made without self-knowledge, from patterns necessary for survival in childhood which have been carried into adult life. They may give temporary respite but usually lead to more serious problems than the immediate one. Suicide means death, loss of control, no chance to change one's mind in favor of another choice.

Such choices as confronting or expressing one's honest feelings may lead to further assault, rejection of the other, or they may open a path of communication by which effects of the assault can be remedied. Self-help can sometimes solve the problem; other times it provides only temporary relief. Turning to others can resolve a problem, but at other times it can lead to dependency.

When each choice and its probable consequence has been examined, the client can decide which appears most suitable, knowing that at any time, he can choose again or return to a more familiar, comfortable response pattern. A system that is generally in a state of equilibrium can usually regain its balance without much effort.

However, repeated assaults to a particular facet or simultaneous and/or frequent assaults on several components can quickly weaken the system, confuse the integration of responses, and mask correct identification of the problem(s). By understanding the basic responses to assaults, we can quickly separate out the various problems and help the client identify priorities. When the client has chosen which problem to attack first, we view together the available choices and carry out the problem-solving process.

In peer practice, the primary focus is on helping clients to learn how they have solved problems in the past and to call this "health"; on presenting a wider variety of available choices; on considering the consequences of each choice; and on continuing our support of whatever decision they make. We have found that, as we support the health and strength the client presents, the client's knowledge, self-reliance, and self-esteem are increased to the point at which future need for health care services is significantly lessened.

In a society in which traditional authority figures are coming under constant attack, we suggest that nursing recognize that each human system has an intellect—one that has kept that human being intact and functioning until our services have been sought, that will continue to integrate that human being long after our services are no longer necessary. As peers, nurse and client can collaborate to strengthen the client's potential for self-direction, knowledge, maintenance of health, and prevention of illness.

Chapter Four

CLINICAL SUPERVISION AS A SUPPORT SYSTEM FOR THE CARE-GIVER

Beverly A. Benfer

CONCEPTUALIZATION, COMPETENCY, AND COMPASSION are the three C's we identified for the title of our 1978 continuing education workshop. These were extracted from the philosophy and practice of psychiatric nursing at The Menninger Foundation. A fourth C, caring, which is one of the C's on which I focus in my paper although not in the title, was added to reflect the support system we attempt to provide through clinical supervision to care for the needs of the care-giver as well as those to whom we give care.

So that we will all be on the same wavelength, I want to share with you some basic assumptions: (1) The psychiatric nurse I am referring to in this paper is a practitioner either engaged in in-depth counseling or in a psychotherapeutic relationship doing on-going individual psychotherapy, or works in a setting with patients who are very ill, such as severe borderline conditions or character pathology, and schizophrenic patients who may be experiencing thought disorders. (2) In our work as psychiatric nurses we are not content to simply "fly by the seat of our pants," or hope that "intuitively" we will know what to do. (3) We wish to study our work carefully, which means making available through clinical supervision

From "Clinical Supervision as a Support System for the Care-Giver," by Beverly A. Benfer, *Perspectives in Psychiatric Care*, 1979, Vol. 17, No. 2, pp. 13–17. Reprinted by permission.

awareness of the feelings aroused in us by patients in our work with them. (4) As professionals, we are willing to scrutinize our work.

Peplau (1977) has pointed out that the development of intellectual competencies, the ability to develop investigative relationships with patients, and the application of theory are the tools of our work as psychiatric nurses. Let me develop this more explicitly in the context of direct patient work and supervision of our clinical work.

Each of us needs a forum or arena to permit careful appraisal of the nurse/therapist behaviors that occur as we participate in the nurse-patient relationship. For instance, if the nurse is not aware of her behavior, and is unobservant of the patient's wish to seek out a relationship that recreates previously experienced and usually problematic relationships, she or he will not be able to intervene or prevent stabilization of problematic patterns of integration that perpetuate pathology in patients. This is where our conceptualization of intrapsychic behavior becomes essential, and the competency of interventions based on understanding theoretical constructs makes the difference. Indeed, it is one of the major differences between professional and technical practice.

Nurses are not just in the treatment business. They are also in the human growth and development business, which encompasses compassion. Compassion is defined by Webster as a sympathetic consciousness of others' distress, with a desire to alleviate it. For our purposes, I suggest we replace the word sympathetic with empathetic. For me, empathy implies that we can hear and understand where the patient is coming from because we have learned to listen to our own feelings, assess our own responses, and recognize our own rational and irrational reactions. In short, we can include our own self-analysis of why we do what we do in our clinical practice.

We can also learn compassion through clinical supervision and, it is hoped, each of us has supervision available. Clinical supervision is having someone who will assist us in studying what we are doing in an investigative, teaching-learning environment. I have been involved in the clinical supervisory role for a few more years than I care to admit, yet, rarely have I had sessions at which I did not learn something new, or was not stimulated to seek further understanding of some aspect of human relations. The same holds true in having my own clinical work supervised. The clinical supervisory relationship must be one in which trust can be built and respect developed. Being able to have one's work scrutinized is difficult enough, but to share one's feelings honestly requires that the supervisee not only be brave but be able to trust as well.

It is not easy to discuss what goes on in the nurse therapist-patient relationship, particularly if we find ourselves relating a little too closely and intimately to the patient, or to look at our own dependency needs when working with a patient whose dependency needs resemble our own, or to share our own need for more support than usual. Nor is it easy to share our feelings of envy of the patient's rich fantasy life or to realize that possibly the practice of psychiatric nursing may require more of us than we can afford to give. To know and to understand the patient's need for nurturing is one thing, but for us, as nurses, to know when we need too much to be able to nurture others is indeed difficult. One of the most significant parts of competency is the competence to know ourselves—our need level, our satisfaction level, and above all, the indirect ways in which our needs get played out.

There is a host of dependency needs to face—needs that create stress in our work as care-givers. The need to be strong, to be the one on whom others lean, may lead to a compulsion to work, and the demanding work ethic "to do good" adds further stress. We may even find ourselves withdrawing from our family or personal life, which adds an additional stress. The need to be needed may be very difficult for us to manage. Mastery of one's own needfulness, as a matter of fact, may have been the very motivation that brought us into our field! One may get caught in the struggle to meet one's own needs through the patient.

As nurses, we have not always studied our own work; we haven't always wondered "why." Why do we react the way we do? Why do some patients we are working with closely get through to us so that we react emotionally ourselves, perhaps not to the point of crying, but at least to the point of tearing? Why? Because we care.

Caring is a scarce commodity. In everyday life there is a great deal of turmoil, conflict, and tragedy. In the face of such conflict and strife, the caring of one human being for another is, at times, usurped by a fight for survival. Yet, both the ability to care for another and to be cared about are of extreme importance for human survival, growth, and development. Nursing is the primary professional discipline that has traditionally been concerned with the caring needs of patients.

Leininger, in a recent article in a series on *The Phenomenon of Caring*, spoke to this point when she wrote: "Indeed, nursing is the profession which should be deeply concerned about and involved with caring behaviors, caring life styles, caring processes and caring consequences." (1977) In her opinion, no construct could be more central, more essential, and more promising for teaching, research, and practice within nursing than ideas related to care and caring. She suggests that concepts and practices associated with caring are rich resources for generating research studies, and we, as nurses, could well study caring behaviors, values, and outcomes for the next two decades and still not tap the full possibilities. We need to heed Dr. Leininger's suggestions as we move toward full professional status. If we do not, inadvertently, caring could be replaced with technology.

Much of what is talked or written about caring is related to the care given to others by the nurse. But what about the other side of the coin— what of the care needs of the care-giver? In other words, who cares for the caring nurse/therapist/therapeutic agent? Where do nurses find support, encouragement, and understanding when they feel drained by needy patients and overextended in their efforts to give to others? It is essential, I believe, to provide a support system for those providing care, for without caring there will be little curative treatment. We must feel cared about ourselves before we can give care to others. We try to teach patients this, but how often we fail to apply what we teach to ourselves!

How do we create a support system? What are the components of such a system? First, for one to be a "people treater" and provide care, he or she must experience being cared for. It is our belief at The Menninger Foundation that a support system can best be provided through clinical supervision; the kind of clinical supervision that embraces an investigative approach toward understanding our interactions and behaviors in working with patients, as well as the human growth and development potential in each of us within our clinical work. The type of supervision I'm referring to is *not* our own little recipes of nursing how-to's, or our own private set of labels by which we stamp out in a neat pre-cut form our own set of expectations of what a nurse should feel, relate to, or say, such as: "the nurse should remain uninvolved and not have any feelings of counter-transference," or "a nurse should never feel anger," or "the nurse must be able to relate to all patients equally well, all the time, without regard for what she or he is feeling."

Unfortunately, nurses have a whole set of internal mental sets which we use to judge our own and others' behaviors. These mental sets in many instances suppress our being open and honest with our own work, deprive us of opportunities to grow and develop in our professional role, hinder our caring capabilities, and cause us to lose sight of the challenge to study our work.

I have noted in my work that whenever I hear nurses on the staff say such things as: "we *really* need to develop a policy about this or that so patients won't pull *that* stunt again," or "these patients are so narcissistic there's no way I can be helpful," or "yesterday the patient seemed to be really working on improving interpersonal relationships but today I can't believe it, he's just the opposite—everything and everyone that was good and worthwhile yesterday is bad and horrible today," or give messages that they, in essence, are feeling "burned out" in their work with difficult patients, I know that we need to be looking at our support system. Something is not working right.

One thing to do in our work is to really study what stresses do occur. When we look at patient behavior let us go further than just say a patient is "acting out" or "is manipulative," or "sexually involved." Let us study what is happening. When we work with patients whose pathology does not permit us to be human with both good and bad points, having a support system where there is care for the care-giver is of paramount importance.

Dealing with intimacy—whether in our work in marital therapy, family therapy, group therapy, or situational counseling, or on a unit involving interaction between patient-patient, patient-visitor, or patient-staff—is yet another example where charged emotions can create conflict for the practitioner. Without a support system available to deal with one's own feelings, or any other emotionally laden human behavior, our work can indeed be draining.

What of our feelings when a patient with whom we have worked intensely commits suicide? How many of us have experienced sleepless nights fearing that call that informs us the patient we have been working with so intensely just took his life? Or have worked with a patient who constantly threatened suicide in such a way as to arouse guilt feelings in us?

Recently, a psychiatrist on the Menninger staff shared his feelings about patients he had been treating who committed suicide, and the feelings he was left with. This is growth in the sense that we, as professionals, are able to share those terrible internal feelings of "where did we fail?" In this type of situation we need to appraise our work, but we also need to work through our feelings of helplessness and, yes, even to mourn. One method of support for the involved staff is to hold a psychological postmortem. It is hard to identify the degree of stress and strain a patient's suicide has on us; suffice to say, at times it may feel like we have reached our stress threshold.

Another stressful situation which acutely affected the staff was shared with us recently by a therapist who was working with a patient who had killed her own child. In such instances, our own moral values become involved when a patient's behavior is not culturally acceptable to us. Do we just shut off these feelings? And if we do shut them off, what happens? How are they played out in other ways?

I would be willing to wager there is not one practicing psychiatric nurse today who hasn't experienced some degree of clinical stress. What about the emotional drain of working with unrewarding patients with whom we experience feelings of hopelessness, yet must do what we can to provide help? How do we feel when we expect more from the patient in the way of some form of increased health which doesn't take place, or we must give up days off or come to team meetings on our time off because of a particular patient—how do these situations affect the nurse-patient relationship and our stress level?

I could give many other examples which point to the need for a good system of clinical supervision and support being available for those who provide care to persons experiencing emotional difficulties, but I will close by saying that after a carefully planned support system is operational, take a moment for the most important non-clinical work of all: say a little prayer that the care-giver feels cared for!

References

Leininger, Madeleine, R.N., Ph.D., "Caring: The Essence and Central Focus of Nursing," "The Phenomenon of Caring," American Nurses' Foundation Research Report, Vol. 12, No. 1, February 1977.

Peplau, Hildegard E., R.N., Ed.D., "The Crux of Psychiatric Nursing," presented at the Visiting Professor Lectureship Series sponsored by the Education sponsored by the Education Department, The Menninger Foundation, Topeka, Kansas, September 19, 1977.

Chapter Five

A CASE STUDY IN THEORY-BASED MENTAL HEALTH LIAISON NURSING

Lynne M. Nickle-Gallagher, R.N., M.S., C.S.

"WHAT EXACTLY IS A clinical nurse specialist?" "What does a mental health clinical nurse specialist do in a rehabilitation center for adults with severe physical disabilities?" These questions have been posed to me numerous times in the several years I have held this position.

The answer must be undertaken on several levels. The first aspect to be emphasized is that, from the beginning, the role was explicitly based on a specific nursing theoretical framework (Nickle-Gallagher, in press). This conceptual base is Orem's self-care deficit theory of nursing (Nursing Development Conference Group, 1979; Orem, 1980). Briefly, the theory postulates that under usual circumstances people perform a wide variety of activities for themselves (self-care) to promote or maintain life, health, and well-being. In the case of children, such actions are performed by adult care givers. When an individual is unable to carry out sufficient self-care to meet his health-related needs, a self-care deficit is said to exist. Nursing is needed for people with self-care deficits.

The second way of describing the role is from the perspective of mental health liaison nursing. Alterations in health state and interactions with a complex, powerful, and often frightening health care system impose demands on patients that many patients are unprepared to handle (Lewis & Levy, 1982). My practice performs the liaison function defined by Lewis and Levy (1982) as "facilitation of the relationship that exists among the patient, the adjustment to the illness, the consultee(s), and the hospital/ward milieu" (p. 13). Consultation services provided in my practice are primarily client centered and secondarily consultee centered (Caplan, 1970).

The language of theory to explain practice is general, even at its most precise. As Benner (1982) observes, "Theory offers what can be made explicit and formalized, but clinical practice is always more complex and presents many more realities than can be captured by theory alone. Theory, however, guides clinicians and enables them to ask the right questions" (p. 407). One way to assimilate and communicate the intricacies of expert practice is by the use of "paradigm cases," those which make a notable impact on the knowledge and understanding of the nurse involved and which readily convey the issues to others (Benner & Wrubel, 1982).

To illustrate as vividly as possible the theoretical issues previously identified, a case has been selected from my practice. It served as a paradigm case for me and has been useful in explaining to others certain aspects of mental health liaison nursing.

A 40-year-old woman with several serious health-related problems was admitted to the rehabilitation center. She had had multiple sclerosis for 25 years and had learned to manage herself very well during the exacerbations and remissions of this frustrating and progressive disease. About nine months prior to her admission, she had developed a severe infection in her left leg. After a long hospitalization that included many treatments and surgeries, the leg was disarticulated at the hip and amputated. She came to the rehabilitation center for prosthesis fitting and gait training. Part of the preparation for these activities was a surgical release of the right knee tendon to gain more movement in that very rigid joint. The surgery was uneventful and minimally painful. Unfortunately, the wound soon became infected. As the infection progressed despite all efforts to check it, her pain increased greatly as did her use of morphine injections. The dressing changes became a focus of intense pain experience.

It was at this juncture that the mental health nurse was consulted. The physician and nursing staff were very concerned about the patient's pain and her narcotic use. Consistent with Lewis and Levy's concept of "diagnosing the total consultation" (1982, pp. 96–99), the case was discussed with the physician and other team members, the chart was reviewed, and the patient was extensively assessed. The major elements of nursing care that I implemented were (a) establishment of a therapeutic relationship with the patient, (b) modification of the pain medication regimen, (c) increased and more systematic communication among the patient and team members, and (d) revision of the dressing change procedure. These are outlined below.

Much time was spent listening to the patient in order to understand her perception of her situation, to gain her trust, and to establish an effective relationship. Important themes that emerged were her long and difficult struggle with multiple sclerosis, her fear of the current infection (because of her recent, devastating experience with infection in the other leg), and her helpless, unassertive behavior with the staff. Progressive diseases, such as multiple sclerosis, impose constantly changing demands for coping on those afflicted. For example, a recent study indicated that multiple sclerosis patients' perceived ability to cope with chronic illness was negatively associated with anxiety, with previous hospitalizations for multiple sclerosis, and with total hospitalizations for all causes (Counte, Breliauskas, & Pavlou, 1983). Listening to the patient and observing her behavior assisted me in evaluation of her capabilities for self-management of her health care. Using self–care deficit theory as the general basis for care meant striving to involve the patient to the fullest extent possible and at the same time insuring her of the necessary assistance.

Although other nurses implementing Orem's framework have encountered some initial resistance to the self–care approach (Anna, Christensen, Hohon, Ord, & Wells, 1978), this patient responded enthusiastically. Indeed, in the large case load of rehabilitation patients in my practice, this is the usual response. Others have likewise found a self–care approach to be effective (Goldstein, Zink, Stevenson, Anderson, Woolery, & DePompolo, 1983), and they have recommended patient involvement and self–management strategies as particularly appropriate for rehabilitation patients (Rheiner, Aslakson, Morin, & Patach, 1981; Sawyer & Crimando, 1984; Smith, 1978).

Modifying the patient's pain medication regimen was the first set of concrete recommendations to emerge from the team consultation. Lewis and Levy (1982) comment on the importance of practical suggestions and note that the very involvement of the liaison mental health nurse often facilitates productive interventions by others. This has been observed time and again in my practice. Lewis and Levy (1982) also recognize that in urgent situations immediate intervention may be needed on the basis of minimal information, with provision for further data gathering and later revisions in the plan. Pain frequently constitutes an urgent problem. Successful intervention requires knowledge of the precipitants, concomitants, and consequences of pain, both physical and mental (Brena, Chapman, Stegall, & Chyatte, 1979; Fordyce, 1976; McCaffery, 1979; Merskey, 1976; Sternbach, 1976; Taylor, Skelton, & Butcher, 1984). Because of the many, complex, and subtle variables in the patient's pain experience and the response of others to the patient in pain, careful assessment is critical (McCaffery, 1979; McGuire, 1981). When medication problems are a prominent feature of a case involving pain, evaluation of medication use must then be a high priority.

In this patient's case, recommendations for alteration of pain medications were generated as early as the first day of the consultation, with continued revision during the following weeks. Based on an assessment of the patient and of the nursing unit situation regarding administration of her pain medications, I consulted with the pharmacist and drew up a list of recommended changes, which the physician accepted and wrote as medical orders. They included increasing the morphine dose to an effective level (Marks & Sachar, 1973; Rodman, 1980), delivering morphine at regularly scheduled intervals (Fordyce, 1976; McCaffery, 1979), switching from injections to oral "pain cocktails," and decreasing the dose gradually to zero (Fordyce, 1976; Rubin & Tomosada, 1981; Tennant & Uelman, 1983).

I taught the patient how to use a numerical rating system to describe her pain (Chapman, 1976). This gave the patient and staff a clear, consistent way to communicate about the "level" of the patient's pain. Although still a subjective description by the patient, it had an objective quality that was easier for the staff to accept. It was also possible to establish at what levels of pain she could tolerate certain activities and at what levels she needed a "time out" for the pain to subside. The nurses administering the pain medication asked for a "pain rating" from the patient before each dose was given and recorded it in the medication record. This provided a helpful, ongoing picture of the patient's pain experience and of her response to treatment.

All of these measures had to be carefully explained to the nursing staff and other team members for several reasons. First, an interdisciplinary approach is by definition collaborative (Lewis & Levy, 1982). Second, the staff nurses and other team members were, at the time of this case, still somewhat unaccustomed and resistant to an advanced nursing practitioner's assertion of authority in these areas (Kohnke, 1978). Finally, this was a very unfamiliar approach for them. It was difficult for them to accept the need for increased doses of medication and a regular schedule of administration. These measures seemed to encourage abuse of narcotics. However, they did approve of the switch from injections to oral administration and the expectation that the dose would decrease over time. These factors made the program a little less threatening. What finally helped them accept the treatment, however, was that the patient experienced less pain and increased her tolerance for dressing changes and other activities. Also, the nurses were freed from having to decide whether or not to give a PRN narcotic, a responsibility which weighed heavily on them. Until the program's effectiveness was demonstrated, my way of dealing with the resistance and fear was to be frequently present on the unit and readily available at other times, even evenings and weekends when needed. The support of the physician and pharmacist was crucial as well.

After the medication program had been instituted, the dressing change procedure was revised. First, I evaluated the procedure by talking to the patient about it, by observing others change the dressing, and by doing it myself. The patient and I worked out a written protocol for the dressing changes to minimize discomfort and maximize patient participation. This was then posted prominently in the chart and at the bedside and taught to the other nurses. In addition, I changed the time of the dressing changes to take advantage of the peak analgesia from the morphine.

The various measures yielded good results. The patient's pain decreased markedly, and her tolerance for the dressing changes increased greatly. Eventually, she "graduated" from the pain cocktail and no longer needed narcotics to control her pain. The infection gradually cleared, and she was able to progress in her rehabilitation program to the point of walking with her new prosthesis. Perhaps most important, a new standard of self-involvement in her own care was established for this patient. Over the course of her lengthy admission, this capacity for self-care and self-determination continued to grow.

Caring for this patient resulted in a paradigm case that helped me realize several important aspects of mental health liaison nursing. Clearly, the mental health liaison nurse's role is unique among mental health providers (Fife & Lemler, 1983). It requires what Lewis and Levy (1982) call "a passion for medicine" along with a knowledge of human behavior and an array of interpersonal skills. A specific nursing theory focus, in this instance self-care deficit theory, facilitated the establishment of the scope, limit, and goals of involvement with the patient and with others in the health care system (Fawcett, 1984; Sullivan, 1980).

The nature of mental health liaison nursing mandates close collaboration with other nurses and health team members. This is especially critical in an interdisciplinary setting like a rehabilitation center. For nurses willing and able to meet the prerequisites of such a practice, there exist many opportunities to make exciting, vital applications of mental health technologies in nonpsychiatric settings and to assist individuals to increase their ability to meet their health-related needs.

References

Anna, D. J., Christensen, D. G., Hohon, S. A., Ord, L., & Wells, S. R. Implementing Orem's conceptual framework. *Journal of Nursing Administration*, 1978, 8 (11), 8–11.

Benner, P. From novice to expert. *American Journal of Nursing*, 1982, 82, 402–407.

Benner, P., & Wrubel, J. Skilled clinical knowledge: The value of perceptual awareness, part 2. *Journal of Nursing Administration*, 1982, 12 (6), 28–33.

Bishop, D. S. (Ed.). *Behavioral problems and the disabled*. Baltimore: Williams & Wilkins, 1980.

Brena, S. F., Chapman, S. L., Stegall, P. G., & Chyatte, S. B. Chronic pain states: Their relationship to impairment and disability. *Archives of Physical Medicine and Rehabilitation*, 1979, 60, 387–389.

Caplan, G. *The theory and practice of mental health consultation*. New York: Basic Books, Inc., 1970.

Chapman, C. R. Measurement of pain: Problems and issues. In J. J. Bonica & D. Albe-Fessard (Eds.), *Advances in pain research and therapy* (Vol. 1). New York: Raven Press, 1976.

Counte, M. A., Bieliauskas, L. A., & Pavlou, M. Stress and personal attitudes in chronic illness. *Archives of Physical Medicine and Rehabilitation*, 1983, 64, 272–275.

Dunham, J. R., & Dunhum, C. S. Psychosocial aspects of disability. In R. M. Goldenson (Ed.), *Disability and rehabilitation handbook*. New York: McGraw-Hill Book Company, 1978.

Fawcett, J. *Analysis and evaluation of conceptual models of nursing*. Philadelphia: F. A. Davis Company, 1984.

Fife, B., & Lemler, S. The psychiatric nurse specialist: A valuable asset in the general hospital. *Journal of Nursing Administration*, 1983, 13(4), 14–17.

Fordyce, W. E. *Behavioral methods of chronic pain and illness*. St. Louis: The C. V. Mosby Company, 1976.

Gans, J. S. Hate in the rehabilitation setting. *Archives of Physical Medicine and Rehabilitation*, 1983, 64, 176–179.

Goldstein, N., Zink, M., Stevenson, L., Anderson, M., Woolery, L., & DePompolo, T. Self-care: A framework for the future. In P. L. Chinn (Ed.), *Advances in nursing theory development*. Rockville, Maryland: Aspen Systems Corporation, 1983.

Gunther, M. S. Psychiatric consultation in a rehabilitation hospital: A regression hypothesis. *Comprehensive Psychiatry*, 1971, 12(6), 572–585.

Kohnke, M. F. *The case for consultation in nursing*. New York: John Wiley & Sons, 1978.

Lewis, A., & Levy, J. *Psychiatric liaison nursing: The theory and clinical practice*. Reston, Virginia: Reston Publishing Company, Inc., 1982.

Marinelli, R. P., & Dell Orto, A. E. (Eds.). *The psychological and social impact of physical disability*. New York: Springer Publishing Company, 1977.

Marks, R. M., & Sachar, E. J. Undertreatment of medical inpatients with narcotic analgesics. *Annals of Internal Medicine*, 1973, 78(2), 173–181.

McCaffery, M. *Nursing management of the patient with pain* (2nd ed.). Philadelphia: J. B. Lippincott, 1979.

McGuire, L. A short, simple tool for assessing your patient's pain. *Nursing 81*, 1981, *11*(3), 48–49.

Merskey, H. Psychiatric aspects of the control of pain. In J. J. Bonica & D. Albe-Fessard (Eds.), *Advances in pain research and therapy* (Vol. 1). New York: Raven Press, 1976.

Moos, R. H. (Ed.). *Coping with physical illness.* New York: Plenum Medical Book Company, 1977.

Nickle-Gallagher, L. M. Structuring nursing practice based on Orem's general theory: A practitioner's perspective. In J. R. Sisca (Ed.), *The science and art of self-care.* New York: Appleton-Century-Crofts, in press.

Nursing Development Conference Group. *Concept formalization in nursing: Process and product* (2nd ed.). Boston: Little, Brown and Company, 1979.

Orem, D. E. *Nursing: Concepts of practice* (2nd ed.). New York: McGraw-Hill Book Company, 1980.

Rheiner, N. W., Aslakson, M. A., Morin, P., & Patach, D. Investigation of compliance in the severely injured: A literature review. *Rehabilitation Nursing*, 1981, *9*(4), 12–15.

Robinson, L. *Liaison nursing: Psychological approach to patient care.* Philadelphia: F. A. Davis Company, 1974.

Rodman, M. J. Drug therapy today. *RN*, 1980, *43*(9).

Rubin, T. N., & Tomosada, W. P. The pain cocktail as an adjunctive agent in the treatment of spine pain patients. *Drug Intelligence and Clinical Pharmacy*, 1981, *15*, 958–963.

Sawyer, H. W., & Crimando, W. Self-management strategies in rehabilitation. *Journal of Rehabilitation*, 1984, *50*(1), 27–30.

Shapiro, L. N., & McMahon, A. W. Rehabilitation stalemate. *Archives of General Psychiatry*, 1966, *15*, 173–177.

Smith, M. C. Self-care: A conceptual framework for rehabilitation nursing. *ARN Journal*, 1978, *2*(2), 8–10.

Sternbach, R. A. Psychological factors in pain. In J. J. Bonica & D. Albe-Fessard (Eds.), *Advances in pain research and therapy* (Vol. 1). New York: Raven Press, 1976.

Strauss, A., Fagerhaugh, S., Suczek, B., & Wiener, C. Patients' work in the technologized hospital. *Nursing Outlook*, 1981, *29*(7), 404–412.

Sullivan, T. J. Self-care model for nursing. In American Nurses' Association, *New Directions for Nursing in the '80s.* Kansas City, Missouri: American Nurses' Association, 1980.

Taylor, A. G., Skelton, J. A., & Butcher, J. Duration of pain condition and physical pathology as determinants of nurses' assessments of patients in pain. *Nursing Research*, 1984, *33*(1), 4–8.

Tennant, F. S., & Uelman, G. F. Narcotic maintenance for chronic pain. *Postgraduate Medicine*, 1983, *73*(1), 81–94.

Zola, I. K. Communication barriers between 'the able-bodied' and 'the handicapped.' *Archives of Physical Medicine and Rehabilitation*, 1981, *62*, 355–359.

Chapter Six

STRESS MANAGEMENT FOR THE PROFESSIONAL NURSE

Reda R. Scott, Ph.D.

EXCESSIVE OCCUPATIONAL STRESS IS one of the most frequently cited reasons for leaving the field of nursing.[1] While it is widely recognized that stress is a natural, unavoidable phenomenon of everyday life, prolonged stressful conditions may produce a number of deleterious psychological as well as physiological effects. Thus, since some stress is inevitable and contributes to professional attrition, it is important for nurses to identify their own stressors and to develop adequate coping patterns. The goal of this article is to provide a working definition of stress, a framework for early identification, and a compendium of practical strategies for successful management.

DEFINITION OF STRESS

Although there are numerous fashionable definitions of stress, it can be simply defined as "the wear and tear of living."[2] Many think that stress results only from serious illness or injury; it may also result from driving in rush-hour traffic, having an assignment due, or even getting a long-desired job offer. Therefore, the common element across stress-producing situations appears to be change, both positive and negative.[3]

The most practical conceptualization of stress is that it is a personal experience rather than something that just happens out there in the environment. In other words, any environmental event that produces a stress response is called a stressor, and an event typically becomes a stressor through cognitive interpretation.[4] Thus, stress represents a reaction to a particular event, and this reaction involves complex psychological and physiological interrelationships. The implication of this is that we are responsible for most of the excessive stress that we experience. Consider this situation:

> Anne is a highly motivated woman who is working part-time while she is getting her master's degree in nursing. She is stunned when she receives a "C" on her latest paper, which she thought was one of the best she had written. She immediately begins to feel that she has let everyone down, and she later questions her career goals. She goes to work that afternoon and discovers that she also forgot to write a progress note on a patient the day before. This becomes further proof of her incompetence, and she begins to panic about "not being able to do anything right." She has difficulty concentrating on her work, and she subsequently experiences shortness of breath and a headache.

Neither of these events (making a "C" or forgetting a task), in and of themselves, will necessarily produce excessive stress. Most of Anne's stress was self-induced through her personal interpretation of events. Instead of confronting these two events directly and planning strategies for preventing their recurrence, Anne interpreted them to mean that she was incompetent not only in nursing but also in life. This interpretation led to increased stress and to further deterioration in performance. Ways of minimizing this circular, wasteful activity will be discussed in a subsequent section.

IDENTIFICATION OF STRESS

Most of us recognize that we experience varying amounts of daily stress, which is manifest in minor physical and psychological symptoms. We often attempt to ignore these symptoms until we begin to suffer prolonged effects, such as chronic fatigue, severe headaches, and depression. Once stress reaches this stage, it is often difficult to discern what situation(s) initially produced the discomfort. Consequently, prompt identification is an important component of effective stress management. You can do this by pinpointing high-risk situations and by increasing your awareness of physicial, behavioral, and psychological symptoms that are secondary to stress.

High Risk Situations

Although inadequate staffing, malfunctioning equipment, and patient emergencies undoubtedly contribute greatly, problems in interpersonal relationships are routinely cited as the greatest source of stress among nurses.[5,6] Such problems include personality clashes with staff, disagreement with physicians concerning patient care, communication problems, and lack of respect from other health professionals. Other high-risk situations involve conflict: contradictory administrative directives and patient care realities; contradictory directions from two different authorities. Consequently, nurses often feel caught in the middle. Although stressful situations will vary across hospital and personal settings, it is essential to identify those situations that cause you the greatest distress. Obviously, you cannot begin to manage a stressful situation until you accurately identify it.

Physical Symptoms

Each individual has a unique way of reacting to stress. For most, physical symptoms can serve as a signal that you are experiencing undue stress. To accurately assess stress, consider the physical symptoms that have occurred during the past week, particularly at work. Ask yourself the following questions:

1. Have you experienced frequent headaches?

2. Have you had any gastrointestinal disturbances?

3. Have you felt tired and sluggish despite adequate sleep?

4. Have you had any difficulty sleeping?

5. Have you had any changes in appetite?

6. Have you experienced shortness of breath or shallow breathing?

7. Have you had any backaches?

If you *have* experienced any of these symptoms, you should consider the possibility that they may be stress related.

Psychological and Behavioral Symptoms

As with physical symptoms, certain psychological symptoms can signal undue stress. For example, in the past week at work or school

1. Have you felt "down" or depressed?

2. Have you been agitated?

3. Have you felt irritable or out of sorts?

4. Have you felt a sense of general dreading?

5. Have you been quickly angered?

6. Have you found it difficult to concentrate?

7. Has your startle reaction increased?

8. Have you felt unusually clumsy or awkward?

9. Have you felt unusually disorganized?

If you have experienced any of these symptoms, you may be reacting to environmental stressors. Both physical and psychological symptoms may be used effectively for early identification of stress.

Using Symptoms to Pinpoint Stressors and Reactions

After identifying potential symptoms of stress, you should take a few minutes to think about the situations that are associated with each. The following situation may clarify:

Three weeks ago Jane was promoted to nursing supervisor on her unit. She was eager to do a good job and was enthusiastic and confident about her abilities. However, today she felt sluggish. She found it difficult to concentrate and had to struggle to complete routine tasks. As the day wore on, she felt anxious and had a tightness in her chest.

All of these symptoms were cues to Jane that she was experiencing stress. However, she could not relate these symptoms to any particular event until she asked herself some questions:

1. What time of day and where was I when I began to feel this way?

2. Who was I with?

3. What was I doing?

4. What did I expect to occur?

5. What did I say to myself at the time?

After asking these questions, Jane was able to remember that she began feeling anxious around midmorning, shortly after an impromptu staff meeting. She had explained some new procedures that had been met with numerous questions and some minor objections. Jane remembered that she had unrealistically expected the staff to fully accept all her suggestions. When they did not do so, she felt defensive and concluded that the staff would never like her. Jane began to question her ability to handle her new responsibilities. Later in the day when she had difficulty completing her work with her usual efficiency, she felt even more convinced that she would fail.

A relatively common effect of stress is that we feel unable to sort out and control what is happening to us.[7] Being able to pinpoint the causes as well as the reactions will make a stressful experience much less frightening and may actually bring about substantial relief.

MANAGEMENT OF STRESS

All of us can adequately manage stress if we use coping strategies that allow problem solving or restoration rather than crisis development. Such strategies may involve either stress reduction or stress resistance and will be described below.[8] Since you will benefit only from those methods you actually put to use, carefully consider which procedures can be realistically adapted to your current lifestyle.

Relaxation Exercises.   You probably think that you already know how to relax. It is important not to skip over this section since many activities that people consider relaxing serve only as pauses.[8] For example, you may feel that you relax every time you stop during the day for a cigarette or a cup of coffee or tea. However, these products contain stimulants, which actually serve in the long run to increase stress. Only activities such as deep muscle relaxation, meditation, imagery, self-hypnosis, deep breathing, yoga, and various types of autogenic training will provide restorative relaxation. Many of these are regularly offered as short courses by community groups or campus organizations. Used consistently, these types of activities can provide both stress reduction and stress resistance.

Cognitive Restructuring.   In previous sections, it was mentioned that we are responsible for much of the stress that we experience. Rather than being discouraged by this, you should think about the implications. If most of your stress is self-induced rather than random, it may be possible to exercise substantial control over it. For example, an environmental event becomes a stressor primarily through our interpretation. If we can change this interpretation, we are likely to prevent or at least minimize a substantial amount of our stress.

Refer to the preceding examples of Anne and Jane. In Anne's case, neither receiving the "C" nor forgetting to write the progress note produced the stress-related symptoms of panic, concentration difficulties, shortness of breath, or headache. Her interpretation that she was incompetent and "unable to do anything right" produced the symptoms. An alternative interpretation could have been that she did not like to make poor grades or forget a task. Everyone makes mistakes, and one mistake or poor grade does not make someone incompetent. Similarly, in Jane's case neither the staff's questioning nor objections alone caused her stress; it was her interpretation combined with these events. Jane had unrealistically expected her staff to love her and immediately comply with her suggestions. When they did not, she interpreted this to mean that she was not qualified to handle her new role. An alternative interpretation could have been that any change, good or bad, is often resisted initially. It would take time for her co-workers to accept her fully as a supervisor, and there would always be times that everyone would not agree with her. This does not mean that she will never be accepted or that she is incompetent for a supervisory role. Just as she has the right to make mistakes, others have the right to dislike her suggestions.

These two examples illustrate that changing our interpretations of events can frequently reduce our stress. Although there are exceptions, whenever you feel physical and psychological symptoms, use the questions for pinpointing antecedents.[7] You will often find that these questions lead you to an earlier, faulty interpretation. If you are able to substitute a healthier, positive interpretation, you can often reduce a substantial amount of stress right away.

Behaving Assertively and Communicating Effectively.   The traditional image of the caring nurse as one who is quiet, agreeable, and vocal only when addressed continues to persist in some settings. However, Donnelly[9] has countered that nurses can be more caring over the long run if they speak up. Assertive behavior and direct communication contribute not only to the welfare of the patient but also to the mental health of the professional. Consider the following situation:

> Louise is a conscientious clinical specialist who has been staying late all week to help out on a short-staffed cardiac care unit. However, her family has begun to complain about her not being able to spend much time with them. On Friday, she is leaving work at her regularly scheduled time, so that she can have dinner and attend a movie with her family. As she is leaving, the nursing supervisor approaches her and requests that she stay a few hours until another nurse can be called in for the evening shift.

A passive response to this situation might include:

"Well. . . uh. . . I guess I could stay for a short time. . . unless you think you could maybe find someone else."

This type of response would probably be detrimental to the nurse, the other staff, and the patients. Violating her own rights by being passive is likely to produce resentment. Louise would probably experience increasing stress, since the longer she stays the less likely she will get home in time to be with her already irritated family. In addition, her increased stress is likely to be perceived by patients as well as other staff who are already anxious about the consistent understaffing. Under these conditions, no one is likely to benefit from Louise's presence. An aggressive response to the above situation might include:

"Get serious! You supervisors are so insensitive to anyone's needs except your own. Why don't you stay if you're so concerned?"

Aggressive responses violate the rights of others because they always involve some form of attack. Such a response might provide immediate relief, but it is likely to increase long-term stress. Aggressive responses rarely promote healthy interaction on any unit and typically create more problems.

An assertive response allows one to achieve some sort of balance between passivity and aggression, although assertion does not guarantee that you will get what you want. An assertive answer to the preceding situation might include:

"I understand that you need someone. However, I have stayed late every night this week, and it is necessary for me to leave right away this evening. I suggest that you try one of the other nurses."

Such a response clearly communicates a position without violating the rights of anyone (including your own). It can be said in a pleasant, courteous manner and is a response that will promote healthy interactions on a unit.

Out of the situational context, being assertive sounds quite easy, but in reality, any new behavior can be difficult. Here are a number of suggestions that might make assertion and clear communication easier:

1. For any new behavior, practice is the key to success. Therefore, you might begin by practicing in front of a mirror, and then with friends.

2. Most people find it easier to begin with positive statements, such as giving a compliment to someone. Then move on to negative statements.

3. Assertive responses usually begin with "I." With these statements, the speaker takes direct responsibility for the

statement. Also, "I" statements are more likely to be clearly communicated.

4. The manner in which a statement is made can be more important than the content. For example, you must be aware of your posture, eye contact, tone of voice, and volume. The nonverbal communication must be consistent with the verbal one in order for a statement to make a clear impact.

5. It is important to be persistent with assertive responses, particularly in the early stages. If you have been passive in the past, people may think that you will acquiesce if they continue to ask. It is crucial to dispel this perception.

While it would be unreasonable to refuse all requests, it is equally unwise to accept them all. Whether or not you are assertive will depend upon the timing of the situation. For example, if the request in the preceding illustration had been made at a less stressful time, Louise may have wanted to stay the extra hours. The decision to be assertive will depend upon one's relationship with the other person(s) involved; being assertive with your colleagues should be considered differently from being assertive with your supervisor.

Day-to-Day Suggestions.   In addition to specific stress reduction techniques that require some skill, you may benefit by trying a few of the following methods for quick, temporary stress reduction. Even on the busiest days it is helpful to get away for just a couple of minutes of quiet, uninterrupted time and take several deep breaths. The bathroom may be the only place for this, depending on your particular setting. Lunch hours and break time should provide some relaxation and should not be used for routinely discussing the day's problems with others. A short, brisk walk may be therapeutic and restorative right after lunch. Finally, taking time to get to know your colleagues is a particularly important part of stress management, since a social support system will allow for therapeutic ventilation and sharing of feelings.[1]

Stress Resistance

An important part of stress management involves building up your resistance, so that you are less vulnerable to stress when it occurs. This can be achieved through adequate diet, exercise, and sleep. Consider your own life style for a few minutes. Did you have only coffee and something sweet this morning for breakfast? Or worse yet, did you skip breakfast altogether? Have you been binge eating highly processed foods? Did you get enough sleep last night? When was the last occasion that you took time for exercise?

Health professionals are often remiss in maintaining a healthful work and recreation balance. When under stress, we tend to give up the very activities that would ultimately provide us with more energy for accomplishing our particular goals. Diet, exercise, and sleep work interchangeably in building reserves. As with other strategies, it is important to be realistic in planning your diet, exercise, and sleep programs, since grandiose plans are likely to be followed religiously for one or two days and then dropped.

CONCLUSION

Stress has been described as an unavoidable phenomenon, and the author has emphasized the deleterious effects of prolonged stress. Effective management of stress can impact therapeutically upon the nursing staff and their patient care. Stress management may also serve to prevent burnout which occurs with alarming frequency among professional nurses. Finally, for students and new graduates, it may be especially important to assess current stress levels and coping strategies, since the patterns being established now will more than likely be carried over to professional nursing roles.

References

1. Ginsberg, E., Patray, J., Ostow, M., & Brann, E. A. Nurse discontent: The search for realistic solutions. *Journal of Nursing Administration*, 1982, *12*(11), 7–11.

2. Gottardi, D. A., & Kidorf, I. W. Team nursing reduces stress. *The Journal of Practical Nursing*, 1982, *32*(6), 34–35.

3. Dohrenwend, B. S. Life events as stressors: A methodological inquiry. *Journal of Health and Social Behavior*, 1983, *14*, 167–175.

4. Everly, G. S., & Rosenfeld, R. *The nature and treatment of the stress response: A practical guide for clinicians.* New York: Plenum Press, 1981.

5. Bailey, J. T., Steffan, S. M., & Grout, J. W. The stress audit: Identifying the stressors of ICU nursing. *Journal of Nursing Education*, 1980, *19*(6), 15–25.

6. Huckabay, L. M. D., & Jagla, B. Nurses' stress factors in the intensive care unit. *Journal of Nursing Administration*, 1979, *9*(2), 21–28.

7. Galano, J., Carr-Kaffashan, L., Ettin, M., Lehrer, P., & Rothberg, M. Handbook of techniques for dealing with stress. *JSAS Catalog of Selected Documents in Psychology,* 1978, 8, 67.

8. Shaffer, M. *Life after stress.* New York: Plenum Press, 1982.

9. Donnelly, G. F. The assertive nurse or how to say what you mean without shaking or shouting. *Nursing '78,* 1978, 8(1), 65–69.

Part Two

MENTAL HEALTH ASSESSMENT OF INDIVIDUALS AND FAMILIES

T he ability to perform comprehensive assessments is a critical nursing skill. Assessment is the basis for therapeutic intervention. Only with adequate assessment can the ensuing steps of the nursing process (that is, planning, implementation, therapeutic intervention, and evaluation) be carried out most effectively. Assessment in mental health may be considered an art; it requires the ability to help clients communicate how they feel about their present situations, perhaps for the first time. Family members too can be helped to look at their sources of pain in the nonjudgmental atmosphere of nursing assessment. The initial assessment lays the foundation for the therapeutic relationship and elicits the data base for a nursing care plan. Finally, the assessment process conveys the nurse's role on the health-care team to clients and families and serves to legitimize future contacts.

The unit comprises five articles: three articles address the initiation and enactment of mental health assessment; the fourth and fifth articles present methods for assessment of alcohol use. Because alcohol abuse is a major health problem in this country, we believe that nurses need to carefully assess clients for alcohol use, not only in psychiatric settings but also on medical-surgical units and in the community.

In the first article, Rapp and Wilcox discuss different methods of data collection, including interviews (client reports), direct observations of behavior, physical examinations, and laboratory reports. They point out that listening to how clients present data is a significant part of assessment. Assessment data may come from a variety of other sources, including spouses, other family members, friends, co-workers, and hospital staff. Data may be either subjective or objective. Rapp and Wilcox stress that comprehensive assessment is an ongoing process, from the initial client contact, through the treatment followup.

Since the individual client is often but one member of a family unit, it is important to understand the interactional dynamics of that unit. Sedgewick discusses the family as a system of relationships and, in doing so, provides five indices to examine these relationships.

Detailed means for family assessment are provided by Morgan and Macey. Family therapists need to assess the family as a whole system, including aspects of their physical health, social, and mental health. The authors present three "family assessment tools" that aid the organization of overwhelming data into comprehensive initial, ongoing, and termination assessment.

Cohn points out that many nurses feel relieved that their hospital does not admit alcoholics, when in fact it actually does under an admitting diagnosis of hypertension, gastritis, or broken arm. Nurses are often reluctant to bring up the subject of suspected alcohol abuse, but the failure to make such an assessment can be catastrophic for the client. Without proper medical and nursing treatment, clients who are dependent on alcohol and not assessed as such may experience withdrawal symptoms and delirium tremens. Cohn presents subjective and objective clues that nurses can use to look for the hidden diagnosis of alcohol use.

Brodsley offers a thorough assessment guide for alcohol use, including questions nurses can ask clients to elicit data. Once the history is obtained, the nursing physical assessment evaluates the objective signs of alcohol-related physical or emotional problems. A data review of the neurological cardiac, blood, gastrointestinal, and liver effects of alcohol is presented in table format.

Chapter Seven

METHODS OF ASSESSMENT IN PSYCHIATRIC NURSING

Stephen R. Rapp, Ph.D. and Sallye M. Wilcox, R.N., M.S.N.

ASSESSMENT, THE SYSTEMATIC COLLECTION of data about the client's problems and resources, is the first step in the nursing process. It provides the basis for the nursing diagnosis, for the formulation of the nursing care plan, and for the evaluation of treatment regimens. It is a continuous process, beginning with the initial client contact and proceeding through the treatment follow up. To be maximally useful, a psychiatric nursing assessment must incorporate several different forms of data gathered from several different sources. The psychiatric nurse, therefore, must become skillful in the use of various assessment methods. This article will review some basic methods of assessment—the structured interview, the unstructured interview, direct observation, and indirect observation—and discuss the advantages and disadvantages of each.

ASSESSMENT BY STRUCTURED INTERVIEW

The most widely used assessment procedure is the clinical interview. An interview may be structured or unstructured. Structured interviews generally involve the use of a standard protocol or guide consisting of a series of questions to be covered. A recently developed structured interview guide for assessing disorders of mood and thinking is the Schedule for Affective Disorders and Schizophrenia (SADS; Endicott & Spitzer, 1978). The SADS lists each of the clinical features for each disorder covered and provides questions the interviewer can ask to obtain data about each feature. Client answers are rated on a 7-point rating scale also provided in the guide. Below is an excerpt from the SADS for the feature of hopelessness or discouragement characteristic of depression:

0 No information

Have you been discouraged (pessimistic, felt hopeless)?

What kind of a future do you see for yourself?

How do you think things will work out?

Can you see yourself or your situation getting any better?

1 Not at all discouraged about the future

2 Slight, e.g., occasional feelings of mild discouragement about the future

3 Mild, e.g., often somewhat discouraged

4 Moderate, e.g., often feels quite pessimistic about future

5 Severe, e.g., pervasive feelings of intense pessimism

6 Extreme, e.g., delusions or hallucinations that he is doomed, or that the world is coming to an end

Another example of a structured interview guide appeared in the *American Journal of Nursing* (August, 1981; pp. 1493–1518). It describes the components of the mental status exam in an easy to learn programmed instructional format.

Structured interviews have the disadvantage of generally restricting questioning to those items listed in the guide. This is especially problematic when the client presents material not covered by the interview protocol. In most instances, additional unstructured interview techniques are needed. Structured interviews have the advantage of making interviews more consistent across interviewers and across time. Thus, Nurse A and Nurse B are more likely to obtain the same information from a certain client if both are following the same structured interview guide assuming the client's condition has not changed during the interim. A second advantage of structured interviews is their value as a means of teaching the skills for the second type of interview: the unstructured interview.

ASSESSMENT BY UNSTRUCTURED INTERVIEW

The unstructured interview gives the interviewer greater flexibility to ask more and different questions, an advantage especially great when one considers the wealth of information provided during a standard nursing interview. With greater flexibility comes, however, the requirement of greater skillfulness on the part of the interviewer. To become adept at interviewing a psychiatric client, the nurse must know both what questions to ask and how to phrase them to yield valuable information. To accomplish this goal, there are several specific skills one must acquire:

1. *Selecting appropriate questions.* Becoming familiar with the different classes of psychopathology or nursing diagnoses will direct one to ask more relevant questions. Also, reviewing the available structured interview guides will familiarize one with standard questions.

2. *Phrasing questions to produce descriptive answers.* For example, instead of asking the depressed client, "Why do you get depressed?" (which presumes he or she is capable of giving an explanation for his or her problem) or "How down do you get?" (which requires the patient to make a difficult comparative statement), one should ask questions like: "Tell me *what* you do when you feel depressed?" and "Tell me *when* you get depressed?" and "Tell me *where* you typically get depressed?" and "Tell me *who* was present when you last became depressed?" Another useful strategy for generating specific, descriptive responses is to have clients quantify their answers. For example, to assess the intensity of the discomfort associated with an anxiety attack, ask the client to rate his or her discomfort on a scale from 1 to 10 where 1 = "no discomfort" and 10 = "the greatest discomfort imaginable." An advantage of quantification in this manner is the nurse has a relatively stable criterion or scale by which to compare the client's state during hospitalization.

3. *Asking easier questions first.* With most psychiatric clients, the treatment team is especially interested in their functioning in four areas or "spheres": behavior, thought, affect (feelings), and physiology. Questions regarding the client's behavior are generally easier for him or her to answer and should be asked first. Somewhat more difficult to describe are thoughts and physiologic responses (e.g., pain or other sensations), so questions related to these areas should be asked next. Most difficulty is

experienced in responding to questions about our feeling states because of their highly complex and subjective nature. Hence, these questions should be reserved for last. By appropriately ordering questions, the client will more quickly feel at ease with the interviewer and interview process. The same *What, When, Where,* and *Who* questions outlined above can be modified to fit inquiries into behavior, physiologic responses, thoughts, and feelings.

   4. *Being an effective listener.* Effective listening implies interacting with the client during the interview process. That is, using the information acquired to influence subsequent questions and hypotheses about the client's condition. Effective listening is active listening as one attends to everything that is said. Without the skill of effective listening, the interviewer is forced to merely recite questions and as such cannot be very helpful to the client. There is another important feature of effective listening. It is as important to listen to the manner with which the client speaks as to what is said. A client's tone of voice, rate of speech, and voice volume can all be significant data. For example, a behavior that typifies a manic state is pressured speech characterized by a faster than normal rate of speech for that person. The observation of this characteristic could be very helpful in making a distinction between a manic client and, say, one experiencing an anxiety attack where speech may also be speeded up.

   5. *Being a vigilant observer of the client's behavior during the interview process.* The interview is a complex social interaction between client and nurse. As in any social interaction, clients will respond to what occurs verbally as well as non-verbally. Their non-verbal responses (e.g., gestures, glances, and posture) are sources of additional data. The client whose eyes tear or dart from side to side, or whose fingers tremble or twitch, or who appears unkempt and dirty, or who is dressed in clothing characteristic of a sub-cultural group is offering valuable data to the alert observer.

   Up to this point, the interview has been discussed exclusively in relation to the identified client. In most cases, the psychiatric nurse will also want to interview a spouse or other family member, an employer, or a friend to gather additional information and to validate the client's report. The same skills described above are also relevant to interviews with significant others.

ASSESSMENT BY DIRECT OBSERVATION

Hospitalization offers the entire treatment staff the opportunity to directly observe the behavior of the psychiatric client over time and amidst situations (e.g., during meals, in group meetings, during visitation hours, on the unit). Since the nursing staff has the greatest amount of direct client contact, they are frequently called upon to make systematic observations of the client's behavior and clearly communicate their observations to the treatment team. Direct observation is an essential part of any assessment and care plan, one which the nurse should learn to do well. To be able to make skillful direct observations, four steps should be taken:

1. *Define that which you wish to observe (i.e., the target) in terms of visible behavior.* Many attempts at direct observation fail simply because the target, though important, was unobservable. For example, while raising the self-esteem of a depressed client is a worthy treatment goal, "self-esteem" is a theoretical concept and, therefore, not observable. Thus, instead of selecting "self-esteem" to observe, the nurse must decide which visible behaviors best represent the concept of "self-esteem." These will vary from client to client but might include initiating conversation with other clients and staff, smiling, or refusing unreasonable requests. Other examples of poorly defined targets are "psychotic behavior," "depression," "anxiety," "adjustment," "resistance to treatment," and "cooperativeness." As a rule of thumb: If your target has not been described in observable terms, you should not attempt to assess it. Rather, redefine it until you have an observable target.

2. *Define the context(s) in which the behavior is to be observed.* Since it is impossible to observe every instance of a particular behavior, it becomes necessary to select those situations or contexts in which target behaviors will be observed. A description of the context generally includes time and place and may include other persons or activities as well. Examples of contexts include "in group therapy," "when alone in his or her room," "when in the dayroom with other clients," or "when asked 'How are you doing?' by staff." Selection of the context(s) will depend upon the individual client's problem and staff convenience. For example, with the paranoid client the nurse may be primarily interested in the occurrence of verbal statements of suspiciousness (the target) directed toward other people during group activities (the context). Or with the depressed client the target behavior may be "sleeping" and the context may be "during scheduled activities."

3. *Select the time schedule for making your observations.* Deciding how often to observe a client's behavior depends, in part, on how often you expect the behavior to occur during the course of a day. If a behavior occurs frequently (e.g., sitting in the dayroom) or if it occurs only in circumscribed contexts (e.g., at meal time) you can easily plan your

observation periods. However, when a target behavior occurs infrequently or in diverse contexts (e.g., a schizophrenic client talking to him or herself) you must plan a schedule that permits you to sample observations across time and contexts. To accomplish this, a procedure called *time sampling* is employed. Time sampling involves the repeated observation of a person for brief periods of time. Observation periods can be as short as two to five seconds. Frequently, ten or more observations are made per day. The exact length and number of observation periods depend on the target behavior(s) and staff time.

   4. *Select a method for recording your observations.* Accurate recording of your observations allows you and other staff to appropriately interpret your findings. When a behavior occurs infrequently, (e.g., vomiting or an act of open aggression) special recording procedures may be unnecessary. However, when a behavior occurs frequently or you are observing several behaviors simultaneously, then you will need a way to record your multiple observations. For a single behavior that occurs with high frequency (e.g., cigarette smoking) a simple tally sheet or mechanical counter is useful. When observing multiple behaviors (e.g., being out of the room, in the presence of other people, and talking) it is helpful to make a *behavior checklist* consisting of a list of the target behaviors with space to make a "✔" if the behavior is present or absent during the observation period. With a behavior checklist each observation period should be clearly separated from earlier periods. In this way changes in the client's behavior can be clearly noted. Several behavior checklists used by nurses have been reported in the literature (Mariotto & Paul, 1974; Rosen, Tureff, Daruna, Johnson, Lyons & Davis, 1980, among others). One example, the Sample Behavior Checklist (Mariotto & Paul, 1974), employs two-second observational periods during which the nurse checks the presence or absence of sixty-nine behaviors. Behaviors are grouped in categories including location, position, awake–asleep, facial expression, normal behavior, social orientation, and crazy behavior. An alternative to the checklist is the *behavior log*. Unlike the checklist, the log does not list different behaviors, rather the observer must write down any behaviors observed during the observational period.

   The major advantage of direct observational procedures is in the quality of the data generated. When properly carried out, direct observation produces objective and verifiable information about the client and reduces the need for subjective inferences (i.e., guesses) by the staff. A disadvantage of direct observation is the increased amount of staff time and energy required. However, once the staff becomes familiar with the steps previously outlined, the procedure becomes somewhat easier. Also, a set of standard behavioral definitions (Step 1), contexts (Step 2), and recording forms (Step 4) can be developed and reused.

ASSESSMENT BY INDIRECT OBSERVATION

Up to this point we have discussed assessment procedures conducted by the nurse. Other procedures are carried out by the clients themselves. Some target behaviors may be easily observed by the client (e.g., cigarette smoking or lying in bed). Other aspects of the client's general behavior may be observable only by him or her such as mood states or intrusive thoughts. In these cases, if properly instructed, some clients can systematically record self-observations. This procedure, called *self-monitoring*, requires that the four steps discussed in the section on direct observational techniques be completed by the nursing staff and then carefully explained to the client.

The obvious advantage of client self-monitoring is an increase of data at little or no additional cost to the staff. A less obvious but important advantage is the increased participation of the client in his or her treatment. Besides being a means for gathering additional data, self-monitoring communicates that treatment is a responsibility shared by the client and members of the treatment team. A third advantage derives from the discovery that self-monitoring of one's behavior may actually increase or decrease its frequency (Nelson, 1977). Thus, asking a client to self-monitor an undesirable behavior (e.g., leaving one's room without combing one's hair) may contribute to its reduction. Conversely, having a client observe a desirable behavior (e.g., eating all one's diet) may cause it to increase in frequency.

The major disadvantage of client self-monitoring is the possibility of unreliable and invalid data. As a precaution, staff should carefully review the data for obvious errors and either train the client further or abandon self-monitoring. Also, clients cannot be expected to continue to self-monitor if staff fails to positively respond to their effort. Therefore, work regularly with clients on their self-monitoring and acknowledge their contribution to treatment.

SUMMARY AND CONCLUSIONS

Assessment is the first step in developing a nursing diagnosis and care plan as well as an on-going part of nursing care. The nurse must obtain as much information about the patient as possible if he or she is to be successful. The methods by which a nurse gathers this information can vary from those that are highly structured to those that are informal and less structured, from those that are direct to those that are indirect. The methods described here are a few of the basic procedures used by mental health professionals. Each assessment method, however, has advantages and disadvantages that must be considered with each new client. As a result, to be effective a psychiatric nurse must become skilled in the administration of each method. In this way he or she can select and employ several assessment methods simultaneously to obtain the most comprehensive picture of the client.

References

Cohen, S. & Harris, E. Programmed instruction: Mental status assessment. *American Journal of Nursing*, 1981, 8r, 1493–1518.

Endicott, J. & Spitzer, R. L. A diagnostic interview: The Schedule for Affective Disorders and Schizophrenia. *Archives of General Psychiatry*, 1978, 35, 837–844.

Mariotto, M. J. & Paul, G. L. A multimethod validation of the inpatient multidimensional psychiatric scale with the chronically institutionalized patients. *Journal of Consulting and Clinical Psychology*, 1974, 42, 497–508.

Nelson, R. O. Methodological issues in assessment via self-monitoring. In J. D. Cone & R. P. Hawkins (Eds.), *Behavioral assessment: New directions in clinical psychology*. New York: Brunner/Mazel, 1977.

Rosen, A. J., et al. Pharmacotherapy of schizophrenic and affective disorders: Behavioral correlates of diagnostic and demographic variables. *Journal of Abnormal Psychology*, 1980, 89, 375–389.

Suggested Readings

Cone, J. D. & Hawkins, R. P. (Eds). *Behavioral assessment: New directions in clinical psychology*. New York: Brunner/Mazel, 1977. An excellent reference text, this edited book has chapters on interviewing, checklists, self-monitoring, and behavioral observations.

Chapter Eight

THE FAMILY AS A SYSTEM: A NETWORK OF RELATIONSHIPS

Rae Sedgewick

IN ORDER TO BETTER understand the family as a unit, let us begin by looking at the family as a system of relationships. Families are made up of relationships between people whose interactions and patterns of living influence each other. A family then, is an integrated system of interdependent structures and functions, is constituted of relationships, and consists of people who must learn to live together.

Each person, in a healthy family, must be capable of transmitting messages and responding sufficiently so that others are aware that a transmission has occurred. Each person responds predictably, with some pattern to the behavior. These patterns of behavior compose a network of relationships which may be referred to as a system. Patterns of behavior may be referred to as components or units which in combination with other components interrelate to produce the overall system known as the family. These units or patterns of behavior reveal via symbols, verbal and nonverbal, what is going on within respective belief systems. These patterns of behavior are transmitted via symbols, from generation to generation. Each member of each generation is, in some way or another, an origin of values, beliefs or attitudes. Each originator or origin acquires tools, skills and expertise which will facilitate or hinder the transmission or articulation of these values, beliefs and/or attitudes.

Since this view of the family differs from traditional approaches and

From "The Family as a System: A Network of Relationships," by Rae Sedgewick, *Journal of Psychiatric Nursing and Mental Health Services*, March/April, 1974. Reprinted by permission of SLACK, Inc., Medical Publishers, Thorofare, NJ.

has concomitant implications for social, psychological and health oriented interventions, it is helpful to describe more fully the family as a network or system of relationships. Viewing the family as a system of relationships can be contrasted with viewing the family as made up of individual people with stereotypic role functions. The latter approach, as is well known, describes the family as a biological unit and calls into play those principles which have been traditionally utilized to understand biological units, i.e., one in which the members are bound by fixed rules and role expectations based on biological functions and explained by historical precedents. The former view entails describing the family as a social unit, and of employing principles and dynamics of group development or social units to understand the overall process.

If we regard the family as a system of relationships, we seek to understand development of relationships, of group norms and expectations, of communication skills, of group decision-making and of group methods of dealing with individual needs and group expectations. If, on the other hand, we regard the family as a biological unit, we seek only to know the traditional expectations of each role or function and any dysfunction is attributed to the individual's inability to properly execute or fulfill those traditional expectations.

A further elaboration is helpful. The family has been traditionally viewed as a biological unit meaning there is a male-father, female-mother and as a result female and/or male offspring. The family is not "complete" without such members. While this is a sound biological description of a "family," parenting is predominately social. Parenting is a process which not only begins with conception but extends throughout the life span. Parenting need not be biological but rather can be quite logically based on social and emotional responsibility. Fathering is traditionally associated with those qualities or characteristics assumed to be typically masculine, i.e., decisive, dominant, aggressive, strong, intellectual and work-oriented. Mothering, on the other hand, is traditionally associated with those qualities or characteristics assumed to be feminine or womanly, i.e., tender, caring, gentle, submissive, cooperative, tactful and home-oriented.

The roles emerging from the traditional biological approach are analogous to the hierarchal structure in industry: manager-policy making and labor-policy implementing. This structure is best understood by knowing tradition and making comparative analyses between what are traditionally or historically acceptable roles and the present role enactments. The understanding gleaned from this approach has very little to do with what actually goes on in any given *group* or family. This approach, while accepted by many lay people, health professionals and behavioral scientists, has added little to our conceptual or practical knowledge of families. It is an approach based on generalities and stereotypes. A family cannot be understood by looking at traditional roles and expectations and inference applying the analysis to all other families.

77

On the other hand, if we approach the family as a system, organizational theory and principles of psychosocial learning become our conceptual framework. The family can be viewed as a social unit made up of interdependent relationships and as a social unit in which decisions must be made, policies determined, feelings honored, skills respected and comfort given. Each person needs space for individual growth and development; but each has group or family obligations as well. Parenting is no less important in this framework. As in every group, leadership is imperative. Those who are best prepared should assume that role. As in other organizational models, there are managerial decisions, labor implementations and consumer/user needs. While traditionally these roles cited above have been filled by father, mother and child, respectively and exclusively, in the systems model these roles need not be so rigidly defined and assigned. Clarity of role is both necessary and useful; however, clarity of role in the traditional approach frequently implies rigidity as well; i.e., one person exclusively fills one role. The social approach allows more flexibility, i.e., one role can be filled by different persons under different situations. The role fulfillment then becomes dependent on an individual's strengths and weaknesses in particular situations. Stress can severely limit one's ability to be protective in one particular instance while that same individual may be very protective and supportive at other times. While roles are necessary for effectiveness, role assignment need not be traditional.

Task and expressive roles are the most commonly agreed upon roles necessary for group effectiveness.[1] Expressive roles are those primarily centered on interpersonal tasks, which are concerned with maintaining and strengthening interpersonal relationships. This is what is meant by being "people centered," so frequently associated with mothering. By contrast, task leaders are primarily involved with task or job accomplishments, with things rather than people and with solutions to problems rather than with interpersonal relationships. Traditionally, it has been assumed that the father will assume a greater degree of leadership in the task area, while mothers tend more often to take the role of mediator, conciliator and comforter. However, regardless of who is assuming a leadership function, effectiveness in group functioning is dependent on a high level of cooperation and support from the partner not assuming that role.[2] This can be contrasted with disturbed families where patterns emerge which are fixed, static and often extreme, e.g., authoritarian, patriarchy. In the healthy family, roles are not fixed and static, but are assumed by the person with the greatest time and inclination for fulfilling that particular role at that particular point in time. Role fulfillment is flexible, e.g., little Diane falls and scrapes her knee, daddy being available picks her up, comforts and soothes, and she's off again. Mother, having taken a course on *Care of Your Car* is making a decision on when and where to have the car serviced.

Dysfunction of the family, using the systems approach, assumes the dysfunction to be either within the particular family system *e.g.*, lack of role clarity, vagueness of expectation, unresolved conflict or some disturbance between the family systems and other systems such as church, police, school. Dysfunction is not taken to be within one individual, *e.g.*, the identified patient, but the result of some system deficit. Additionally, a dysfunction in any one part of the family system or any impinging systems, *e.g.*, school, has an effect on all systems involved. The child who demonstrates behavioral problems in the classroom or at home is frequently an indication that something is amiss in one of the systems, *e.g.*, parental disharmony, teacher-principal conflict, vagueness of policy or inadequate role definition.

Several indices can be employed to examine relationships within a group, social unit or family.³ Five common yardsticks are: productivity, decision-making, utilization of information or data, implementation of decision-making and resolution of conflict or disagreement.

Productivity relates to a family or group's ability to complete a task. For example, if a family has defined priorities for itself, how able are the members as a group to carry them out? Observation should be made of how the family decides what a task will be, who decides how a task will be carred out and who participates in the task solution.

Decision-making is inextricably linked with how the family utilizes information in their environment, how they refer to each other and how they identify, mobilize and utilize their own resources within the family. It is undoubtedly obvious that the healthy family is better at making decisions than unhealthy families. How these decisions are reached is also more apparent in the healthy family. In the effective group and healthy family, there emerges a pattern of decision-making which is observable. It is one in which a leader assumes final responsibility. I would interject that while ideally each member has input, parents act as ultimate leaders or responsible people in the process. There must be a point, it seems to me, at which the parent or leader assumes a firm-footed stance, based on experience, expertise and justice. While each member in the family should be heard and allowed decision-making responsibilities for which they are prepared, there are certain times and particular areas for which parents or leaders should assume final responsibility and assume leadership in the implementation. I would suggest that in unhealthy families roles of adultness are not assumed by the parents and frequently fall to the children, who are ill-prepared for the roles and responsibilities. In terms of decision-making, one would want to observe who takes responsibility for making decisions, who initiates, who follows, who suggests, who addresses whom and who listens.

Utilization of information means seeking, sharing, listening and utilizing each other, outside agencies and other people, to achieve the best decision, *i.e.*, how open is the family to outside influence? Here one would want to observe what kinds of information are useful to the family; with regard to that information, who seeks, sends, clarifies, inquires and deciphers the data. It is important to observe whether the family seeks information which supports what they already know or which raises questions which allow for growth or change.

Implementation of decision-making is barely separable from gathering data and making decisions. However, we all know families or groups who make decisions, but who never seem to carry them out. This may be related to: (1) the decision-making process, (2) who feels and who assumes responsibility in the group, (3) lack of specification about who is supposed to be doing what, or (4) uneven allocation of responsibilities within the family.

Resolution of conflict is an extremely important index because unhealthy or ineffective groups tend to ignore, deny and push under the surface any conflict, thereby failing to identify problem areas and hence solutions. This type of behavior is somehow based on the mythical notion that harmony is characteristic of healthy families and that conflict is an adaptive failure. Harmony is *not* equivalent to stability nor is conflict necessarily a sign of dysfunction.[4] A family, as a group, which does not deal only with conflict, problems or disagreements, may resort to backbiting, deception, undermining and disillusionment. Careful observations to make here are how able the family members are to challenge one another's ideas, how open and honest they are, how often deception must be resorted to in order to maintain pseudo-harmony and how able they are to seek differing opinions and utilize information available to them. Don't be surprised if you find that the mode most frequently employed is denial that any conflict exists. To many people, conflict means denial of love or potential rejection and while it need not be so, it is a very real fear of many people.

We have thus far explored the family as a psycho-social unit of relationships, affected by and having influence on other systems. Maladjustment is taken to be a manifestation of dysfunction within the system itself or in some system influencing the family, thereby removing the blame or responsibility for the "problem" from the "identified patient." One implication of the psycho-social approach is that the counselor, public health nurse, community mental health nurse or other health related personnel operates from a knowledge base of organizational and group dynamics, and learning theories of behavior. The role of such an intervener becomes one of consultant and of social change agent in an ever evolving, ever changing family unit or system. Applying the social system approach to the family implies some changes in traditional role assignments, some rethinking of traditional givens for men and women, an expanded role for the mental health nurse and can result in greater effectiveness in identifying solutions for social and family problems. Some indices of effective family behavior have been identified, with some specific references to important observations and assessments for the health professional to make. Attention must now be turned to explicating effective health interventions.

References

1. Johnson, M., Martin, H.: A sociological analysis of the nurse role. *Amer J. Nurs,* March 1958, pp. 373-377.
2. Murrel, S.A., Stachowiak, J.G.: Consistency, rigidity, and power in the interaction patterns of clinic and nonclinic families. *J. Abnorm. Psychol.* 72:265-272, 1967.
3. Cartwright, D., Zander, A. (eds): Group Dynamics: Research and Theory. New York, Harper and Row, 1968.
4. Kelly, J.: Make conflict work for you. *Harvard Bus. Rev.,* July/August 1970, pp. 103-113.

Bibliography

Bell, J. E.: A theoretical position for family therapy. *Family Process* 2:1-14, 1963.

Laing, R.D.: *The Politics of the Family.* New York, Vintage Books, 1972.

Satir, V.: *Conjoint Family Therapy.* Palo Alto, California, Science and Behavior Books Inc., 1967.

Chapter Nine

THREE ASSESSMENT TOOLS FOR FAMILY THERAPY

S. A. Morgen and Jane Macey

FAMILY THERAPY, A RELATIVE newcomer to the practice of psychotherapy, has been increasing in popularity since the 1950s.[1] Therapists are becoming more cognizant of the fact that coping with life is much easier when the entire family is made aware of dysfunctional behavior. The family therapist often serves as the catalyst for bringing about awareness of this dysfunctional behavior. As a member of the mental health team and a systems analyst, the therapist is responsible for comprehensive family assessment before she can proceed with family therapy. It is from this viewpoint that the literature has been researched, clinical data have been collected, and family therapy tools have been developed.

REVIEW OF THE LITERATURE

Many authors simply include family concepts in the body of their papers without mentioning family assessment.[2-4] There are, however, several definitions of assessment in the literature on family therapy. For the

From "Three Assessment Tools for Family therapy," by S. A. Morgen and Jane Macey, *Journal of Psychiatric Nursing*, March, 1978, Vol. 16, pp. 39–42. Reprinted by permission of SLACK, Inc., Medical Publishers, Thorofare, NJ.

purpose of this paper the following definition of assessment is to be applied.

> Assessment is a process that includes the collection of data regarding family health, health habits and health behavior, as well as factors in the community that affect these things. . . . The assessment process can be compared to the life process itself—a constantly interacting, fluctuating, and changing phenomenon.[5]

Also in the literature there is little categorization or consistency of approach to the use of terminology for family therapy. Donald A. Bloch affirms this fact by stating that "there are no clearly defined exclusive tools or techniques" for family therapy.[6] Hopefully the assessment tools to be presented will represent pertinent familial information in terminology that can be synthesized by all persons interested in family therapy.

Family therapists must be concerned with an assessment of the family as a whole system, which includes physical health, social, and mental health aspects. For example, in assessing the family, the therapist takes into account each member of the family *and* how that member affects and interacts with all the other family members. This is done with each member and with the family unit as a whole in its community relationships. Therefore, the following assessment tools combine Sobol and Robischon's health aspects, Lickorish's psychological assessment, Westley's emotional aspects of the family, Rice's economic assessment, Ruesch's communication assessment, Ehrenwald's patterns of interaction and other assessments that are important to family therapy.[5,7-11]

THE ASSESSMENT TOOLS

As stated in the definition of assessment, the process of life itself is constantly changing; therefore, the assessment tools must be flexible and fluid in carrying out the process of implementing family therapy. In the process of family change and growth, marked reactions from each family member will occur which may result in the therapist's need to implement an initial or primary assessment, an ongoing assessment, and a summary or termination assessment.

THE INITIAL ASSESSMENT

In the initial session with the family, the therapist must assess as much of the family system as possible in order to arrive at a better understanding of the family's ability to function. The therapist needs to obtain information concerning the family's background: social, cultural, religious, financial, emotional, psychological, educational, and occupational. She also needs to acquire information concerning the present status of the family. The present status includes patterns of interaction, family constellation, relationships, living conditions, assets, liabilities, roles, norms and rules, and family functioning. The therapist collects the data, analyzes and assesses this knowledge imaginatively and, in collaboration with the family, they arrive at treatment goals and a prognosis relating to the family's needs. The therapist also keeps in mind that the assessment tools are applicable to all families, but not all sections are necessarily utilized in every case. The family therapist uses her creativity in applying the necessary tools for each individual family assessment.

One of the pitfalls that the therapist must avoid is the overzealous approach to family therapy without adequate assessment of the family's willingness and readiness to participate. The therapist's entry into a situation may be solicited by only one member of the family. The question may then arise as to whether or not that one member is the family spokesman. The therapist must assess the willingness and readiness of the other family members to participate in therapy. If the therapist's assistance is solicited *en masse*, further assessment of the family's common effort in therapy may not be necessary. Also the family's cooperativeness in setting up appointment times may be an indication of their desire to participate in therapy. The proposed Initial Family Assessment Tool is shown in Figure 1.

FIGURE 1

Proposed Initial Family Assessment Tool

I. Background Data

   A. Family compositions — members
1. Ages (ordinal position of children)
2. Marital status
3. Personality
4. Intellect (level of education)
5. Physical health status
6. Culture
7. Number of persons living in the home
8. Extended family

   B. Material dimensions
1. Income (source, amount, and management)
2. Occupation
3. Size and nature of house
4. Neighborhood
5. Socioeconomic status (number of cars, dishwasher, etc.)

C. Family-community interaction
   1. Political
   2. Educational
   3. Religious
   4. Recreational activities (entertainment, television, etc.)
   5. Relationship with neighbors

II. Present Situation

A. Visual data
   1. Dress
   2. Posture
   3. Subgrouping (clingers and loners)
   4. Similarities in appearance (facial expressions, body language)
   5. Initial greeting (verbal/nonverbal)

B. Number of persons participating in therapy

C. Communication patterns and levels
   1. Inferences
   2. Affect
   3. Motivation

D. Relationships
   1. Degree of warmth and affection
   2. Clients' balance of dominance
   3. Role reciprocity
      a. Kind
      b. Degree
   4. Sexual
   5. Stability
   6. Expectations
   7. Acceptance of responsibility

E. Social functioning
   1. Marital patterns

2. Childrearing and development (socialization process)
3. Family norms
4. Role of pets
5. Extrafamilial socialization agents
   a. School (teacher, principal)
   b. Community center
   c. Religious group
6. Geographical boundaries (family's world of experience)

F. Psychological-emotional health integration
   1. Status
   2. Power
   3. Acceptance and fulfillment of roles
   4. Autonomy of members
   5. Level of trust
   6. Members' self-esteem
   7. Congruence of family and societal values
   8. Attitudes toward self and others
   9. Reality orientation
   10. Tension management (mediating conflict)
   11. Adaptability (principal defensive operations)
   12. Flexibility

G. Physical health
   1. Conditions or illness
      a. Acute or chronic
      b. Disabling defects
   2. Growth and development disorders

H. Stress vulnerability

I. Assets and liabilities

J. Family's objectives and
    goals (individual
    and family)
    1. Immediate
    2. Intermediate
    3. Long-term
K. Prognosis for family
    therapy

1. Willingness for family
    therapy
    a. Family initiated
    b. Referred
2. Readiness for family
    therapy
    a. Cooperativeness
    b. Resistance

THE ONGOING
ASSESSMENT TOOL

Ideally, the initial assessment is completed as early as possible in family therapy. It is realized that much of the intial data collection goes on throughout therapy. Therefore, in addition to the initial evaluation, an Ongoing Assessment Tool (Figure 2) is proposed as a means of identifying the changes that take place during therapy. During this phase of

FIGURE 2

Ongoing Assessment Tool

I. Communication Patterns
    A. Active or passive
    B. Ability to express
        selves
    C. Verbal assessment
        (coding, example:
        identifying defense
        mechanisms)
    D. Nonverbal assessment
    E. Complete-incomplete
    F. Distinctive features
    G. Timing
    H. Effects of interaction
    I. Changes in interaction
    J. Limitations
    K. Direction and response
II. Themes
    A. Recurring

    B. Dominating the
        session
III. Family Functioning
    A. Sharing
    B. Resistance
    C. Complementary
    D. Contagion patterns
    E. Decision-making process
    F. Functioning as a
        system
IV. Emotional Overtones of
     Session
V.   Roles
VI. Assets and Liabilities
VII. Seating Arrangement
VIII. Ability to Bargain

assessment, it is imperative that at least one home visit be made to promote a realistic evaluation of the home environment and to decrease the artificiality of the interactions which take place in the office visit.

TERMINATION ASSESSMENT

The two previous assessment tools focus on the active role of the therapist in the evaluation process. The Termination Assessment incorporates the therapist's identifying with the family their perceptions and progress in therapy. The Termination Assessment is shown in Figure 3.

FIGURE 3

TERMINATION ASSESSMENT TOOL

I. Notable Changes
  A. As seen by family
  B. As seen by therapist

II. Identified Alternatives for Adaptation

III. Areas in Need of Refinement
  A. As seen by family
  B. As seen by therapist

CONCLUSION

In this paper the authors attempt to utilize existing knowledge of the family and family therapy in order to develop a universal tool for family analysis. The assessment tools represent a conceptualization of the three phases of family analysis. Using a simplistic guide, such as these assessment tools, should aid the therapist in organizing the overwhelming volume of information that is obtained in a short amount of interviewing time. Again, the assessment tools are only as applicable as the family therapist is imaginative and creative.

References

1. Miller J C: Systems theory and family psychotherapy. *Nurs Clin North Am* 6:395, 1971.

2. Knox D: *Marriage Happiness.* Champaign, Illinois, Research Press Co, 1971, pp 1–144.

3. Bernardo F: The anthropological approach to the study of the family, in King RJR (ed): *Family Relations: Concepts and Theories.* Berkeley, California, Glendessary Press, 1969, pp 55–78.

4. Handel G: Psychological study of whole families, in Handel G (ed): *The Psychosocial Interior of the Family.* Chicago, Aldine Publishing Co, 1967, pp 517–550.

5. Sobol E G, Robischon P. *Family Nursing.* St. Louis, CV Mosby CO, 1970, p 6.

6. Bloch D A: *Techniques of Family Therapy.* New York, Grune & Stratton, 1973, p 17.

7. Lickorish J R: The psychometric assessment of the family, in Howells JG (ed): *Theory and Practice of Family Psychiatry.* New York, Brunner/Mazel Publ, 1968, pp 553-585.

8. Westley WA, Epstein NB: *Silent Majority.* San Francisco, Jossey-Bass, Inc, Publ, 1970, pp 26–66.

9. Rice AS: An economic framework for viewing the family, in Ivan F N, Bernardo F M (eds): *Emerging Conceptual Frameworks in Family Analysis.* New York, Macmillan Co, 1966, p 255.

10. Ruesch J: Synopsis of theory of human communication, in Howells JG (ed): *Theory and Practice of Family Psychiatry.* New York, Brunner/Mazel Publ, 1968, p 227-266.

11. Ehrenwald J: Family diagnosis and mechanisms of psychosocial defense, in Howells J G (ed): *Theory and Practice of Family Psychiatry.* New York, Brunner/Mazel Publ, 1968, pp 390–399.

Chapter Ten

THE HIDDEN DIAGNOSIS

Lucile Cohn

MANY NURSES BREATHE A sigh of relief that their hospital doesn't admit alcoholics. But, of course, it does. The admitting diagnosis, however, may be hypertension, pneumonia, gastritis, hepatitis, malnutrition, or a broken arm.

When nurses discover that a patient is alcoholic, they resent the feint—the passing of the buck. The physician, in an attempt to maintain the fictitious diagnosis, often relies on narcotics and sedatives to ensure that the patient causes as little disturbance as possible. Such subterfuge often evokes anger and hostility among the nursing personnel, lowers the patient's self-esteem, and frequently aggravates his or her behavior problem. Too often the physical complications of alcoholism are treated and the patient is discharged without the subject of drinking ever having been raised.

The patient who is obviously intoxicated when admitted to the hospital is not necessarily an alcoholic, but you should be alert to the possibility. Unless the admitting nurse documents alcohol on the breath or signs of intoxication when the patient is admitted, one or two shifts later, the nursing staff on the unit may be puzzled and totally unprepared when the patient becomes anxious and disruptive "for no apparent reason."

Many nurses admit they do not know how to bring up the subject of suspected alcohol abuse. Of course, the most direct method of uncovering alcoholism is to ask patients about their drinking habits as factually as you ask them about their allergies. True, alcoholics frequently lie about the amount they drink—many even deceive themselves. But you may be surprised by how open a response you can get with a nonjudgmental inquiry. Even a nonalcoholic who has a regular drinking pattern can experience the agitation of mild withdrawal when that pattern is disrupted by hospitalization. For the alcohol-addicted patient, the staff's failure to assess alcohol use can be catastrophic.

It certainly was for Alice, the 32-year-old wife of a prominent philanthropist, who was admitted for a minor operation. The surgery was uneventful except that she required additional anesthesia, had an unusually prolonged recovery from it, and was returned to her room with a hold on sedation. A few hours later, she developed elevated vital signs and mental confusion that progressed to hallucinosis and aggressive behavior.

Alice was an alcoholic. Without proper medical management, she had progressed into withdrawal and delirium tremens.

If her condition had been recognized and reported on or before admission, her surgery would have been delayed until she completed alcohol withdrawal. Or if the situation had been an emergency, the choice of a different anesthetic agent and postoperative management would have reduced the chance of DTs.

Taking an alcohol history is part of a complete nursing assessment. Sharing a potential diagnosis of alcoholism with colleagues is collaboration and communication, not betrayal of a confidence.

A staff nurse on a surgical unit stated that a 50-year-old man was admitted from the emergency department late one night with a scalp wound, allegedly due to a fall in his basement. He was lethargic and confused and slept for long periods. Sedation was withheld and his neurologic status was checked every 15 minutes. A few hours after admission, he had full-blown DTs. Though one of the nurses in the emergency department was aware that this patient was an alcoholic, she knew he was trying to cut down and felt she would have betrayed his trust had she revealed his alcohol problem. But knowledge of the crucial fact of his addiction, together with the observation of his vital signs, would have led to the proper diagnosis of alcohol withdrawal. Sedation would probably have prevented the DTs.

When you believe the patient has a drinking problem, discussing the possibility does the patient a favor. Remaining a "hidden" alcoholic is exhausting and frightening—a dreadful secret.

Ms. D, age 39, was hospitalized after she lost control of her car and crashed into a fence. She had fractures of the leg, pelvis, and arm, as well as bruises and superficial abrasions. Nevertheless, she was considered to be in good condition. She was cheerful and compliant, and nurses enjoyed talking with her.

On the third day postadmission, Mr. T, the evening nurse, entered the room to ask Ms. D if she needed anything for sleep or for pain. The room was dimly lit. Ms. D was restless and agitated. In a caustic tone, she asked that he "make the orchestra go away." She complained that the musicians were being rude and watching her. Mr. T told the patient that she must have been dreaming. At that point, Ms. D became abusive and demanded that the nurse "warn the musicians." Unless they left immediately, she said, she would call her doctor.

Mr. T was perplexed, but realized that Ms. D was frightened and seemed to be disoriented. He turned on the bright light, gently touched Ms. D's arm and tried to reassure her. Mr. T notified the attending physician, who diagnosed delirium tremens. The physician admitted that he had known of Ms. D's drinking problem but said he hadn't thought of it as serious.

An examination of Ms. D's bedside table revealed two bottles of liquor. She was started on a detoxification regimen with chlordiazepoxide (Librium). She was also put on a high fluid intake of water and juices, as well as a high protein, high-carbohydrate, low-fat diet, supplemented with multivitamins and vitamin B-complex.

The nursing staff kept Ms. D under close observation to ensure her security and allay her anxiety. Her room was kept adequately lit to prevent shadows from increasing the possibility of illusions. Nurses spoke often, and calmly, and distinctly to her. Low-voiced conversations of personnel within her hearing were avoided to prevent her from misinterpreting anything she might over-hear.

Her history of drinking was elicited after the acute episode. She said she was relieved that her secret was out, that she could speak of her dependency without the fear that her loved ones would discover her disease and abandon her.

Some "problem" patients have problems precisely because no one recognizes or admits that they are alcoholics. Once nurses become alert to this possibility, the problems are less likely to be mismanaged.

Clues that should alert one to look for the problem include:

- A patient's failure to respond to standard doses of tranquilizers or sedatives. A regular drinker who has developed tolerance isn't going to sleep after one sleeping capsule.

- Mood swings. A patient may grow agitated and tremulous before visiting hours, then become calm, even euphoric, afterward.

- Frequent treats of beverages liberally laced with alcohol.

- Overabundance of mouthwash or toiletries. (One patient on a medical unit developed DTs after two weeks in the hospital; the source of his alcohol was after-shave lotion.)

- Physical signs of chronic alcohol use, such as tremors or periorbital and pretibial edema caused by fluid retention after a drinking bout.

- Frequent references to alcohol or alcohol use, indicating the importance of alcohol in the individual's life.

- Physical signs of current drinking, such as alcohol on breath or flushed face caused by the vasodilative effects of alcohol.

- Multiple bruises, burns, or abrasions at different stages of healing. These are most frequently at table-top height or on hands and face and are caused by falls and accidents when intoxicated.

- Slash marks on wrists from suicide attempts associated with the depression of chronic alcoholism.

- An older appearance than stated age. The debilitating effects of prolonged, excessive use of alcohol can result in premature signs of aging.

Chapter Eleven

AVOIDING A CRISIS: THE ASSESSMENT

Laurel Brodsley

ONE-THIRD TO ONE-HALF OF hospitalized medical-surgical patients have problems with alcohol. Yet nurses who work in a hospital setting rarely evaluate their patients for alcohol use or look for its physiological and psychosocial health effects.

When I do an admission assessment, I ask the question, "Do you drink alcohol?" immediately after another common query, "Do you smoke?" If the answer is yes, I ask further questions about what the patient drinks, when he or she drinks, and how much he or she drinks. I also look for effects of alcohol use and signs of withdrawal.

Another way I sometimes broach the subject of drinking is to ask about it as part of my assessment of the patient's prescription and nonprescription drug use. Alcohol can be seen as a commonly used, rarely reported, self-prescribed, over-the-counter medication.

When the nurse asks, "What medicines do you take at home?" patients usually list the pills prescribed by a physician. When asked, "What over-the-counter medicines do you take?" they may mention sleeping pills, antihistamines, or laxatives. To elicit information about other medicines, the nurse must ask directly, "Do you also take vitamins, hormones, or birth control pills? And do you drink alcohol?"

If the patient seems surprised by the last question, the nurse can explain that since all of these substances have physiological effects that can affect treatment, the staff needs to know about them.

BE DIRECT

If the patient reports drinking alcohol, ask the usual questions about medication use: dose, frequency, side effects, and most recent use. The necessary questions are very simple and direct:

1. What do you like to drink?
2. How much do you take?
3. How frequently do you drink?
4. When you drink, about how much do you usually have in 24 hours? What is the *most* you can drink in 24 hours?
5. When was your last drink?
6. What was it, and how much did you have?

When asked what they drink, patients sometimes respond as if they think beer and wine are as innocuous as soft drinks: "I like a glass of wine now and then." "I only drink beer."

Keep in mind that alcohol—whether in beer, wine, or hard liquor—has the same effect. One twelve-ounce can of beer or one four-ounce glass of wine have the same alcohol content as one ounce of scotch, bourbon, vodka, or gin. A six-pack of beer delivers the same amount of alcohol as six highballs.

When asked about quantity and frequency, many patients will say that they drink only small amounts in social settings. Others will reveal a longstanding pattern of moderate drinking. Others will admit periodic bouts of heavy drinking. But often, these questions elicit general replies: "Oh, a few beers on the weekends." "I like a nice tall bourbon-on-the-rocks when I get home from work." "A bit of wine with dinner is nice." "Sometimes when I can't sleep, I'll have a drink or two."

BE SPECIFIC

Try to help the patient be more specific: "When you say 'a few drinks,' do you mean two or three? Or perhaps you finish a six-pack on a Sunday?" "How many shots do you put in your glass? And how much ice?" "Do you drink about a half-liter carafe òr more, or only a glass of wine?"

LET PATIENT ADMIT
TO HEAVY DRINKING

Give the patient room to admit to heavy drinking without forcing a confession of excessive alcohol use. Many people, but especially alcoholics, do not realize how much they really do drink, or do not want to admit it to anyone else.

Gently elicit the truth through open and easy questions. Try not to push the patient or engage in confrontation. At this point, the task is simply to gather as much data as possible. Later, when you evaluate the case as a whole, the patient's evasiveness or denial during questioning may be considered a symptom of possible alcohol abuse. But such judgments ought not creep in during the assessment.

The quantity of alcohol the patient can drink may indicate whether or not the liver has been affected. If the patient seems to be able to drink a great deal, he or she may have developed alcohol tolerance over years of drinking. The ability to drink three or four bottles of wine, a quart of hard liquor, or a case of beer in a 24-hour period is a sign to the nurse to be attentive for other symptoms of alcohol abuse.

A recent decrease in tolerance is another sign of alcohol-related physical damage. Some patients may admit to a long history of heavy alcohol consumption and then say, "Lately I just can't drink as much as I used to." A decrease in alcohol tolerance may indicate liver damage, and the patient may be in the late stages of the disease of alcoholism.

AVOID A CRISIS

The most important information to elicit, in terms of immediate intervention, is the time of the last drink: "I had a couple of swigs in the parking lot before I came in, maybe a half pint of vodka. Boy I sure needed it. Am I nervous!" "Hmm, not for a few days. The doctor told me to cut out booze before surgery, so I guess my last drink was Friday. I sure celebrated though—finished off almost a bottle of scotch!"

If there has been any alcohol use within five days of the patient's admission, be sensitive to signs of alcohol withdrawal.

Alcohol, a sedative, has a short-acting depressant effect on the brain, followed by rebound irritation in the nervous system. In addition, alcohol directly damages the brain cells. These two physiological effects cause the blackouts, memory lapses, hallucinations, and seizures experienced by heavy drinkers. They forget what happened at the party; they cannot remember where they left the car; they see "pink elephants" or spiders crawling up walls; they feel bugs on their skin; they hear voices.

Minor symptoms—nervousness or irritability, mild tachycardia and hypertension, flushed face, gastrointestinal irritation, insomnia—are common during the first 24 hours after the last drink. Even nonalcoholics can experience these signs of psychomotor agitation after one night of heavy drinking. The situation is much more serious for the alcohol-addicted person.

If the patient's history points to heavy drinking, ask about problems commonly resulting from it: "When you drink or stop drinking, do you ever have blackouts (that is, memory lapses)? Hallucinations? Seizures? DTs?"

Untreated alcohol withdrawal can progress to life-threatening DTs within 12 to 36 hours after the last drink. The usual symptoms are severe agitation, copious diaphoresis, markedly elevated vital signs, muscle spasms, frightening hallucinations, confusion, and disorientation; these can lead to myocardial or cerebral infarctions, vascular collapse, and death.

This brief drinking history can give you some insight into the patient's pattern of alcohol use. Next, you can assess whether alcohol is affecting the patient's health.

A long history of heavy drinking will probably lead to physiological damage. However, a binge drinker—one who imbibes a great deal in short episodes between periods of sobriety—can suffer the same deleterious effects from alcohol as a steady drinker. And, steady regular drinking, even in relatively moderate amounts, can be dangerous for some people.

Patients do not have to be diagnosed alcoholics for the chemical to endanger their health. A patient with pancreatitis or infectious hepatitis cannot drink at all without life-endangering consequences. If such a patient cannot restrain himself even from such "small" indulgences as a few weekend beers or an evening nightcap, he can still kill himself with alcohol. In such cases, it is not just quantity or frequency of alcohol use that is dangerous; *any* alcoholic intake is signficant.

LOOK FOR PHYSICAL EVIDENCE

Once you have obtained a history, you can look for objective signs of any alcohol-related physical or emotional problems.

The nursing physical assessment is completely adequate for this. You just have to keep in mind the wide variety of diseases and conditions that may be associated with alcohol use and the signs and symptoms of alcohol intoxication and withdrawal. Evaluate the patient's status by physical examination and history, as follows:

Head

Skull for concussion, contusion, fractures, abrasions, and wounds caused by falls and accidents under the influence of alcohol.

Eyes for red conjunctiva and jaundiced sclera.

Face for "alcoholic nose" caused by capillary fragility from chronic alcohol use; for flushed skin and diaphoresis associated with intoxication or withdrawal.

Breath for odor of alcohol.

Verbalizations for slurred speech, inappropriate responses, contradictory replies, evasion, long rambling stories, memory lapses, emotional lability (especially anger and tears), irritability, confusion, anxiety, depression, guilt, suicidal ideation, lethargy.

Chest

Fractured ribs or bruises from falls.

History of pulmonary problems—TB, COPD, pneumonia—from debility associated with chronic alcohol use.

History of cardiovascular problems—CHF, hypertension, tachycardia, and arrhythmias—from cardiovascular effects of alcohol or from alcohol intoxication or withdrawal.

Abdomen

Signs of liver damage: protruding abdomen ("beer belly"), enlarged liver, peripheral edema, systemic jaundice, history of diagnosed fatty liver or cirrhosis.

Signs of damage to intestinal tract: history of gastritis, hemoptysis, melena, pancreatitis, malabsorption syndrome, ulcers, colitis; signs of dehydration, malnutrition; complaints of nausea, vomiting, anorexia, diarrhea.

Extremities

Fractures and wounds at various stages of healing.

Circulatory and neurological deficits, weakness, dermatitis, pruritus, ataxia, edema (especially of feet and lower legs).

Fine or gross tremors (or shakes); muscle spasms associated with intoxication or withdrawal.

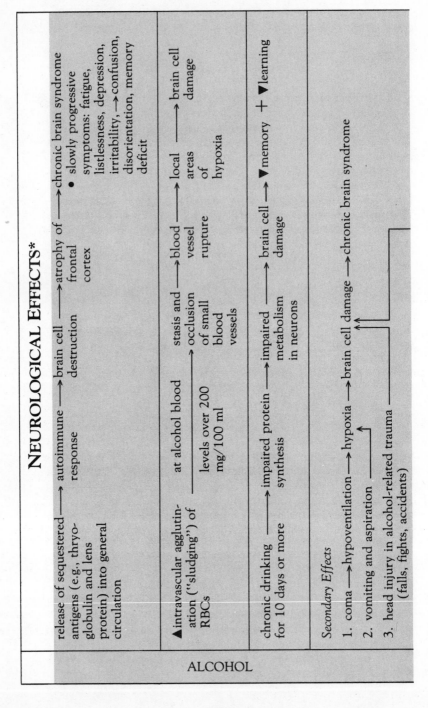

NEUROLOGICAL EFFECTS*

ALCOHOL

release of sequestered → autoimmune → brain cell → atrophy of → chronic brain syndrome
antigens (e.g., thryo-   response   destruction   frontal   • slowly progressive
globulin and lens   cortex   symptoms: fatigue,
protein) into general   listlessness, depression,
circulation   irritability, → confusion,
                                                                           disorientation, memory
                                                                           deficit

▲intravascular agglutin-   at alcohol blood   stasis and → blood → local → brain cell
ation ("sludging") of   occlusion   vessel   areas   damage
RBCs   levels over 200   of small   rupture   of
                            mg/100 ml   blood   hypoxia
                                                 vessels

chronic drinking → impaired protein → impaired → brain cell → ▼memory + ▼learning
for 10 days or more   synthesis   metabolism   damage
                                        in neurons

Secondary Effects

1. coma → hypoventilation → hypoxia → brain cell damage → chronic brain syndrome
2. vomiting and aspiration
3. head injury in alcohol-related trauma
   (falls, fights, accidents)

98

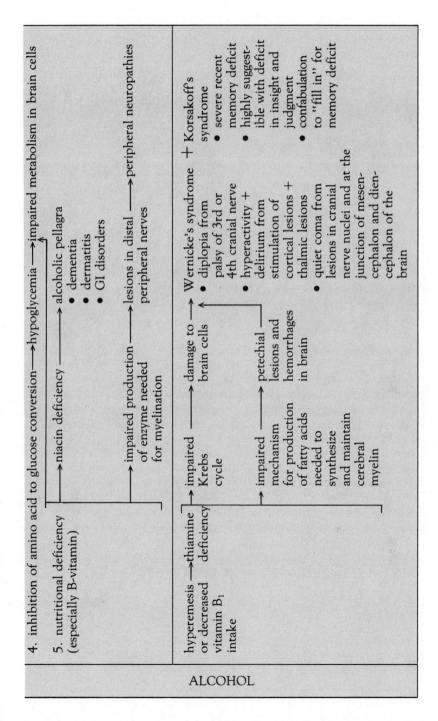

4. inhibition of amino acid to glucose conversion ⟶ hypoglycemia ⟶ impaired metabolism in brain cells

5. nutritional deficiency ⟶ niacin deficiency ⟶ alcoholic pellagra
(especially B-vitamin)
 • dementia
 • dermatitis
 • GI disorders

⟶ impaired production ⟶ lesions in distal ⟶ peripheral neuropathies
of enzyme needed   peripheral nerves
for myelination

hyperemesis ⟶ thiamine ⟶ impaired ⟶ damage to ⟶ Wernicke's syndrome + Korsakoff's
or decreased   deficiency   Krebs   brain cells   syndrome
vitamin B₁   cycle   • severe recent
intake   memory deficit
                                     • diplopia from   • highly suggest-
          ⟶ impaired ⟶ petechial   palsy of 3rd or   ible with deficit
            mechanism   lesions and   4th cranial nerve   in insight and
            for production hemorrhages • hyperactivity +   judgment
            of fatty acids in brain   delirium from   • confabulation
            needed to   stimulation of   to "fill in" for
            synthesize   cortical lesions +   memory deficit
            and maintain   thalmic lesions
            cerebral   • quiet coma from
            myelin   lesions in cranial
                                        nerve nuclei and at the
                                        junction of mesen-
                                        cephalon and dien-
                                        cephalon of the
                                        brain

ALCOHOL

NEUROLOGICAL EFFECTS

ALCOHOL			
demyelination of optic → alcoholic amblyopia nerves	toxic effect on pons → destruction of myelin → central pontine myelinosis sheaths of nerve fibers in pons	▲levels of acetaldehyde → ▲concentration of acetaldehyde → corticocerebellar lesions and degeneration (from metabolism of in cerebellum ethanol)	interference with biochemical → sleep brain substances (e.g., de- fragmen- struction of serotonogenic tation neurons → ▼serotonin → ▲wakefulness)

demyelination of optic → alcoholic amblyopia
nerves
• painless, bilateral blurred vision
• decreased visual acuity, but peripheral vision intact
• scotomas

toxic effect on pons → destruction of myelin → central pontine myelinosis
sheaths of nerve fibers
in pons
• dull mental state pro-
gressing to coma in one
to two weeks
• quadriparesis
• signs of bulbar paralysis but
sensation in mouth and face intact

▲levels of acetaldehyde → ▲concentration of acetaldehyde → corticocerebellar lesions and degeneration
(from metabolism of in cerebellum
ethanol)
progressing to cerebral atrophy
• broad-based, unsteady gait
• impaired coordination
• fine tremors

interference with biochemical → sleep
brain substances (e.g., de- fragmen-
struction of serotonogenic tation
neurons → ▼serotonin
→ ▲wakefulness)

+ ▼REM sleep at sedative → sleep → depression
levels of alcohol followed disorders
by ▲REM (rebound as
alcohol/sedative level
drops)

LIVER EFFECTS

ALCOHOL

oxidation in alcohol dehydrogenase system → hydrogen-bound nicotinamide adenine dinucleotide (NADH) → ▼glycogen formation, ▲lipid formation, + ▼lipid oxidation ⟶ hepatic fat (fatty liver)

damage to mitochondria of hepatic cells (site of fatty acid oxidation) → ▲beta-oxidation of fatty acids ⟶ ketogenesis ⟶ ketoacidosis

oxidation in microsomal fraction of liver cell (microsomal ethanol oxidizing system) → hypertrophy of smooth endoplasmic reticulum (SER) of hepatic cells → ▲metabolism of drugs and alcohol → ▲tolerance to sedatives, alcohol, etc.

inflammation of hepatic cells (hepatitis) → necrosis of hepatic cells → fibrosis → cirrhosis + obliteration of hepatic central veins → collection of hepatic lymph in peritoneal cavity ⟶ ascites

*Mechanisms of damage have been identified on the basis of animal studies, observations of humans, and theories of pathophysiology. Information here and on the charts in the following four pages is derived from *Alcoholism: Development, Consequences, and Interventions* by N. J. Estes and M. E. Heinemann, St. Louis: The C. V. Mosby Co., 1982, pp. 136–143 (GI and Liver Effects), pp. 144–167 (Neurological Effects), pp. 168–184 (Cardiac and Blood Effects).

COMMUNICATE FINDINGS

Once you complete your collection of data, evaluate it. If you identify alcohol use as a problem, check to see if the physician is aware of the patient's secondary disease. If the physician is not aware of the disease, communicate the findings from your assessment—just as you would for any other condition.

Alcohol affects people of any age, sex, race, or income level. The teenager who miscarried may have been a heavy drinker; her infant, a victim of fetal alcohol syndrome. The little old lady who broke her hip may have had one too many sips of Nyquil. The young man on the motorcycle, too many beers. The physician's wife with the bleeding ulcer, the young woman with severe depression, the successful corporate executive with the heart attack may all have been moderate to heavy drinkers.

And some of those difficult, nervous, and anxious patients who seem so demanding and annoying in the hospital may be missing their usual tranquilizer—alcohol.

The nursing assessment for alcohol use gives the health team a clearer understanding of the patient's use of alcohol and its effect on his or her life-style and health. It also gives the staff more insight into the problems of the patient who suffers from the chronic and debilitating disease of alcoholism.

Part Three

INTERVENTIONS WITH INDIVIDUAL CLIENTS

W hat do you do when you're talking to a client and he suddenly announces, "I think I'll take my clothes off"? Nurses, in their effort to show acceptance and nonjudgmental attitudes toward clients, often find it difficult to set appropriate limits. The severely depressed client offers a very different set of problems for nursing management. Such a client may say and do very little yet provoke anger and frustration in the nurse who initiates efforts to help. This unit contains ten articles about nursing interventions for problem behaviors observed primarily in interactions with manipulative, noncompliant, depressed, and psychotic clients.

As King and Morrell suggest in their article on working with the depressed client, it is often necessary to take the initiative and break into the depressed client's world, in order to help him or her to begin interacting positively with the environment once again. Daily contact with hospitalized depressed clients gives nurses a critical role in facilitating recovery. King and Morrell offer a number of specific suggestions for management of these clients.

Kroah attempts to classify and clarify the disordered language and thoughts of clients with schizophrenia. The strategies she suggests for intervention, based on the theories of Sullivan, Haley, Kasanin, and Whorf, have been applied to psychiatric nursing by Peplau. Kroah gives examples of actual dialogue, demonstrating language and thought disorders such as scattering, circumstantiality, and idiosyncratic language, and presents nursing interventions for these behaviors.

Schwartzman uses Sullivanian theory to analyze the hallucinatory process and attempts to answer such questions as why does the person show this behavior? what needs is this person meeting by using hallucinatory behavior? what does the experience mean for this person? how should the nurse respond? The author presents a detailed account of her relationship with a client who had hallucinatory behavior. Medications, group therapy, and family involvement also play important roles in the treatment of these clients.

It should be noted that the theoretical bases of Kroah's and Schwartzman's articles are not the only accepted positions and that there is extensive research support for a biological/organic etiology for the thought disorders these authors describe. We believe their suggestions for intervention can be helpful, even if one subscribes to an alternative theory of the etiology of the problem behaviors. Biological intervention in the form of neuroleptic medications would be part of the total treatment plan for these clients.

Manipulation can be a losing game for staff, clients, and everyone concerned. McMorrow uses a troublesome ICU client as the subject of her article on the manipulative patient. Specific suggestions for nurses include taking coffee breaks or other "mini vacations" to get control of one's own emotions before going back to help clients gain better control of theirs.

Underwood discusses how role playing can facilitate communication between nurses and clients. Role playing is a learning experience in which nurses and clients act out a situation, either past or expected, as if it were actually happening. Dialogue from several role-playing sessions illustrates how this technique can be used. The article also points out how the nurse-client relationship helped one client develop appropriate assertiveness.

Treatment of the borderline client has not received much attention in the nursing literature thus far. Castelli and Delaney discuss the role of the psychiatric nurse as administrator in the therapeutic milieu. Psychodynamic theory related to the treatment of borderline clients is presented in some detail; this theoretical rationale can help in understanding the clients' behavior and the nurses' role in the treatment process. These authors believe the milieu provides the context in which the client can best test out healthier interpersonal behavior.

The anguish of the loss of a client through suicide is usually exacerbated by the question, was this suicide preventable? Hoff and Resing carefully analyze one case and, in doing so, discuss the specific assessment and intervention activities that might have prevented this man's death. Their recommendations should be extremely helpful to practitioners working with depressed clients.

What is an appropriate intervention if a client takes off his clothes, gives you a gift, or kisses you? Lyon's article gives helpful suggestions; it explains why there is a need for limit setting and how limit setting can be used as a therapeutic tool. She shows how, when used properly, limit setting helps reduce clients' anxiety and allows them to function in a more comfortable and acceptable way.

Buckwalter and Kerfoot's article concerns actions that nurses can take to improve clients' chances to stay in the community after their discharge. The "revolving door" situation (that is, high discharge rates followed by high readmission rates) brought about by deinstitutionalization is at least partly the result of families' and clients' lack of coping skills. The authors' approach to discharge planning is designed to provide clients and their families with the information they need to deal with minor crises, detect early signs of potential relapse, and initiate appropriate action.

In the final article of this unit, Brief and Dorman discuss in some detail the problem of noncompliance, the failure of clients to follow the prescribed treatment plan. Noncompliance is a common and frustrating problem in most mental health settings. The article analyzes the common causes of noncompliance and offers a number of practical intervention strategies that can be tried when the client fails to comply. Ideally, compliance problems can be prevented by anticipating where difficulties are likely to occur and by tailoring the treatment plan to the client's ability to collaborate with the practitioner.

Chapter Twelve

HELPING THE HOSPITALIZED DEPRESSED CLIENT

Abby C. King, Ph.D. and Eric M. Morrell, Ph.D.

ALL OF US EXPERIENCE bouts of depressed mood from time to time. However, when the depression becomes severe enough to require hospitalization, the experience can be extremely upsetting both for clients and for those around them. One notable aspect of such depression is its pervasive effect on all spheres of the person's life. Mood is strongly affected, and a host of physical symptoms is often noted—such as psychomotor retardation or agitation, loss of appetite, sleep disturbance, constipation, and fatigue. In addition, the individual's thinking is typically affected. Self-devaluative, pessimistic, or suicidal thoughts as well as feelings of inadequacy, helplessness, and hopelessness may be present and may persist in the face of seemingly positive events. The apparent loss of motivation and interest in their environment, along with the attendant social withdrawal evidenced by depressed clients, make them particularly difficult to deal with on a day-to-day basis.

Because depressed clients tend to be far less animated and verbal than others on the ward, it may seem easier to leave them on their own, as they frequently request. However, to facilitate improvement in mood and behavior, it is often necessary to break into the depressed clients' world and to encourage them to interact positively with their environment. The daily contacts psychiatric nurses have with hospitalized depressed clients provide nurses with unique opportunities to intervene in important ways. There are many things that the nurse can do throughout the day in interacting with the client that can help to speed recovery. These include (a) *acknowledgement of the client's concerns and communication of understanding these concerns*, (b) *active facilitation of positive or realistic thoughts or behaviors* (e.g., encouraging positive rather than deprecatory self-statements), and (c) *rewarding of efforts to engage in positive behaviors and self-statements.*

When they occur consistently throughout the day, these three types of nurse-client interactions can help the client focus on positive or productive, rather than negative or unproductive behaviors and thoughts. This, in turn, can lead to constructive behavioral change that facilitates improvement in mood and attitude (Lewinsohn, 1974). The relationship between changes of behavior and changes in mood and attitude is important to realize. Many clients feel, erroneously, that only when their mood lifts will it make sense to begin engaging in their normal, daily routine again; in actuality, engaging in activities can spur a positive change in mood.

In order to clarify how the nurse can interact with depressed clients in the most helpful way, we are going to discuss symptoms typically presented by depressed clients in terms of a specific plan the nurse can use to help relieve each symptom. Following each plan, we will present examples that focus upon communicating understanding to the client, facilitating a positive or productive client response, and rewarding the client's effort.

PHYSICAL AND BEHAVIORAL SYMPTOMS

Sleep Disturbance

Sleep disturbance in the depressed client consists of difficulty in initially falling asleep or early-morning awakening. With both types of sleep disturbance, the client often ruminates over feelings of self-doubt, failure, helplessness, or guilt.

Plan. Reality testing, which involves reflecting back to the client whether the self-doubts or concerns are realistic, interrupts the rumination. The best way of doing this is *not* to argue with clients about these concerns but simply to give them positive feedback concerning how they appear to the nurse (e.g., "You say you are an insensitive, mean person, but you always seem to be quite sensitive to my feelings"). If the client remains unable to sleep, it may be helpful to encourage him or her to do something other than ruminate or feel sorry for him- or herself (e.g., read a book or magazine, walk).

Example:

Communicate under-standing, with intent to help	"I know how hard it can be to sleep when something's on your mind. What I find helpful is to try to do something about it rather than to keep thinking about it. It would be good for you to get some sleep, but if you can't you might want to try...(reading, getting up and walking, taking a shower, etc.)."
Facilitate the response	"Here, let me...(get you your robe, get you a magazine, help you out of bed, get your slippers, etc.)."
Reward the effort	"That's great that you tried this. It will take a little while, but the more often you try to do something when you're feeling this way, the more it will help you feel better. You look much better when you...(read, keep busy, etc.)."

Lack of Appetite

Depressed clients may reduce their food intake, complaining that the food is tasteless or bland.

Plan.   While acknowledging that that may indeed be the client's perception, it is important to actively encourage eating behavior. If possible, talk to the client during meal times and try to make it a more pleasant experience. In addition, praise efforts to eat. If weight loss becomes a particular problem, making the client more aware of this by taping a simple, daily weight chart or graph by the bedside may help. Each day the client's weight can be recorded and any weight gains praised.

Example:

Communicate under-standing, with intent to help	"Sometimes hospital food does taste a little bland, Mr. Franks, so I know how you feel. The important thing to remember is that you need to eat it to help you feel better."

Facilitate the response	"Let's see if I can't make this a little more appealing. Do you have enough pepper (margarine, etc.)? Why don't you try a little bit of this?"
Reward the effort	"Very good. You're going to be feeling better very soon if you keep eating this well."

With a daily weight chart, give feedback and praise each time improvement occurs. Example: "Look at this. You've gained——pounds. That's great! You're well on your way."

Psychomotor Retardation and Fatigue

Depressed clients will often state that they do not have the energy or desire to ambulate. They may attempt to remain in bed for most or all of the day. Such inactivity should be actively discouraged, since there is evidence to suggest that positive moods will increase as the client engages in a greater amount of activity (Lewinsohn, 1974). In addition, physical activity can help to decrease feelings of fatigue and, if maintained, in some cases may help to reduce constipation.

Plan. A problem with such increases in activity is that clients typically will not get relief right away. They may complain initially that increased walking just makes them feel worse or more tired. Clients should be informed from the beginning that this is to be expected and that they will begin to feel better if they consistently maintain these activities for awhile.

Walking can be facilitated through use of a pedometer, which can be attached to the person's clothing and records how much the client has walked during a set period of time. From the pedometer readings a simple chart can be kept by the client's bed to give the client, as well as the staff, feedback as to activity level. The staff should enthusiastically praise all instances of walking or activity. Clients who are particularly averse to leaving their rooms may be locked out of their rooms during portions of the day to help them make the first step toward increased activity.

In addition, encourage regular participation in formal occupational therapy (OT) and physical therapy (PT) classes and other recreational activities. It must be kept in mind that the client will probably not feel like attending ordered activities and may try to cajole or persuade the nursing staff to be excused from such activities. Although the client might perceive forced attendance as cruel, the nurse must keep in mind that participation in activities is important to the client's eventual recovery.

Example:

Communicate understanding, with intent to help	"Mrs. Stewart, I understand that you don't really feel like walking around, but it is important for you to try. If you keep at it, it will help you to feel better."
Facilitate the response	"Here, let me...(help you up, get your slippers or robe, etc.). I'll walk with you down the hall (to the lounge, etc.)."
Reward the effort	"Great! You're really making progress." *Specific Feedback:* "You seem to be moving more easily, and your face has much better color. Your distance is improving too. From your pedometer chart I see that you walked 200 feet more today than yesterday. I heard that you're making a nice-looking leather pouch in OT."

Psychomotor Agitation

Sometimes a client will show agitation instead of psychomotor retardation. Agitation is expressed by continuous pacing, hand rubbing or wringing, outbursts of complaining or shouting, or continual pulling or rubbing of clothes or other objects.

Plan. Behavioral methods of decreasing a client's agitation include helping the client to relax by breathing slowly and deeply as well as helping the client to engage in an alternative, constructive activity.

Example:

Communicate understanding, with intent to help	"Mr. Jones, you seem a little upset today. You might feel better trying to use some of that energy."
Facilitate the response	"First, let's see if I can help you to relax some. Sometimes it helps to take some slow, deep breaths. Ready? In...Out...In...Out...Good.

	How are you feeling? Why don't you walk with me. . .(to the lounge, down the hall, etc.); or how about playing Ping-Pong with me?"
Reward the effort	"Excellent, Mr. Jones. You're looking better to me."

Poor Personal Hygiene

When an individual is depressed, attention to and interest in personal hygiene and grooming will often decrease. Since how we present ourselves reflects how we feel about ourselves, increased attention to one's grooming and hygiene can help spark renewed interest in oneself and one's activities.

Plan. In order to encourage daily grooming and hygiene, rules can be established addressing the types of behavior expected daily from the client, such as getting dressed, showering, brushing teeth and hair, shaving. It should be explained to the client that keeping a daily routine of personal grooming is essential to returning to a normal, active life. Because the client's tendency is to do as little as possible, it will be up to the nurse to actively encourage such behavior on a daily basis. This may be done by setting up goals whereby the client must complete certain activities (dress, shower, shave) before other activities such as watching television are allowed.

Example:

Communicate understanding, with intent to help	"I know it's difficult to get going sometimes, Mrs. Fredericks, but I believe you will feel better if you try."
Facilitate the response	"Let's keep a record of when you. . .(shower, get dressed, etc.). I'd like to see how many of these things you can do each day. What would you like to wear today?"
Reward the effort	"You look great today, Mrs. Fredericks! I really like that dress. All you need to do now is brush your hair to get your TV privilege."

112

Lack of Social Interaction

Evidence from a variety of sources suggests that a lack of positive social interactions can play a major role in causing and maintaining clinical depression (Coyne, 1976; Libet & Lewinsohn, 1973). Social interaction can help to divert the depressed client's attention away from negative ruminations, and can help to increase the individual's self-esteem by giving social approval, acceptance, and recognition. The nurse's daily contact with the hospitalized client offers an excellent opportunity to encourage positive social interactions.

Example:

Communicate understanding, with intent to help	"It's nice to see you today, Mr. Smith. I know that it can be hard to mingle with others sometimes, but a lot of us around here would enjoy seeing more of you."
Facilitate the response	"If you'd be interested, some of the others would like to have you join them. Mr. White (another patient), why don't you take Mr. Smith to the lounge and have some coffee?"
	Or "Several of the others are looking for someone to play cards with. Do you play?"
Reward the effort	"Mr. Smith, it's good to see you doing some more things with some of the other people here. It looks like they're enjoying your company."

Habitual Mild Chronic Hyperventilation (HMCH)

Habitual mild chronic hyperventilation is sometimes seen in depressed clients who are tense or anxious. Such symptoms may enhance feelings of fatigue and exhaustion and exacerbate the depression in other ways (Damas, Patel & Jenner, 1977; Gibson, 1978). The client's physician should be consulted about the diagnosis of HMCH.

Plan. The nurse can help by making the client aware that he or she is doing this and by encouraging diaphragmatic breathing.

To summarize briefly, it is important to remember that preoccupation with physical and mood-related symptoms is commonplace for depressed clients and that they will frequently use such symptoms as a reason for remaining inactive or not complying with previously agreed-upon plans. It typically helps to explain to the clients that they can expect to have such symptoms until they begin carrying out the activities and tasks that are important for normal daily living.

SYMPTOMS OF THOUGHT AND FEELING

Self-deprecation

Although it is important for the nurse to remain sympathetic to the client's problems, the nurse should help the client avoid continuous "wallowing" in self-pity. Attempts should be made to redirect negative, self-deprecatory thoughts to more realistic, positive thoughts about self. For instance, in response to a client's statement of being the most useless person in the world, the nurse may point out that the client was quite useful earlier that day with a particular task or activity on the ward. Although one cannot expect to obtain dramatic changes in mood or verbalization with one such statement, the cumulative effect of consistently administered reality-oriented statements can aid in changing some of the irrational beliefs and unreasonable demands depressed clients often place on themselves.

Example:

Communicate understanding, with intent to help	"I know how it's easy to feel useless or like a failure sometimes. However, I think that you sell yourself short when you say that you do nothing right. I was very impressed with how well you were able to...(discuss politics with Mr. Jones, make those drawings in your OT class, etc.). This is only one of many things you've done well."
Facilitate the response	"The next time you find yourself putting yourself down, try to remind yourself of the things such

114

	as...and...that you do well. I think it will help you feel better."
Reward the effort	"I'm glad to hear you give yourself some credit, Mr. Kent. You deserve it."

Helplessness, Hopelessness, Pessimism

Depressed clients often feel that they are completely helpless when it comes to making changes in their lives. They are often inclined to try to solve problems with wishful thinking rather than with action. Encouraging clients to become more active and to set daily goals for the day's activities can help them feel in better control of their lives. Daily goals might include spending a specific amount of time walking, conversing with a particular client or staff member, or engaging in a similar activity.

Example:

Communicate understanding, with intent to help	"I bet you're feeling like you can't win when it comes to making the changes you'd like to. A way out of that may be to take small steps."
Facilitate the response	"For example, I'd like to see you try...(walking down the hall twice a day, cleaning up each morning, reading the newspaper each day, etc.). Small things lead to bigger things. Let's see if you can't try...(one of above examples)."
Reward the effort	"Great! I really like seeing you...(one of examples above). You're doing well. Pretty soon you'll be ready for the next step (walking outside, going to the cafeteria, etc.). Keep up the good work. You're making great progress."

Feelings of Being "Abnormal" or "Crazy"

Depressed clients will benefit from the knowledge that other people experience the same types of feelings, thoughts, and behaviors that they do. Reminding depressed clients about this can be of great help to them. By emphasizing that depression is often a reaction to stressful events in the environment and is influenced by behavior as well as perception of such events, clients can be encouraged to reduce the stress by modifying their behavior. In contrast, an approach that states or implies that the individual is "mentally ill" fosters feelings of abnormality and helplessness, which can discourage efforts to make behavioral changes. In fact, there is evidence to suggest that a social learning explanation of psychological disturbance, which focuses on the interaction of an individual with the environment, fosters self-help behaviors more than a mental illness explanation (Farina, Fisher, Getter, & Fisher, 1978).

Example:

Communicate understanding, with intent to help	"I think all of us at times feel a little strange or different from the rest of the crowd. I know I do at times. Your being in here is all the more likely to lead you to feel that way. This doesn't mean you have no control over your feelings, thoughts, or behavior, though. You can take steps to improve so you'll be ready to start again."
Facilitate the response	"One way to help you feel like you're not alone is to talk more to others on the ward."
Reward the effort	"Terrific. I'm glad that you're talking more to others on the ward. You look better to me."

Suicidal Thoughts

Methods of dealing with the suicidal client are addressed elsewhere in this book. Suffice it to say that the presence of suicidal thoughts should be taken seriously and brought immediately to the attention of the attending psychiatrist, physician, or primary therapist. In dealing with depressed clients, of whom a significant number will report suicidal thoughts, it is important to know that caring and supportive interactions have been considered a crucial aspect of successful treatment (Linehan, 1981). The importance of supportive interactions extends to the nursing staff as well as to other significant individuals in the client's life.

SOMATIC TREATMENTS

Drug Therapy

The depressed hospitalized client will typically receive one or more types of pharmacological treatments for depression, including tricyclic compounds, monoamine oxidase inhibitors (MAOIs), lithium carbonate (Mendels, 1976), and phenothiazines (Nelson & Bowers, 1978). Because all of these treatments have a number of potential side effects, the nurse should become familiar with possible side effects from each treatment. By doing this, the nurse can readily provide important reassurance to clients, who may be prone to focus upon somatic concerns. Such information can help put some otherwise distressing symptoms into more realistic perspective.

Because the most frequently used antidepressant drugs are the tricyclics, such as imipramine and amitriptyline, it is especially important to be fully aware of the course and side effects of these powerful drugs. In particular, clients should be cognizant of the fact that it may take as long as ten to fourteen days after first being placed on tricyclic medication before its antidepressant properties will be felt. For depressed clients, this length of time may seem an eternity. Therefore, reassurance that they will begin to feel better and encouragement to reinstitute a daily routine independent of the drug effect are imperative.

Side effects produced by other drugs used must also be closely monitored; in particular, incompatibility reactions, such as hypertensive crises or headaches, may be caused by eating certain foods while on MAO inhibitors. The nurse can help by making certain that the client and the family members are knowledgeable about which foods to avoid.

Electroconvulsive Therapy (ECT)

In addition to drug therapy, severely depressed clients will at times be given electroconvulsive therapy (ECT), in which a mild electric current is administered to produce a seizure. Although ECT administration has been made progressively safer over the years, fear of complications or of negative side effects is often the most distressing aspect of the procedure for the client. The most common side effects of ECT are memory loss and confusion. Memory loss generally becomes noticeable after the third or fourth treatment and becomes worse as the number of treatments increases (Gulevich, 1977). Following the end of the ECT series, memory gradually returns over three to six weeks, depending upon the number of treatments delivered. Given these side effects, the nurse who has established a rapport with a client scheduled for ECT can play an invaluable role in helping to allay fears prior to the treatment and in supporting the client through the trying period of memory loss and confusion that develops after treatment. The nurse who is knowledgeable of the course and side effects of ECT can also be extremely helpful to concerned family members of the client. Again, the communication of understanding and support prompts the return to normal activities, and the reward of efforts to do so can go far in facilitating recovery.

CONCLUSIONS

The major point of this paper is that psychiatric nurses in their daily contacts with depressed clients can have an important impact on the clients' recovery. This is particularly so if the nurse focuses upon encouraging and supporting positive action and verbalizations on the part of the depressed person. However, several caveats must be mentioned.

First, nurses may find that many of their prompts, suggestions, or supportive statements are ignored or strongly rebuffed by some clients. This does *not* mean that these comments or statements are inappropriate; it indicates that the depressed individual is not ready at that time to take responsibility for feeling better. Such comments are frequently stored away to be thought about at a later time. Although such negative reactions on the part of clients can be quite discouraging for the health professional, it is important to recognize that frequent prompting and support does help to assist recovery. In fact, clients who struggled to remain immobilized while their nurses continued to coax them to begin to walk or care for themselves have later reported how helpful they found the nurse's efforts, even though they were unable to verbalize this at the time.

Second, it may be useful for nurses to explain to clients that recovery from depression is a slow process that takes *time*. Because of this, the setting of short-term, daily goals can be particularly helpful in bridging and at times shortening this period for the clients.

A final point as essential to providing quality client care as other points listed throughout this paper is the nurse's own support from co-workers who understand the stressful nature of the psychiatric nurse's position. Because interacting with depressed clients can be frustrating and disappointing, the presence of co-workers who can be used as a "sounding-board" and support for day-to-day events on the ward can be crucial. Such support helps nurses personally and allows them to maintain the best care possible for their clients. Therefore, we strongly urge frequent supportive interaction and discussion among nurses and between nurses and other health professionals responsible for client care.

References

Coyne, J. C. Depression and the response of others. *Journal of Abnormal Psychology*, 1976, *85*, 186–193.

Damas, M. J., Patel, M. K., & Jenner, F. A. The effect of mild hyperventilation on red cell sodium. *British Journal of Psychiatry*, 1977, *130*, 459–462.

Farina, A., Fisher, J. D., Getter, H., & Fisher, E. H. Some consequences of changing people's views regarding the nature of mental illness. *Journal of Abnormal Psychology*, 1978, *87*, 272–279.

Gibson, H. B. A form of behavior therapy for some states diagnosed as "affective disorder." *Behavior Research and Therapy*, 1978, *16*, 191–195.

Gulevich, G. D. Convulsive and coma therapies and psychosurgery. In J. D. Barchas, P. A. Berger, R. D. Ciaranello, & G. R. Elliott (Eds.). (Eds.). *Psychopharmacology, from theory to practice*, New York: Oxford University Press, 1977.

Lewinsohn, P. M. A behavioral approach to depression. In R. J. Friedman & M. M. Katz (Eds.). *The psychology of depression: Contemporary theory and research*, Washington, D.C.: Winston-Wiley, 1974.

Lewinsohn, P. M., Biglan, T., & Zeiss, A. Behavioral treatment of depression. In P. Davidson (Ed.). *Behavioral management of anxiety, depression and pain*, New York: Brunner/Mazel, 1976.

Libet, J., & Lewinsohn, P. M. The concept of social skill with special references to the behavior of depressed persons. *Journal of Consulting and Clinical Psychology*, 1973, *40*, 304–312.

Linehan, M. M. A social-behavior analysis of suicide and parasuicide: Implications for clinical assessment and treatment. In J. F. Clarkin & H. I. Glazer (Eds.). *Depression: Behavioral and directive intervention strategies*, New York: Garland Publishing, Inc., 1981.

Mendels, J. Lithium in the treatment of depression. *American Journal of Psychiatry*, 1976, *133*, 373–378.

Nelson, J. C., & Bowers, M. B. Delusional unipolar depression. *Archives of General Psychiatry*, 1978, *35*, 1321–1328.

Chapter Thirteen

STRATEGIES FOR INTERVIEWING IN LANGUAGE AND THOUGHT DISORDERS

Janet Kroah

ANYONE WHO WORKS WITH a schizophrenic person sooner or later experiences bafflement. It may seem that both you and he are talking about the same subject and yet as the exchange continues it becomes clearer to you that neither is understanding what the other is saying. As a therapeutic person you know that both the therapist and the client must understand what this individual is trying to communicate if you are to help him overcome the obstacles that prevent him from becoming a functioning member of the community. As Cameron has suggested, it is easy to conclude that even though your communication is not always clear, the primary difficulty lies with this other individual; that something has gone wrong with the schizophrenic person's machinery of communication, although it is difficult to pinpoint the trouble. The client arrives at conclusions that you cannot share, by logical methods that you cannot follow. He uses words in a way that you cannot understand.[1]

In order to classify and thus move toward clarification of the language and thought of the schizophrenic individual, this paper will include three foci. Initially, some theories explaining the language and thought process of the schizophrenic will be reviewed, forms of the schizophrenic's speech will be identified and illustrated, and finally

From "Strategies for Interviewing in Language and Thought Disorders," by Janet Kroah, *Journal of Psychiatric Nursing and Mental Health Services*, 1974, Vol. 12, No. 2. Reprinted by permission of SLACK, Inc., Medical Publishers, Thorofare, NJ.

strategies that the therapeutic person might use to intervene in the language and thought disorder will be suggested.

SOME THEORIES ABOUT THE LANGUAGE AND THOUGHT OF THE SCHIZOPHRENIC

Sullivan says that the young child uses "private language" and at some point undergoes revision because the child discovers that he is better able to get what he wants from the adult if he uses their language.[2] Throughout life language is largely an instrument for getting what we want. Generally, according to Sullivan, this is obtaining satisfaction and preserving a feeling of personal security. Sullivan concludes that most children learn to use language more to preserve security than to obtain satisfaction.[2]

The schizophrenic individual uses language primarily because of an extreme need for personal security. The individual who becomes schizophrenic is one who early in his life has had many, repeated traumatic experiences which generate a continuing insecurity. In accommodating these experiences, and in an attempt to gain personal security, he uses language exclusively for counteracting his feelings of insecurity among other people. Thus he uses words as protective mantles or shields rather than as a means of communication. What further compounds the difficulty between the schizophrenic person and someone else is that the former has not learned to consensually validate, or to use language as a device for checking up on things.[2]

Miscommunication leads to increased anxiety on the part of the "listener." This increased anxiety is felt by the schizophrenic individual. He in turn gets more anxious, needs more security, but gets more "schizophrenic" in the process. In other words, the initial use of language to gain security becomes, later on, a way of perpetuating his insecurity, and thus the language becomes more problematic as its use to counteract continuing insecurity escalates and becomes more widespread.

Haley presents his explanation of what happens to the schizophrenic individual when he attempts to relate to another person but miscommunicates instead. Haley indicates that when any two persons meet each other for the first time and begin to establish a relationship, any range of behavior is possible. As they define the relationship they work out what type of communicative behavior is to take place in this relationship. They decide what is and what is not to take place. In this way the relationship is mutually defined by the presence or absence of messages interchanged between two people. Messages are not always verbal. Tonal qualities or bodily movement (away or toward) also convey a message.[3]

When assessing the schizophrenic individual's difficulty in getting into a relationship, Haley indicates that this person has been in an extremely dangerous or painful or disorienting family situation in which it was impossible for him to attain a positive health relationship. Thus when he encounters a therapeutic person, he tries many language maneuvers to avoid defining the relationship. Haley says that he may do this in any one of four ways: (1) the individual can deny that he communicated something, "The voices told me," "God is speaking through me," "It's the alcohol or drugs that made me say that"; (2) he may deny that something was communicated, "I don't remember saying that" or "You don't understand what I said"; (3) he can deny that he was communicating to another person, simply that he was talking to himself; or (4) he can deny what he says is said in this situation by labeling his statements as referring to some other time or place, "My parents treated me badly before and will probably when I go home."[3]

Thus, Haley is suggesting that because talking "straight" would be too threatening or because he has never learned to do so, that when the schizophrenic person gets into any interpersonal setting he tries to avoid defining the relationship and in so doing his language sounds "crazy," illogical or autistic.

Another theorist, Kasanin, has described the development of the thought process. First what Kasanin describes and defines as the normal thought process will be presented and then how he sees the thought process in the schizophrenic.

Kasanin defines three stages in the normal development of thought: physiognomic thinking, concrete thinking, and abstract thinking. In the first state the child animates an object, and projects his ego into it (when a child plays with a chair and calls it a horse). He then advances to the level of literal or concrete thinking. At this point, when the child says table or chair, he does not mean table or chair in general, but the particular table or chair which is in his house, or belongs to him. The third state, abstract thinking, usually occurs after the individual has acquired formal or informal education.[4]

After testing the levels of thought that the schizophrenic individual obtains, Kasanin's conclusion was that the schizophrenic has a reduction in abstract thinking and that his thought process was at a more concrete, realistic, matter-of-fact stage which had a personal rather than a universal value.[4]

There would seem then to be a relationship between both Sullivan's and Haley's ideas about the highly personal language of the schizophrenic and Kasanin's ideas about the personal concrete level of thought process that schizophrenic individuals exhibit.

One may then wonder if one process, language, affects the other process, thought? Whorf[5] says that it does. He proposes that all higher levels of thinking are dependent on language, and that the structure of language a person habitually uses influences the manner in which he understands his environment and behaves with respect to it.[5]

FORMS OF SCHIZOPHRENIC SPEECH

After having reviewed some theorists' explanations of the language and thought process of the schizophrenic person, I will now identify some patterns in the schizophrenic's language.

Concrete rather than abstract. A colleague of mine related an incident which is a good example of this. She had just met this person and told him her name and then said "Give me your name." The person responded by saying "No, I need mine. You have your own."

The schizophrenic's language contains many private meanings as evidenced in neologisms or symbolism.

Perseveration of sounds. "The Purple Paulist priests pushed, pulled, and provoked parishioners, poorly, piously, and proportionate to propriety."

Coded mechanisms. For example, in *I Never Promised You a Rose Garden*, Land of Ur, Mapmaking, and list making.

Mixed "C"s. Frequently the language of the schizophrenic gives evidence of his confusion when the person mixes the command, context, and content.

Word salads. Scattering, prototaxis, circumstantiality.

VARIANTS OF LANGUAGE AND THOUGHT DISORDERS AND STRATEGIES OF INTERVENTION

Initially I mentioned that if the nurse (or other therapeutic person) is to help the schizophrenic individual become a functioning member of society, she must make every effort to understand his language and help him become understandable to others. This is no easy task. But there are strategies that you can use to help him communicate in a clearer manner. The strategies that I will talk about are based on Sullivan's, Haley's, Kasanin's, and Whorf's ideas which have been applied to psychotherapeutic nursing by Peplau. Peplau firmly believes that the corrective language the nurse uses will directly affect the language of the schizophrenic individual. In turn this will have a positive effect on his thought processes and behavior.[6,7]

It should be pointed out that change does not occur overnight. The nurse may use a strategy over and over again before the language of the schizophrenic individual changes, but it will change.

Now, to make things clearer, I will focus on variants of language and thought disorders, describe each, and show interventions appropriate to each that either my students or myself have had with schizophrenic individuals.

Scattering

Mr. W's initial session was characterized by scattering or "looseness of associations," prototaxis and parataxic associations. However, what I want you to listen for is the scattering. After the nurse had introduced herself and told the patient why she was there, he said:

> P: *Insemination, Rugers—The State University. If you are outside for inquire, I won't lie for you. I will lie in bed for you. Age, money, worry about war, government circumstance and his son, kerchief, nice hair-do, oh is good hair-do, Irma.*
>
> N: *Who is Irma?*
>
> P: *Might be our own daughter?*
>
> N: *Who is Irma to you?*
>
> P: *Can you think? Strong good features. I will shrink for her. I will solve Germany's problems.*

The patient's initial response seems scattered, although there are other elements present. It is quite difficult to determine what he is talking about. This is the function of scattering. The hearer will not understand and may become disoriented. Anxiety increases scattering. In this instance the nurse told the patient that she would be seeing him twice a week for 15 weeks. This fact alone tends to increase anxiety on the basis that most schizophrenic patients do not expect such attention. Thus one strategy of intervention has to do with anxiety reduction. If the anxiety is reduced the scattering will also be alleviated in some degree.

A second strategy, based upon the assumption that the focus of the patient's attention is more likely to be sustained on the last thing in the scatter sequence, is to ask about the last word or phrase. In this instance when the nurse asked, "Who is Irma," he gave an answer (distorted) but did not scatter. After the second question, "Who is Irma to you," the patient began to scatter again.

The first few sessions were characterized by scattering. However, the nurse continued using the same strategy of exploring or focusing on the last thing the patient said or occasionally she would interrupt his string of associations by saying: "Before you go on, tell me more about X." By the sixth session, it seemed that the patient had begun to feel more "safe" in the relationship, could sustain a focus, and the security derived from these two newly generated behaviors obviated the former language usage called scattering.

Improvement in the patient's language behavior is illustrated by the following data from the sixth session.

N: *Tell me one thing that has happened since I was here two days ago.*

P: *I took a shower today. We had a Christmas party. Ice cream, cake. They put the curtains up.*

N: *When was the Christmas party?*

P: *Yesterday.*

N: *What was one thing you did at the party?*

P: *I ate, sang songs.*

In this excerpt, when the nurse asked for one thing, the patient gave her two or three answers. The nurse then explored the one which she thought had the most interpersonal content. The patient was able to offer a brief description of the party. This was a noticeable difference from the first few sessions.

Circumstantiality

When the patient uses a language pattern called circumstantiality, there is usually an idea or event that he wants to talk about, but finds the material too threatening to his self-system. He is in conflict about this and goes around the problem attempting to reduce his anxiety and to lose you, the hearer.

A patient in a Community Mental Health Center that I have been seeing in individual therapy opened the session a few weeks ago like this:

P: *Mothers shouldn't take sides. I don't think it's right that mothers favor one son over another. It's not fair. My brother's coming home this weekend. I should be able to also. Dr. X said I could go home.*

N: *What are you trying to say Mr. P?*

P: *Mothers shouldn't take sides.*

N: *But what's the issue?*
P: *(angry) She said I couldn't come home this weekend 'cause my brother is.*

Then I focused on the actual incident that occurred and the patient's thoughts and feelings about not going home.

When the patient is being circumstantial, that is, talking around the issues, the nurse must abstract the theme or decode what the patient is saying and help him get to the main idea and stick to it. Strategies like: Describe one time your mother took sides; What are you trying to say? What's the point you are trying to make? What's the issue? Force the patient to stop being circumstantial and begin dealing with the anxiety also. Once the issue is apparent, further exploration of the patient's thoughts, feelings, and actions is necessary.

Idiosyncratic Language

Another aspect of a schizophrenic individual's language usage and thought process that can be extremely difficult to understand is symbolism or idiosyncratic wording. When you hear this language being used it is necessary for you to decode this language in order to understand what the patient is saying.

Umland defines decoding as the process of reclassifying key symbols in a sentence by using synonyms to a given word to rephrase the sentence to show its meaning.[8] To further clarify what I mean I will decode a proverb: "When the cat's away, the mice will play." (1) Pick out the key symbols in the proverb ("cat's," "away," "mice will play"); (2) list synonyms for each of the words (*Note:* Do not impart sex where there is none. Do not change the tense of the verb. Do not add value judgments):

When the cat's	*away the mice*	*will play.*
authority gone	*subordinate will have fun.*	
superior absent	*inferior*	*will frolic.*

Now translate the decoded proverb: "When superiors are absent the inferiors will frolic" or "When authority is gone the subordinates will have fun." Now let's do the same process with a patient's symbolic data. One of the nurses was working with a paranoid woman who said: "The *witch is going to try me* because *they say I am a war monger*. You are a war monger, you are going to have a witches trial." Synonyms for the italicized words (in order of appearance) are:

female	*judge*	*female*	*I'm bad.*
mother	*question*	*mother*	*I'm wrong.*

126

nurse	punish(?)	nurse
person		person

The decoded message becomes, "What person punished you because she said you did something wrong?" Now what the patient seems to be saying is a lot clearer than her initial symbolism. The second half of the message the patient gives to the nurse is also threatening(?) her and subsequently the nurse was going to be punished, by whom is not clear. After the nurse decoded the message, she recognized that she had been pushing the patient too hard to make a decision about staying in or leaving the hospital. The nurse then began to deal with this issue with the patient who was indeed angry at her. Now the nurse did not ask the patient what female had punished her because the patient's anger with the nurse was very apparent. The nurse first focused on the patient's anger toward her. After the patient has sufficiently dealt with her angry feelings towards the nurse, then the initial message can be decoded and dealt with (who in the past had punished the patient because she thought the patient was wrong).

There are times when it is not always necessary to go through this process to decode symbolic or idiosyncratic language the patient uses. If you have been working with a patient in therapy for a time and have a fairly good idea of what the symbolic language represents, you may interpret what you hear and then validate your perceptions with the patient. I'd like to explain how I did this with a 15-year-old patient I am presently seeing in therapy.

During the first five sessions Barbara had been describing her life style, her friends and problems with parents. I thought I had a fairly good idea of her thoughts on these topics. She opened the sixth session with the following words: "Last night as I lay awake in bed I sent a rocket off to chip away at something that's around the world."

N: *What do you think is around the world?*

P: *I put a glass ball around the world two weeks ago when I was tripping. I planted rockets around the world and set them off at night to chip away at this glass ball so I won't suffocate now. Last night I knocked a big chunk off but man came and replaced part of it.*

N: *I wonder if you put the glass ball around the world for protection?*

P: *I'm afraid I'm going to die. I keep seeing a coffin close in on me. I can't sleep. I get up and have peppermint tea with my father. I'd like to go away where nurses and doctors can check up on me to be sure I'm alright. I'm afraid I'm going crazy. I'm losing control of my thoughts.*

N: *Are you saying that two weeks ago you wanted someone to protect you and help you control what was happening?*

127

P: Yes. *Another girl went on the trip with me and I couldn't leave her—
     she got scared. I had to spend all my time with her—no one helped
     me.*

N: *So you created something artificial to help you (a fantasy). Now
     something has happened within the last two weeks that you feel
     trapped or alone.*

P: *No one is helping me. My father listens at night. I'm losing control of
     my thoughts. I'm afraid I'm going crazy.*

As a strategy, when you hear indefinite pronouns ask the patient
whom he means. For example: Who are you talking about? What is her
name? Who is we? Name one person. By forcing the individual to present
real names, the therapist gets the patient to think more particularly about
specific people and his relationship with them. The therapist needs to
influence the person to think in terms of relations and connections and
not to incorporate others in a roundabout way.

Overgeneralizations

Frequently, what you will often hear from a patient is not a description of
an experience or observation of the situation (raw data), but a conclusion
he has already formed about an experience or situation. (The nurses don't
like me around here, Mary is jealous of me.)
     When an individual draws conclusions the next step is some
behavioral pattern in response to this conclusion. What has usually
happened with the hospitalized patient is that his conclusions about his
experience can get him to adopt behavioral patterns that society labels as
deviant or sick.
     Thus when an individual makes assertions or draws conclusions
without giving the description or raw data, the hearer cannot check the
validity or accuracy of the incident. An example is global vagueness:
everything happened today, everybody hates me around here. The strategy
for encountering this is to: (1) ask for an example of one thing, What's
one thing that happened?; or (2) cast doubt—Everything? Everybody?

Erroneous Misclassification of
Experience

An individual, instead of describing, classifies a situation or draws a
conclusion. An example: "Mary is jealous of me." The strategy: Where
did you get that idea? Tell me one time you thought that Mary was jealous
of you.
     By using the various strategies suggested you are forcing the

individual to be specific. You also are assisting him to recover, review, and recheck instances from which he drew the conclusion. The therapist cannot validate the patient's perception unless she knows all the facts.

Non-Actual Experience

The individual most likely to exhibit this type of language and thought disorder is the obsessive-compulsive or someone who is guilt-ridden. The problem with the non-actual experience is that it has never really occurred and time is spent in talking about what hasn't happened unless she [the nurse] intervenes.

Examples of this are: (1) *Future* oriented: I will do it tomorrow; (2) *If* oriented: If I could get out of this situation; (3) *Negative* oriented: I don't think I can do that; (4) *Compulsive* oriented: I should go home.

The most obvious strategy the nurse uses in this type of language and thought disorder is to get the patient to say what he *did* do today, or the reality is he can't get out of this situation and what *is* he going to do about it *now*. One other strategy that is useful for the compulsive oriented patient is to say: Who *said* you should go home?

Now, I might point out that there is a great deal of anxiety and psychotic behavior occurring in Barbara [the patient]. Thus, I did not decode a lot of what she said. Primarily because during this session I did not know how much stress she could handle and I heard the message that she felt alone and was fearful of losing control. Thus to prevent any more psychotic material from coming into awareness I only decoded what the glass ball represented to her. This was enough to get her talking about what she perceived happening to her then.

The following variants of language and thought disorders occur frequently in patients as well as in people who are not labeled patients.

Automatic Knowing

In automatic knowing the individual assumes that the therapist knows what he means or is thinking without his having to tell her. There is a quality of mind reading and taking for granted that the hearer knows what the user is thinking without any data. With the constant use of this problematic language the individual begins to think others know about him without any information. This is a major problem you may hear with a paranoid patient. Expressions like: *you know* how it is; *you see* how it is, indicate this disorder.

Strategy: No, I don't know. What are you assuming I know? Tell me what you want me to know. I don't know how it is, tell me.

Inability to Name Referents to Pronouns

Psychiatric patients use pronouns to conceal themselves from others and to hide information that is being conveyed. Eventually they lose the ability to recall names and thus never deal with people on an individual basis. The identity of the people to whom the pronouns refer is lost and communication is ultimately hampered. Example: they did it to me; she said so; we went downtown.

I have talked about eight variants of language and thought disorders that have already been defined in literature. I think it is extremely important for nurses to continue observing patients' communication patterns, to compile these observations and from them develop appropriate strategies.

SUMMARY

In this paper I have attempted to clarify the communication patterns of the schizophrenic person by looking at various theorists' descriptions of the language and thought process and by identifying and illustrating specific forms of schizophrenic speech. I hope to build on your therapeutic communication by suggesting strategies to intervene in the language of the schizophrenic individual.

References

1. Cameron, N.: Experimental analysis of schizophrenic thinking. In Kasanin, J.S. (ed): Language and Thought in Schizophrenia. New York, W. W. Norton and Company, 1944, p. 50.

2. Sullivan, H. S.: The Language of Schizophrenic. In Kasanin, J. S. (ed): Language and Thought in Schizophrenia. New York, W. W. Norton and Company, 1944, pp. 4–7.

3. Haley, J.: Strategies of Psychotherapy. New York, Grune and Stratton, 1963, pp. 6–8, 89–90.

4. Kasanin, J. S.: the disturbance of conceptual thinking in schizophrenia. In Kasanin, J. S. (ed): Language and Thought in Schizophrenia. New York, W. W. Norton and Company, 1944, pp. 41–43.

5. Whorf, B., Carroll, J. B. (eds): Language, Thought, and Reality. Cambridge, Massachusetts, M.I.T. Press, 1956.

6. Peplau, H.: Psychotherapeutic strategies. *In* Perspectives in Psychiatric Care VI(6):264–270, 1968.

7. Peplau, H.: Steps in the Causation of Anxiety. New Brunswick, New Jersey, Rutgers—The State University (unpublished papers).

8. Umland, T.: A Manual for the Evaluation and Development of Intellectual Competence. New Brunswick, New Jersey, Rutgers—The State University, 1961, p. 14 (unpublished papers).

Chapter Fourteen

THE HALLUCINATING PATIENT AND NURSING INTERVENTION

Sylvia T. Schwartzman

A BEHAVIOR PATTERN WHICH I have observed in working with mentally ill persons that seems especially problematic is that exhibited by the hallucinating patient. From various observations it appears that nursing staff, other professional personnel, and paraprofessionals find it difficult to work with the hallucinating patient and sometimes quite frustrating. It was this that spurred me to investigate the hallucinatory process more in depth. Furthermore, the fact that an hallucination is the form that dissociated material of the self has taken and hence is representative of a partial psychological death of the individual's self-system, perhaps as a last-ditch mechanism against actual physical self-annihilation, has intrigued me for a number of years.

The mental anguish that many acutely hallucinating people display compelled me to make an in-depth analysis and appraisal of this process to find answers to the following questions: Why does the person manifest hallucinatory behavior? What need(s) does this behavior serve for the individual? What does the patient mean by this behavior? What is the nurse's role in relationship to this behavior? In this way, it is hoped that this paper will transmit a notion of hallucinatory behavior and the nursing

From "The Hallucinating Patient and Nursing Intervention," by Sylvia T. Schwartzman, *Journal of Psychiatric Nursing and Mental Health Services*, November/December, 1975. Reprinted by permission of SLACK, Inc., Medical Publishers, Thorofare, NJ.

intervention required to effect a well integrated plan of care for the patient. There will be examples of nurse-patient encounters cited from my own professional experiences which will serve to illustrate various points. In no way will the identity of the patient be made directly so as to insure anonymity and respect the confidentiality of the patient.

In order to try to make some sense of the hallucinatory process and its significance for the patient, it is first necessary to define an hallucination. Gravenkemper states:

> . . . an hallucination is an inner experience expressed as though it were an outer event. It arises out of the dissociated motivations of the self-system and is an uncanny, yet real, experience for the person. [1:86]

To know what is meant by "dissociated motivations of the self-system," one must first gain some understanding of the self-system itself. As Sullivan has viewed it, the self-system originates from early childhood in which the child becomes aware of himself through the appraisals of the significant others in his life. The child comes to internalize these appraisals accorded him into a formulation of self—the self-system. This development involves beginning personifications of "me" as the good-me, the bad-me, and the not-me. [2:161]

> . . . The good-me is the personification that organizes experience in which satisfactions have been enhanced by rewarding increments of tenderness, which come to the infant because the mothering one is pleased with the way things are going; therefore, and to that extent, she is free, and moves toward expressing tender appreciation of the infant. Good-me, as it ultimately develops, is the ordinary topic of discussion about "I." Bad-me, on the other hand, is the beginning personification which organizes experience in which increasing degrees of anxiety are associated with behavior involving the mothering one in its more or less clearly comprehended interpersonal setting . . . with increasing tenseness and increasingly evident forbidding on the part of the mother. [2:162]

Sullivan continues to state that:

> . . . For the expression of all things in the personality other than those which were approved and disapproved by the parent and other significant persons, the self refuses awareness. . . It does not accord awareness, it does not notice; and these impulses, desires, and needs come to exist disassociated from self, or dissociated. When they are expressed, their expression is not noticed by the person. [3:21]

This essentially is the not-me, which develops out of experiences with significant others that have been fraught with intense anxiety. This overwhelming experience of anxiety prevented the developing individual from developing any grasp of or making any sense out of the particular circumstances which dictated the experience of this intense anxiety.

> . . . Thus while the self-system excludes from awareness clear evidence of a dissociated motivational system, that which is dissociated is represented in awareness by some group of ideas or thoughts which are marked uncannily with utter foreignness—they have nothing to do with oneself. [2:361]

H. S. Sullivan posits that the next step in this sequence is the actual occurrence of the hallucination, which the individual perceives as deriving outside himself, alien to himself and engendering feelings of terror, hatefulness, fear, or something like this.

Before I can cite examples of an encounter with the patient demonstrating hallucinatory behavior, it is necessary first to provide a brief background history of the selected patient before the reader will be able to grasp the significance of the hallucinatory behavior for the patient. The patient was a twenty-nine-year-old, Caucasian woman, henceforth designated as P. (for "patient"). She was diagnosed as "acute schizophrenic." She was born of Catholic parents and was one of five children. At the age of two it was noted that her father had inflicted beatings upon her. Because there were marital difficulties between the parents and because of the father's frequent abandonment, the mother placed P., then a child of eight years, into an orphan home for approximately five years to be cared for by religious sisters. The patient stated that these nuns showed her many injustices. For example, she had recollection of their forcing her to eat her own vomitus on an occasion when she refused to do more work than some of the other girls in the home and she became upset to her stomach as a result. The patient was returned to her natural home at the age of thirteen, and recalled that living there was intolerable. That is, she had to assume a great deal of the work around the house and there were many ill-feelings among family members. She completed school to the eighth grade, began drinking and engaging in sexually promiscuous activities thereafter. She was married at the age of seventeen, "to get away from home." She married a manual laborer, who was alcoholic. They had six children, but, the paternity of the children was questionable.

The patient characterized her marital life as "beautiful at first"— approximately for the first two years—but later, as the husband subjected her to many abuses, she became more unhappy. When he began to engage in extramarital relationships, she believed he no longer cared for her but was only exploiting her. She then resorted to drinking and engaging in her own extramarital affairs for outlets to her feelings. Because of her various acting-out behaviors, the children were not being adequately cared for and as a result, all six of them were taken from the patient and her husband

and placed in different foster homes by the court. The patient was twenty-six years of age at this time. Shortly after the placements, the patient made a suicide attempt, without success, by drowning. As a result of this attempt, she was hospitalized for a period of six months of continuous treatment followed by her release and readmission approximately one year later for a second suicide attempt.

It was during this second hospitalization that I met P. who was very verbal throughout meetings but her main manner of relating was quite psychotic. That is, she related auditory hallucinations, which she had continually been experiencing for two months prior to hospitalization. P. related that the voices were "a thousand of my voice. I can't fight them anymore." If one looks at P.'s above brief developmental history sketch, it becomes apparent that she experienced early in her life:

> . . . a self which arose through derogatory experience, hostility toward the child, disapproval, dissatisfaction with the child, then this self more or less like a microscope tends to preclude one's learning anything better, to cause one's continuing to feel a sort of limitation in oneself, and while this cannot be expressed clearly, while the child or the adult that came from the child does not express openly self-depreciatory trends, he does have a depreciatory attitude toward everyone else, and this really represents a depreciatory attitude toward the self.[3:23]

Thus, P., with early childhood rejections and injustices by parents—her father beat her; she was placed in an orphan home; she stated that her mother neither held nor cuddled her much as a child; her father called her a "tramp" and "bum" as she got older; neither parent came to visit her while she was hospitalized; and later injustices inflicted by her husband—she became one of, ". . . those people with chronically low self-esteem who have advantage taken of them, and who may later go on to plunge into the bad waking dream of schizophrenia attendant with all its uncanny emotions of awe, dread, loathing, and horror."[2:359]

An example of P.'s early dealing with anxiety, precipitated by her separation from her family at the age of eight to go to an orphan home, is that she began to have "visions" at that time of the Blessed Virgin Mary and God whom she related were "the only ones I have been close to." On a superficial glance one might be inclined to label these visions as part of the normal fantasy life of a child. And yet, because of the abrupt development of the visions approximating the separation of the patient from her family, and the extreme detail with which she described them— for example, the physical attire and characteristics of the Blessed Virgin Mother were identical with the patient's own mother and the God figure was her father's chronological age—the visions appeared to be more than merely childhood fantasy. Rather, the visions seemed reminiscent of Phase I in the development of an hallucinatory process as outlined by Janice

Clack in "An Interpersonal Technique for Handling Hallucinations."[4] In this Phase I, the person first experiences mounting stress and severe anxiety (for P. this was separation anxiety), or loneliness (for P. this was rejection by her parents both physically and emotionally). The patient then willingly and wittingly focuses on certain personal thoughts (in this case, P. focused on the holy figures) that to some degree are comforting. These figures seemed to represent substitute parents for the eight-year-old girl who had been separated from her own biological parents.

Apparently, the patient did not re-experience any more "visions" after being returned to her natural home until the time just prior to hospitalization but, of course, the available information of this is limited and at best subject to speculation. I have given this brief account of an early experience to point out: (1) the extreme vulnerability of this patient's self-system by virtue of her past history to future evolution or predisposition to an hallucinatory experience—actually, a schizophrenic process; (2) a way in which this individual attempted to deal with mounting anxiety in her earlier years; and so provide the reader with some indication of her ego functioning.

In adult life P. apparently was finding it more difficult to deal with her rising anxiety so that by the time I met her she was blatantly hallucinating. She exhibited flight of ideas—mostly of religious, sexual, and aggressive themes. She stated the voices told her to "do all sorts of awful things." An example she gave was "to roast my children; put my bottom in God's and the Virgin Mother's faces; urinate in people's mouths," and engage in assorted sexual activities. She stated, "I'm no lesbian, don't be afraid of me." Thus, as the unconscious feelings and thoughts which the self-system tends to keep dissociated are recalled—the hallucinations—the individual experiences renewed anxiety and much psychic pain as demonstrated by the content of the hallucinations cited.

Sometimes P. would cock her head to one side and assume the "listening attitude" that Clack describes in Phase II of the hallucinatory process. Another characteristic of this Phase II which P. demonstrated was P.'s attempt to place distance between herself and the hallucinatory phenomena by projecting the experience outward as if the sounds were coming from another person or place. For example, as P.'s anxiety increased when I was touching on material too emotionally laden for P. to deal with at that time, she stated, "Oh, they just told me to pee in your mouth. My golden mind (she saw this as her healthy mind) would never tell me to do that. I'm sick of this disgusting mind!" Here she has projected the hallucinatory phenomena outward as not belonging to her being. She assumes possession of the "golden mind" as part of her former real self as opposed to not assuming possession of "this disgusting mind," which is dissociated and separate from her.

Another indication that P. was in Phase II of the hallucinatory process occurred when she related that two months before, when the hallucinations had first begun, the voices were "friendly." That is, she experienced thoughts that were "happy—of the holy people and not dirty." She also (two months before) had more control over focal awareness of these thoughts. That is, she was better able to control them stating, "I'd think of pleasant thoughts or sing happy songs instead to fight them, but now they're getting bad and harder to fight!" Thus, the nature of the hallucinations was changing and becoming more controlling, indicative of Phase III described by Janice Clack. It must be added that P. did not advance further into the various remaining phases as a result of the therapeutic relationship she and I had developed. P. seemed to want to exercise and/or regain control of herself. She had not given up forming or wanting to form satisfying relationships with real people in favor of the hallucinations—unlike some of the more chronically institutionalized patients one sees lining the walls of state hospitals today. In fact, two episodes during the course of P.'s hospitalization—one episode in which she eloped from the hospital, went to a tavern, was picked up by two men, and then submitted to sexual advances; and the other episode in which she left the hospital with a fellow patient to get inebriated at a local tavern—although demonstrating the inappropriateness of P.'s actions and her apparent lack of ego controls also revealed that on both occasions the patient went out to have "fun" and "try to lose the voices," as she related. One can interpret this behavior as Sidney Levine does in *The Meaning of Despair*, "... Many patients seek relief from depression by acting out sexual impulses."[5:371] There seems to be a parallel here between Levine's statement and the patient, who attempted to seek relief from the constant bantering, persecutory, and accusatory voices by engaging in rather tenuous relationships with others.

If one looks at P.'s life in operational terms to understand the evolution of the hallucinatory experience, first the patient probably had feelings and thoughts that were disapproved of by significant others in her life resulting in the formation of the bad-me personification. These negative standards and appraisals were next incorporated by the patient. Sometime later in her life she experienced one of these disapproved feelings causing a rise in her anxiety level to severe proportions. If she could not handle the anxiety via healthy security mechanisms, pathological ones came into play. When the mechanisms worked effectively she was free from the disapproved occurrence, thought, or feeling in that it had been adequately banned from awareness with a subsequent decrease in anxiety. But, gradually, the dissociated content continued to appear in disguised forms—that is, hallucinations.[6:138]

For the purpose of example, I would now ask the reader to focus back into the childhood of P. when she was two years of age upon the occasions of her father beating her. Hypothetically, this two-year-old child probably expressed anger by perhaps hitting back, kicking, saying "No" to him. Now, it must be remembered that shortly after this, the father abandoned his wife and children. The departure probably engendered a great deal of anxiety and guilt in the child, for her unconscious wish to kill

father, in her child's mind, had been attained. Hence, any future
expression of hostile feelings, actions, or thoughts—which seemingly had
been so destructive and overpowering to effect father's disappearance
and her usual methods of coping with the anxiety—(1) confession of her
wrongdoings/thoughts to an authority confessor figure; (2) repression; (3)

Whenever feelings of anger toward parents, husband, or children
entered awareness in the adult P., anxiety and guilt concomitantly arose
and her usual methods of coping with the anxiety:—(1) confession of her
wrongdoings/thoughts to an authority confessor figure; (2) repression; (3)
substitution of happy, pleasant, unrelated thoughts and feelings for the
anxiety-provoking ones; and (4) fabrication of fantasies—no longer proved
effective in decreasing the anxiety such that, hallucinations ensued.
Furthermore, "a hallucinating patient is generally unaware of the
dissociated, disintegrating, unconscious material. When it bursts through
into awareness, it produces anxiety; it seems foreign; it is 'not-me.'"[4:17] A
most fitting example of this from interaction with P. occurred in relation
to an hallucination she was experiencing in which she was "told" that she
had inflicted harm upon her children. Whereupon, after relating this to
me, she immediately added, "I would never do those things to my
children. I would kill myself first. I love my children. It's them voices!"
One could say the voices were representative of a rigid, punishing
superego. P. seemed to have had little opportunity to freely express her
feelings towards the significant others in her life as evidenced by the
parents' use of physical rather than verbal discipline meted out to P.
during the course of her life. It is noteworthy that whenever I interpreted
or labeled an affectual display, which the patient exhibited when talking
about her parents and which obviously was fraught with much hostility, as
"anger" the patient immediately denied this threatening interpretation but
would ask immediately afterward, "Do you get angry with your parents?"
This response is reminiscent of a child who seeks and tests for the
reassurance of a parent for possession of hostile feelings. At times I had
the impression that P. was asking for permission to safely express these
pent-up feelings of hostility without fear of condemnation or retaliation by
me.

It is most significant to comment that P. could not differentiate
thought content of the auditory hallucinations from actions and often
times she would believe that the hallucinations were facts and had meaning
for her in reality. But, since she was convinced that the hallucinations were
not-me, she could not be held responsible for her "evil thoughts/actions/
feelings." One can see then that the voices were of social
significance to P. in that she dissociated the voices from belonging to
herself and so she became socially inculpable of any enactment of the
voices' demands. For example, if the voices told her, "You are a whore,"
and the patient then proceeded to engage in endless promiscuous activity,
she might, for awhile at least, believe she had no responsibility for her

actions but rather the voices, which she perceived as external to herself, would be the culprits.

Another social function that the hallucinatory behavior served for P. was to ward off loneliness. From the "visions" experienced at the age of eight and in adulthood where the patient heard the holy voices "singing songs to me" two months prior to hospitalization, it appears that the hallucinations provided her with a fantasy world of "loving" others away from her world of loneliness where she described herself as "starved for love." The patient described two other visual hallucinations she experienced prior to entering the hospital. One was of a "holy man with a bald head and a kind face who kissed me" and another of a "man burned in the fires of hell who came to give me comfort"—which, by their described loving and comforting natures, one must seriously consider the need for contact and tenderness. That is, for P. these hallucinations served a need for interpersonal intimacy. Therefore, this woman, who as a child was lonely and resorted to substitute satisfactions in fantasy did not fully as an adult, ". . . despite the pressures of socialization and acculturation. . . sufficiently learn to discriminate between realistic phenomena and the products of (her) own living fantasy."[7:4]

As evidenced from the brief developmental history presented earlier, P. probably experienced loneliness which in a Sullivanian sense can be described as an extremely uncomfortable experience connected with an insufficient discharge of the need for human closeness. For Sullivan, real loneliness in infancy appears as a need for contact. P. stated that her mother rarely cuddled or held her but was too busy with the other children. Might not this early deprivation of maternal tenderness have planted the seed of loneliness within this patient? According to Sullivan, in childhood the need extends to adult participation in activities. As previously stated, the patient's father was frequently out of the home and the mother was "busy" and likely not free to engage with the patient in any expressive play activities so that P. was deprived of learning ". . . how to express emotions by successes and failures in escaping anxiety or in increasing euphoria; in various kinds of manual play in which one learns coordination, and so on; and finally in verbal play—the pleasure giving use of the components of verbal play speech which gradually move over into the consensual validation of speech."[2:261]

After the orphanage experience, P. reportedly quit school, started to drink, and began engaging in sexually acting-out behavior. In these ways the patient seemed to have been attempting to satisfy the need, of which Sullivan speaks, for an interpersonal relatedness with a fellow human being to gain a sense of personal satisfaction and security. That is, not having had her need for contact and freedom from interpersonal loneliness ever met from infancy onward, the patient resorted during her teen-age years to socially unacceptable ways, knowing little else. Her unbearable need for interpersonal intimacy culminated in her marriage, but the need was met only momentarily until the time her husband became abusive and unfaithful to her. The children provided her with some comfort but only sporadically because the patient was such a deprived child herself, who saw her children as "my dollies that I used to play with." The patient's later extramarital relationships plus the two elopements from the hospital represent her reaching out to anyone—strangers—and anything—alcohol—in an attempt to search out a loving, caring relationship that would provide her with safety from loneliness despite how transient the relationship. By these examples, one can see that loneliness played an important role in the genesis of P.'s mental disorder.

When Sullivan points out that people will even resort to any anxiety arousing experiences in an effort to escape from loneliness, even though anxiety itself is an emotional experience against which people fight, as a rule with every defense at their disposal, one can perhaps see parallels with P. whose hallucinations, at least early in their development, served as defenses against loneliness![2] The hallucinations not only have social significance for the patient but also dynamic significance as well.

When one examines P.'s hallucinations in a dynamic context, it becomes apparent that they contain elements of a triple wish as Freud had posited. There is the pleasure-seeking, libidinous wish; an aggressive wish exists; and an undoing of the erotic/aggressive components as expressed by a punishment component. The content of most of P.'s hallucinations consisted of primary process (Id) preoccupations where the voices told her to engage in all kinds of sexual pleasures with others so that, here the voices served to fulfill an unconscious libidinous wish. The hallucination in which the patient was told to "urinate in people's mouths" illustrates one way in which the hallucination is symptomatic of an unconscious aggressive wish. The patient related this very hallucination during a meeting immediately after I had attempted to structure the patient's activity, which was not in accordance with her wants at the moment. This demonstrated P.'s attempt to tell me in the language of "schizophrenese" that she was angry with me and not in agreement. The patient could only relate such "forbidden" feelings via the hallucination and not on a more direct communication level. In like fashion she could only tolerate talking lucidly about her parents for brief intervals and then would say that the voices told her to put "my bottom in God and the Blessed Virgin Mary's faces." This translated communication meant that P. was telling her parents, as signified by God and the Virgin Mother, to kiss her derriere—a most aggressive wish indeed! The hallucinations, centered on harming her children, are also a reflection of her aggressive wishes toward them. Once her husband could not come to visit her because, "He had to see the kids in the homes. The kids are more important to him than me. No one gives a damn for me!" This example provides some indication of the aggressive competitiveness she had felt with her children for her husband's attention.

The hallucination is symptomatic of a third wish as well—that of undoing the erotic/aggressive components through punishment. This was displayed in the example just cited in that, after P. expressed that her children were more important to her husband than herself, she experienced increased anxiety as evidenced by her outward restlessness as well as by the content of the voices. The voices then said she was not a good mother to her children and that the children were better off without her. The patient then stated that she believed the children were more important than herself and that her husband *should* be visiting them instead of her. Thus, one can see how an hallucination can consist of a punishment component as well. It is interesting to note that P. perceived the later developed and more "disgusting" hallucinations as punishments for her "sins," and for her entire life stating, "I was born to be punished; my life's been so rotten that I think God chose some people to suffer all their lives with no love." These statements are representative of the patient's need for self-punishment. And, an interesting side note to this is that, according to Sandor Rado, self-punishment is a way of winning love. "It is an expiatory act, a plea for forgiveness for the attack of rage (that is, aggressive wishes harbored toward significant others) in order to reconcile with the mother, toward whom the depressed person is still resentful for the deprivations suffered from the mother."[8:98] So, in a way, when P. stated, "God chose some people to suffer all their lives with no love," she was speaking of herself and the self-punishing aspect of the hallucinations as, in Rado's terms, a means of achieving love from the mothering one. Thus, the hallucinatory behavior pattern is a manifestation of a person's mental suffering and indicates often times a desperate need for help.

With these understandings of the social and dynamic significance of the behavior for the individual and the possible developmental processes contributing to the person's utilizing such problematic behavior, what then is the nurse's role in relation to the patient's behavior? Gravenkemper cites:

> . . . The patient who hallucinates has a strong need to believe in the reality of the hallucination. . . The patient will not begin to doubt the reality of the hallucination until the need that the hallucination is fulfilling has begun to be met in some other way. To discover the purpose of the hallucination and to satisfy the need in another way are the functions of the nurse. . .[1:86]

Arteberry adds:

> . . . The need may be for dependence or to be rejected, or it may be a more personalized need such as for reassurance, self-esteem, acceptance. The nurse should be alert to these cues of needs, and should provide for means to meet them, if meeting them seems to be the therapeutic goal.[9:35]

For the nursing intervention then, the nurse must first know the purpose(s) which the hallucinatory process serves for the patient. That is, she must know the need(s) the hallucinations meet before she can satisfy the need(s) in other ways. In the case of P. the need was to escape from loneliness and rejection and to obtain some degree of interpersonal intimacy. With this understanding then, the first step in working with the patient is to begin establishing an interpersonal relationship with her. In this way, the nurse's "love" toward the patient as exemplified by the nurse's "recognition of the patient as a total being (hallucinations and all) with acceptance and no strings attached,"[10:165] would help the patient escape from loneliness, the subjective state of illness most productive of psychic pain. In such a relationship, the patient would be given the opportunity to begin to develop trust and closeness with the nurse in her capacity as a benevolent, non-punishing authority figure. But, the nurse must be cautioned not to encourage too much dependency of the patient upon her, especially where the patient's ego strengths are tenuous as in the schizophrenic and the patient may strive to engage in therapy beyond the need for such intervention.

Once the patient is provided with a reliable relationship with the nurse, he may no longer need to burst through the particular dissociated material, which the hallucination arouses, because, the patient will have "lost" the hallucination in favor of more interpersonal and more reality-based situations. With the hallucinating patient, the nurse requires an understanding of interpersonal techniques she can use in handling the hallucinations. Foremost, the nurse should recognize and acknowledge the feeling (affectual) tone behind the patient's experience of the voices—to the patient directly—in order to convey to the patient her understanding for what it must be like to be hearing voices, seeing visions, feeling crawling objects, and so forth. For example, when P. related she was hearing "a thousand of my voice," the nurse, after also noting the panicked expression on the patient's face and her agitated, restless body movements, should say, "I can see you are frightened by the voices you seem to be hearing so I will stay with you now."

Secondly, the nurse should be alert to not only the verbal but also the non-verbal cues (for example, the patient moving his lips, or placing his head to the side as though listening intently) that the patient is experiencing hallucinations. In this way, the nurse can use such observations to elicit the patient's descriptions of the hallucination. The rationale for this nursing measure is based on the guiding principle that, "whenever the patient is anxious, the nurse assists the patient with the recognition and naming of the anxiety in order to initiate the patient's learning and/or problem solving."[11:311] The hallucination is an example of a dissociated perception by the patient of his own anxiety so that, by questioning the patient and eliciting observation and description of the hallucination, the nurse helps to bring this aspect of the situation into the patient's perceptual range. As in the case of P., by encouraging description of the hallucination in its fullest context—the thoughts, feelings, and actions attendant with it—the nurse can help the patient to differentiate between thought, feeling, and action reality. At times P. believed the hallucinations were fact, and she required frequent pointing out that the hallucinations did not necessarily have basis for her in reality.

Thirdly, as Grosicki and Harmonson point out, the nurse must present reality to the patient by simply pointing out to the patient that she, the nurse, does not experience the hallucination. In doing this, the nurse must be very careful not to deny the existence directly of the hallucinations since, for the patient, the "voices" are very real. The nurse must avoid conveying to the patient that she believes the voices are real or that she hears them too. She does this by using such terms as, "the voices you say you hear."[12] By so doing, the nurse refrains from entering into the psychotic process with the patient; nor does she reinforce the hallucination's reality for the patient. Rather, the nurse consensually validates what is real in her sensory awareness. In this way, according to Clack, doubt and question is raised regarding the reality of the hallucination without directly denying the patient of its reality. The nurse attempts to introduce her own reality in lieu of the reality which the hallucination has for the patient.

Fourthly, the nurse should provide protection when needed to prevent patient self-injury or injury to others in the environment if the hallucinations are accusing, frightening, or commanding the patient to harm himself or others.

Fifthly, as Grosicki and Harmonson further state, the nurse should respond verbally to anything that is real that the patient talks about in an effort to reinforce reality away from the hallucinatory experience. Another help for the nurse is to avoid non-verbal approaches such as shaking her head, gesturing with her hands that may add to the patient's hallucination. The nurse should ask the patient to let her know when the auditory or visual hallucinations intrude into his conversation with the nurse so the nurse can attempt to structure the conversation to some topic of interest to the patient in his immediate environment—that is, in reality. Another guide for the nurse is to help the patient focus on and identify current situations and/or people that evoke anxiety and lead to hallucinatory development. It is the nurse's task to identify the triggering mechanism of the hallucination if one indeed exists. Peplau comments:

> . . . Counseling in nursing has to do with helping the patient to remember and to understand fully what is happening to him in the present situation, so that the experience can be integrated with rather than dissociated from other experiences in life.[13:64]

A good example of this with P. would be for the nurse to help the patient realize the connection between going home on weekends, outside the protective hospital setting, and coming back to the hospital on the following Monday with an increase in the hallucinations, which the patient described as "harder to fight when I'm home." It would be helpful for the nurse and the patient to consider this "differentness" in the intensity of the hallucinations whenever the patient was placed in the family situation with all its conflicts for her. By looking at the home environment with the patient, the nurse can help the patient identify anxiety-arousing situations, which are particularly bothersome and contribute to an increase in hallucinatory activity, and so help the patient seek alternative, less anxiety-provoking methods of dealing with these situations.

As the nurse continues to work with the hallucinating patient, she should gradually increase social interaction in the patient's environment. That is, by introducing others into the patient's interpersonal world by moving from one person (the nurse) to small group activities such as conversation groups, or games, such as cards, ping-pong, to interaction with large numbers of people (patient government groups; and eventually perhaps some form of group therapy) as the patient is able to tolerate this, the nurse is, according to Clack, assisting the patient in increasing his interpersonal relationships and identifying other helpful means of satisfying his persistent needs for interpersonal closeness.

It is well for the nurse to remember that there may be and probably is more than one underlying problem deriving from a single need, as in P.'s case. Eventually the nurse in working with the patient may move to help the patient see the linkage between the hallucinatory experience and the need(s) that it serves. As Clack observes, the nurse and patient may discuss the outcomes of using the hallucination to meet the particular need, but the patient may not recognize all aspects of the hallucination so that some of the learning and self-integration involved in abandoning the hallucination are outside the patient's awareness.

Some other objectives the nurse must consider in working with the hallucinating patient but which are not directly related to dealing with the hallucinations *per se* are the following: (1) to provide greater alleviation of the hallucinations—that is, the anxiety—through prescribed dosages of medication in order to decrease this anxiety to workable levels which allow the patient to engage more psychotherapeutically with the nurse; (2) to consider the possibility of entering the patient into a group experience within the hospital and perhaps eventually on an outpatient basis, which would be conducive to the patient's forming new relationships to help replace overwhelming feelings of loneliness and gain new insights into self (In this way, the patient can gain group support, which if adequate, can lead to an increase in self-love and esteem by the patient and an elimination of the intense loneliness.); (3) to enlist family cooperation into the patient's treatment plan. This would be accomplished by having meetings with the spouse primarily, and perhaps other family members in order to provide some educative measures regarding the patient's illness so they may come to understand the behavior more clearly. Eventually lines of communication between them could be improved. In this way, continuity of treatment which originated in the hospital with the nurse could be effected into the home setting.

By way of summary, this paper has been concerned with a patient's problematic behavior pattern, namely hallucinations. The social and dynamic significance of the behavior for the individual have been explored and analyzed and a formulation of possible developmental processes influencing the patient to utilize hallucinations has been discussed. On the basis of these analyses, formulations for a psychiatric nursing treatment plan of intervention have been presented.

In conclusion, it is well to bear in mind that the schizophrenic patient who is hallucinating, is striving to communicate in as clear and a straightforward way as he knows, the nature of his anxieties and expriences, despite how radically different they are from the nurse's, with speech content that is difficult to follow. Thus, with this understanding, it behooves us as nurses to intervene accordingly and "decode" the hallucinated messages and thereby assit in breaking into the third stage in the evolutionary cycle of a psychosis, as cited by R. D. Laing: Stage 1 = Good (me); Stage 2 = Bad (me); Stage 3 = Mad (not me).[10:13]

References

1. Gravenkemper, Katherine H.: "Hallucinations," in *Some Clinical Approaches to Psychiatric Nursing,* edited by Shirley F. Burd and Margaret A. Marshall. New York: The Macmillan Company, 1963, pp. 184–188.

2. Sullivan, Harry Stack: *The Interpersonal Theory of Psychiatry.* New York: W. W. Norton and Company, 1953.

3. Sullivan, Harry Stack: *Conceptions of Modern Psychiatry.* New York: W. W. Norton and Company, 1953.

4. Clack, Janice: "An Interpersonal Technique for Handling Hallucinations," in Monograph No. 13, *Nursing Care of the Disoriented Patient.* New York: The American Nurses' Association, 1962, pp. 16–26.

5. Levine, Sidney: "Some Suggestions for Treating the Depressed Patient," in *The Meaning of Despair,* edited by Willard Gaylin. New York: Science House, Inc., 1968, pp. 353–386.

6. DeAugustinis, Jane: "Dissociation and Memory Gaps," in *Some Clinical Approaches to Psychiatric Nursing,* edited by Shirley F. Burd and Margaret A. Marshall. New York: The Macmillan Company, 1963, pp. 137–142.

7. Fromm-Reichman, Frieda: "Loneliness," *Psychiatry,* XXII (1959), pp. 1–16.

8. Rado, Sandor: "Psychodynamics of Depression from the Etiologic Point of View," in *The Meaning of Despair*, edited by Willard Gaylin. New York: Science House, Inc., 1968, pp 96–107.

9. Arteberry, Joan K.: "The Disturbed Communication of a Schizophrenic Patient," *Perspectives in Psychiatric Care*, III (1965), pp. 24–37.

10. Laing, R. D.: *The Divided Self*. Baltimore: Penguin Books, 1960.

11. Burd, Shirley F.: "Effects of Nursing Intervention in Anxiety of Patients," in *Some Clinical Approaches to Psychiatric Nursing*, edited by Shirley F. Burd and Margaret A. Marshall. New York: The Macmillan Company, 1963, pp. 307–322.

12. Grosicki, Jeanette P. and Harmonson, Marguerite: "Nursing Action Guide: Hallucinations," *Journal of Psychiatric Nursing and Mental Health Services*, VII (May-June, 1969), pp. 133–135.

13. Peplau, Hildegard E.: *Interpersonal Relations in Nursing*. New York: G. P. Putnam's Sons, 1952.

Chapter Fifteen

THE MANIPULATIVE PATIENT

Mary Ellen McMorrow

"MARY ELLEN! MARY ELLEN!" shouted Gary from the corner bed of the large ICU.

If I hear him call my name one more time, I thought, I'm going to scream.

"Mary Ellen!"

I finished suctioning Mr. Cook and stomped over to Gary.

"Gary, if you dare to call me again when I'm caring for another patient, I'll throw you out of this 15th-story window. Is that clear?"

"What kind of nurse are you? Don't you have any feelings?"

"And Gary, stop playing games with me. From now on if you call me when I'm not at another patient's bedside, I'll come, but not when I'm with another patient. If you do, I'll stop coming over here just to talk."

"You're only saying that because Welfare's paying for me. If I was a paying patient. . ."

"Baloney and you know it!"

Gary laughed.

What brings a nurse to the point of threatening, even as a joke, to throw a patient out the window? The answer is not simple, but no one ever accused Gary of being simple. He would find a person's weak spot and attack. The weakness he found in me was my perception of myself as a nurse. I saw myself as kind, supportive, and caring, but Gary told me and everyone within a hundred miles that I was rigid, unfeeling, and sadistic.

I felt guilty every time I suctioned a trach because Gary would scream across the room, "You really enjoy gagging that little old lady,

From "The Manipulative Patient," by Mary Ellen McMorrow. Copyright © 1981, American Journal of Nursing Company. Reproduced with permission from *American Journal of Nursing*, June, Vol. 81, No. 6, pp. 1188–1190.

don't you?" Every time I gave him an injection he would scream and complain to everyone about my poor technique.

I had known Gary before this admission to the hospital for an aortic valve replacement. He had been a client in the methadone clinic where I was counseling as part of my training as a rehabilitation counselor. At the clinic, Gary and I had been able to communicate, so why couldn't we establish a therapeutic relationship in the ICU? Gary was the same: manipulative, hostile, and frightened. But I was different.

My perception of my role as nurse was making me act differently in the ICU. As a nurse I was being kind, supportive, and false. I was false in not expressing my feelings honestly to Gary. As a counselor, I had set strict behavioral limits, identified manipulations, and accepted persons for themselves. But Gary was now "my patient," and I responded to him as a patient, rather than as Gary. After my outburst of anger at him—my first honest expression of feeling—we began to understand each other again.

Gary continued to test me, but since I no longer felt guilty or manipulated, I could recognize his machinations and use them to set limits and initiate a more honest communication.

Gary was one of those patients nurses have nightmares about. Within three days of his admission to our hospital, every nurse, doctor, and aide in the place had heard about his antics. After all, it's not every patient who will start fires if you're late with his 9 P.M. medications or who has fist fights with fresh post-MI patients.

Once, on the evening shift, the nurse was alone in the unit with approximately 30 patients. It was before Gary's surgery. Besides threatening to jump out the window, Gary started a fire in the patient lounge and then disappeared from the unit for several hours. He became verbally abusive when the nurse was unable to take time to chat with him. When the nurse walked away, Gary clutched his chest, writhed in pain, and fell to the floor. The nurse, thinking he had arrested, responded dramatically. Gary jumped up laughing, "Ha, ha, I fooled you."

This became Gary's favorite attention getter. Soon the staff were watching his act and grading it for realism and then, gradually, ignoring it altogether. Visitors must have thought the staff were crazy as they stepped over Gary lying in the hall as they went about their tasks.

After his open heart surgery, Gary was transferred to the ICU because the nurses on the unit that usually took the open heart cases threatened to quit en masse if Gary came to their unit. Naturally, Gary's reputation preceded him to the ICU. The nurses there had premonitions of disaster. I was one of them, and Gary lived up to our worst expectations.

Not only were we prophets, we were also martyrs. Few can be martyrs like nurses.

"Why us?" was the plaintive cry. However, unlike the early Christian martyrs going quietly to the lions, we let everyone know how we were suffering.

At first Gary was prejudged and our responses were stereotyped, whether those responses were rejection or nonfeeling sweetness. Gary was manipulative and showed self-destructive tendencies. When he expressed real problems, however, our responses did not change.

On several occasions Gary talked about his fear of death. When I spoke with him about dying, he seemed genuinely relieved. Afterwards Gary said I was the only one who "really talked."

When I finally did what we should have done initially—assess Gary's behavior—I noticed a pattern. He was most abusive and demanding after the surgeon's visit each morning. Gary responded to increased anxiety by increasing his negative behavior. After this simple discovery, I made it a habit to be with Gary when the surgeons came, and as soon as they left, I would reexplain what the physicians had said in positive terms that he could understand.

Another behavior pattern also emerged. Gary wasn't abusive to everyone. Gary never put one nurse and one physician through the verbal wringer. Both, however, were known for their own abrasive personalities. Gary seemed to attack only those who would not fight back.

After Gary was transferred and the anxiety level of the staff returned to normal, we agreed that we had not met Gary's needs nor our own needs during his admission. We also had to accept responsibility for this rather than blame Gary. The staff conceded that Gary needed consistent structuring. Behavioral expectations should have been realistic and clearly defined to Gary and accepted by him. These behavioral expectations should have been enforced by all the staff, giving positive reinforcement for acceptable behavior.

During his ICU stay we did the exact opposite: when Gary was quiet, we ignored him; when he screamed and refused care, he had all our attention.

Gary was discharged from the hospital 97 days after admission. Follow-up was done by the cardiac clinic. He was readmitted three weeks after discharge for complaints of chest pain. The third day after his readmission Gary suddenly clutched his chest, writhed in pain, and fell to the floor. All resuscitation efforts were unsuccessful. Gary expired at the age of 29—with no one to cry for him.

THE ROOTS OF MANIPULATION

Everyone learns early in life to manipulate. In a healthy sense, manipulation refers to purposeful behavior directed at getting needs met. The manipulator, however, does not say, "please," to get a cookie, but to make the other person do what he wishes.

A manipulator is an individual who exploits, uses, and controls others as objects in certain identifiable, self-defeating ways.[1] He uses manipulation to control others rather than to reach a goal of fulfilling real needs.

The manipulative person does not trust his own emotions and, therefore, cannot trust others. The manipulator tries to control himself by controlling others.

What can a nurse do with a manipulative patient? The major problem for the nurse is to get the manipulator to establish trust in his true feelings, so he or she can learn to trust him/herself. Establishing such trust is difficult. The characteristic behaviors of a manipulator are diametrically opposed to trust. Deception is a way of life. Thus, instead of expressing himself, the manipulator creates impressions. Expressed feelings are deliberately planned to fit the occasion and to obtain a desired effect.

The manipulator is always "wheeling and dealing." This person is fearful of expressing feelings, and may even have lost touch with honest emotions. Berne sees the manipulator as one fearful of intimacy who uses games as an alternative to no interaction with others.[2]

Manipulative behaviors may take many forms, from violent threats, to shallow erudition, to helplessness. As a recurrent pattern of dealing with others, manipulation is characterized by a lack of concern for others as people and by a desire to meet one's own immediate wants and needs, whatever the effect on others or even on one's own long-range goals.

The manipulator seeks out others' weaknesses and uses these weaknesses to gain control. His behaviors may be active: making demands, violating rules and routines, or making threats. Behaviors may also be passive: self-pity, procrastination, ingratiation, and tardiness. The manipulator will use emotional blackmail, create guilt feelings, and abuse compassion.

Frequently, manipulative behavior results in unpleasant responses from those being controlled, which include anger, frustration, indifference, and withdrawal. These responses are enjoyed by the manipulator as signs of his power.

The manipulative personality is interested in control. The end result of controlling others is self-defeat. The manipulator eventually alienates everyone, which supports his basic distrust of others. The alienation reinforces the manipulative person's belief that if he expresses his true feelings, people will reject them.

Since manipulative behavior varies with the situation, the best barometer of these behaviors is the nurse's own affective state. If the nurse is feeling angry or frustrated, the situation must be assessed. Who is in control? Is the nurse reacting to having his or her emotional strings pulled?

Establishing a therapeutic relationship with a manipulator is difficult. Distrustful and cynical, the manipulative person cannot understand the reality of the nurse's caring attitude, but will interpret it as the nurse's desire to control. Real personal contact requires openness and spontaneity.

The manipulator avoids personal contact, since it involves risk.

The nurse's goal, then, is to discover the person's true feelings by showing concern and by providing an environment for the safe expression of these feelings. However, this cannot be accomplished if the nurse is being controlled by the manipulator, for allowing herself to be manipulated supports the unhealthy behavior.

The nurse can only help the manipulator by setting firm and clearly defined behavior. Consistency is essential. The nursing staff must be united, since the manipulative person will play one staff member against the other.

If, when caring for a patient who is manipulative and abusive, you begin feeling angry, depressed, or confused, the patient is manipulating. I have found the best thing to do is take a mini-vacation. Go for coffee. Get control of your emotions and try to determine why he is manipulating you. Is it because you are false with him? Could it be because you are reaching him, and it scares him? Then, you can go back to your patient and respond to him rather than be controlled by the emotions he arouses in you.

Analysis of the manipulative behavior will help the person see his own manipulations and will let him know you recognize his attempt to control. When the manipulator is seeking to control, encourage expression of feelings. This can be done simply by asking him what he feels right now.

If the manipulative person refuses to recognize the inappropriateness of his controlling behavior, refuse to play the game. Change the subject or leave the situation. Not supporting manipulative behavior tells the manipulator you cannot be used as an object and protects you from being used. Allowing yourself to be used can only lead to negative feelings toward the manipulator.

Group therapy can be an effective method for helping develop congruence between feelings and behavior.[3] It enables the manipulator to recognize his machinations and permits the expression of feelings in an atmosphere of trust and security.[4]

The manipulative person must learn to feel secure about himself and trust his own emotions before he can learn to control himself and give up controlling others.

References

1. Shostrom, E. L. *Man, the Manipulator.* New York, Abingdon Press, 1967, p. 15.
2. Berne, Eric. *Games People Play.* New York, Grove Press, 1964, p. 18.

3. Rogers, C. R. *Carl Rogers on Encounter Groups.* New York, Harper & Row, 1970, p. 118.

4. Burgess, A. W., and Lazare, A. *Psychiatric Nursing in the Hospital and the Community.* 2nd ed. Englewood Cliffs, N.J., Prentice-Hall, 1976, p. 255.

Chapter Sixteen

COMMUNICATION THROUGH ROLE PLAYING

Patricia R. Underwood

TAKE A NURSE WHO grew up in the little New England town in which her family lived for generations. Put her to work in a big-city hospital in the Middle West. Give her a patient from the Southwest, of immigrant parentage. That nurse is likely to run into communication barriers that make providing adequate care more than a little difficult. But role playing can serve her well in breaking down those barriers.

Role playing might best be defined as a learning experience in which the nurse and the patient act out a situation, either past or expected, as if it were really happening. They might act out a discussion the patient has already had with a family member or a job interview the patient is anticipating. The situation to be acted out depends on the needs of the patient. I found it valuable in working with Mary.

Mary was a 20-year-old, unskilled factory worker with nine years of education, a history of immature acting-out behavior, and limited communication with her family. She had immigrated to the United States 11 years ago.

I saw Mary shortly after her admission to a residential home for unwed mothers, angry, frightened, unable to adjust to the residential center. After several meetings with her, I found she thought there was something wrong with her or her unborn baby. Our discussion revealed an underlying fear of doctors and nurses based on a few unhappy encounters. She was unable to ask questions of the doctor or nurse and left each antepartal examination frightened and certain she was ill. To help her overcome her fears, I tried role playing.

MARY: I have an itch down here. (She indicated the pubic area.)
NURSE: That is something the doctor should know.
MARY: You know I can't tell him.
NURSE: Let's try. I'll be the doctor and you be you. O.K., tell me.
MARY: I have an itch down here. (She laughs and blushes.) That sounds funny. What do you call this?
NURSE: It's the pubic area.
MARY: I have an itch in-on-which is it? (laughs)
NURSE: Try "around."
MARY: I have an itch around the pubic area.
DOCTOR: (as played by the nurse): How long have you had it?
MARY: (relaxing): About two weeks.
DOCTOR: Can you show me exactly where it is?
MARY: Right here.
NURSE: Good, that's it. You'll be able to talk to the doctor and tell him how you feel.
MARY: Hey, it's not too hard once you know what to say.

Mary had numerous other questions about her pregnancy that had been on her mind for weeks, questions that could easily have been answered by the nurse. But role playing with less complicated questions helped her to learn to express herself more directly. Over the weeks we worked on more difficult areas until she was able to talk to the doctor with ease. Her sense of well-being increased as her self-confidence increased, and this encouraged her to try talking more directly not only with me and the physician, but also with other staff members and with patients in the residence.

Mary had difficulty in communicating with her family and rarely disagreed or openly resisted decisions they made. She simply did not comply with decisions she did not like. That usually got her into trouble. Although she did not really want to relinquish her child, Mary agreed with her family's decision that she should. She said her family made her depressed. Believing they did not understand her, she felt angry and resentful toward her family. However, she did not recognize the anger she felt. Again role playing helped.

MARY: I wish they would quit asking about what I'm going to do and then saying what I have to do.
NURSE: That must make you angry.
MARY: No! I just feel low.
NURSE: What do you do when they start telling you?
MARY: Nothing, just listen.

NURSE: *What would you like to do?*
MARY: *I don't know.*
NURSE: *Let's role play. I'll be your brother Joe and you be you.* (I had
seen the brother once, and Mary had talked about him quite
often. Even if the nurse doesn't know the person she is playing,
the situation will build as one gets into it.)
JOE: *Well, Mary, what have you decided? Have you seen the adoption
lady? You should begin to plan.*
MARY: *Just shut up! I don't want to plan anything. I don't know what
to do.*
JOE: *Why are you yelling at me? I asked you a simple question.*
MARY: *Nag, nag, nag. That's all you ever do. I hate you and I'm tired
of it all.* (The patient looked at me bewildered.) *What did
I say?*
NURSE: *You seemed to be saying what you felt. You're pretty upset
with your brother who is pushing you.*
MARY: *But I don't hate him. He has been good to me.*
NURSE: *It's all right to be angry. You can love and hate at the same
time.*
MARY: *I shouldn't have said that.*
NURSE: *It was the way you were feeling.*
MARY: *But that would just make him mad at me.*
NURSE: *What might you say that would get the point across without
making him angry? I'll be Joe again.*
JOE: *Well, what are you going to do? You should be thinking about
what to do with the baby.*
MARY: (looking straight at me, speaking with a calm, confident
voice): *I don't know. I haven't decided. When I do, I will tell
you.*
JOE: *O.K., Mary. As long as you're thinking about it.*
NURSE: *That's it. There is nothing left to say. Now you be your
brother, and I'll be you, Mary.*

We exchanged roles and repeated that conversation. Mary had the same
feeling I had had: She had made a final statement that left no room for
further questioning. Mary then used this approach with her brother. He
responded by telling her to let him know what she decided. He did not
question her further. Shortly thereafter, Mary was able to begin to work
on her feelings about the child she was expecting and to decide what she
was going to do.

Mary's sister planned a large church wedding the month following
Mary's delivery due date. Mary wanted very much to be in the wedding;
however, her family felt she would not be well enough. Although Mary
knew otherwise because of her antepartal classes, she did not assert herself,
but went along with the family's decision. She was hurt and felt the family
did not want her. She said she really didn't care about the wedding, but as

the date drew near and plans were being made, she finally admitted that she cared very much but didn't know how to tell her sister. Role playing helped her decide how to express herself after she had decided what needed to be said. I played Mary while she played her sister, Lynn.

MARY: *(as played by the nurse): Lynn, I have been thinking, and I really want to be in the wedding.*

LYNN: *But you won't be well enough.*

MARY: *Yes, I will. The baby is due a month before the wedding, and I know from my classes that I will be fine in about two weeks.*

LYNN: *How will we ever get a dress for you? When will you be able to be fitted?*

MARY: *I get discharged four days after the baby is born, and I can go then.*

LYNN: *How will I know what kind of dress to get?*

MARY: *Well, it is your wedding, and you know what you want. You and mother know what I like. I really just want to be in the wedding.*

LYNN: *What will we say to the relatives if you don't get there? If the baby is late?*

MARY: *I can have the flu, or something.*

That sounds like a question and answer session, but it allowed Mary, by playing her sister, to ask a lot of questions about what she herself was thinking that she had been unable to ask before. We then discussed the questions and answers until she felt she could answer anything her sister might ask. She left the session feeling that she could talk to her sister and that she could also take part in the wedding.

The actual encounter with her sister was much easier than she had anticipated. Lynn agreed immediately and was very pleased that Mary had asked to be in her wedding; she had believed Mary was not interested. Thus, when some of her fears had been acted out in role playing, Mary was able to discuss the matter and discover that her sister wanted her in the wedding as much as she wanted to take part.

As the delivery date approached, Mary began to think about being discharged from the residential center and returning home and to work. We used role playing to clarify her feelings regarding what to say if she met someone who was a patient with her in the residence; what to say if Aunt Sally remarked that she was fat; how to tell her mother that she wanted to use contraceptives, and how to ask the doctor for contraceptives; how to obtain information about enrolling in a school of beauty culture rather than returning to the factory to work.

When the baby was about seven days overdue, Mary began to feel helpless and depressed. She cried, was despondent and unable to talk about her feelings. Her anger seemed to be directed toward the baby and herself. She berated the unborn child and would then feel guilty and still more depressed. I tried a different version of role playing.

MARY: (looking at her abdomen): *You stupid thing. Why don't you come out? I hate you. You are seven days late, and you just sit there.*

NURSE: *If the baby could talk to you, what would he say?*

MARY: (after some hesitation, surprised at the question, responding in an angry voice): *It's not my fault. I didn't put me here; you did. I don't know why you yell at me. I'd like to get out too.*

NURSE: *The baby seems angry too.*

MARY: *Why shouldn't he be? He's right! I put him there. It's all my fault. God is punishing me.*

That allowed the whole area of punishment to surface, and Mary could talk about fears previously expressed only in tears and berating of the baby. She could recognize that the anger she felt was actually toward herself rather than the child. She was able to verbalize rather than internalize her anger.

The foregoing are only a few examples of how effective role playing can be. It allowed me to utilize rather than overlook basic differences—in this instance socioeconomic differences. I could work at the educational level of the patient without embarrassing her. On the other hand, Mary got immediate satisfaction, quick results. Role playing added action to the interview sessions, and Mary felt she was getting something done, not "just talking." And it opened areas that might otherwise have remained closed to both the nurse and the patient.

As with any other interpersonal technique, role playing is not appropriate for every situation. It can, however, be a very simple and effective tool for improving communications, understanding, and treatment.

References

Corsini, R. J., and Cardone, Samuel. *Role Playing in Psychotherapy: A Manual.* Chicago, Ill. Aldine Publishing Co., 1966.

Edwards, G. Role-playing theory vs. clinical psychiatry. *Int. J. Psychiat.* 3:203–205, Mar. 1967

Gould, R. E. Dr. Strangeclass: or how I stopped worrying about the theory and began treating the blue-collar worker. *Amer. J. Orthopsychiat.* 37:78–86. Jan. 1967.

Hersch, C. Mental-health services and the poor. *Psychiatry*. 29:236–245, Aug. 1966.

Riessman, Frank. Role-playing and the lower socio-economic group. *Group Psychother*. 17(1):36–48, 1964.

——. and others. *Mental Health of the Poor*. New York. The Free Press of Glencoe, 1964.

Suchman, E. A. Social patterns of illness and medical care. *J. Health Hum. Behav*. 6:2–16. Spring 1965.

Chapter Seventeen

IN-HOSPITAL NURSING CARE OF THE BORDERLINE CLIENT

Carolyn Cathey Castelli and Jeanne R. Delaney

INTRODUCTION

THE TERM BORDERLINE IS often confusing to nurses, because of the myriad of definitions and explanations found in the psychiatric literature. In the 1940s and 1950s the diagnostic terms used to describe those clients with weak egos who did not fit neatly into the neurotic or psychotic categories were *borderline schizophrenia* or *borderline state*. In the 1960s, Dr. Otto Kernberg developed the psychostructural conception for what he called *borderline personality organization* (BPO):

> A *specific, stable, pathological personality organization which is neither typically neurotic nor typically psychotic. It is characterized by a typical constellation of symptoms (such as those exhibited by persons with infantile personality disorder and the schizoid, paranoid and hypomanic personalities), typical defense mechanisms (such as splitting, projective identification, and omnipotence and devaluation),*

by a typical pathology of internalized object relationships, and by genetic-dynamic features. Identity diffusion is evident and reality testing is generally intact, except under stress, when the person may experience transient psychotic episodes.[1]

In addition to this generally accepted definition, the *Diagnostic and Statistical Manual*, third edition (DSM III), provides us with a descriptive and clinical formulation of *borderline personality disorder* (BPD).[2] According to this definition, at least five of the following eight characteristics are required within the current and long-term functioning of the individual, causing either significant impairment in social or occupational functioning or subjective distress: (1) impulsivity or unpredictability; (2) a pattern of unstable and intense interpersonal relationships; (3) inappropriate, intense, uncontrollable anger; (4) identity disturbance manifested by uncertainty about several issues related to identity; (5) affective instability; (6) intolerance of being alone; (7) physically self-damaging acts; and (8) chronic feelings of emptiness or boredom.

When considering nursing care planning and intervention, it is important to understand both theoretical frameworks. In our experience, a combination of the psychostructural and descriptive definitions has been useful. Thus, along with considering the client's current and past behavior, an assessment of the client's degree of reality testing (especially when under stress) and of the defense mechanisms utilized is helpful.

This paper will address the psychodynamic issues underlying borderline personality as well as an organizational structure that facilitates nursing management of milieu activities and is especially effective in work with borderline clients.

PSYCHODYNAMICS

Development and object relations theories contribute heavily to the discussion of etiology of borderline personality organization. As opposed to a psychotic personality organization that results from a fixation in ego development during the normal symbiotic stage of an infant's emotional growth (2–8 months), people with borderline disorders seem to have a fixation in ego development in the next stage—the normal separation-individuation phase (6–36 months). People with neurotic personality organization have had difficulty with the last stage in ego development—the integration of self and object relations (36 months to early childhood).

Why does ego development for clients with borderline personality become fixated at the separation-individuation phase?

One theory is that these infants are born with unusually strong aggressive tendencies[3] that increase the child's frustrations and lead to frequent feelings of rage toward the mother, making normal conceptions of her impossible to internalize. Another viewpoint is that the mother (or primary person/object in the infant's life) encourages the symbiotic union and dependency to continue beyond its normal time, never allowing emotional separation and individual identity to develop.

During the normal separation-individuation phase of ego development, a child is beginning to crawl and walk, literally taking autonomous steps away from the mother. Emotionally, there is a parallel process as the child begins to see himself or herself as a separate individual from the mother. At this point, the memory is rudimentary, and the infant begins to organize it by associating good or pleasant feelings and experiences with a *good-self* and *good-object* and by associating bad or painful feelings and experiences with a *bad-self* and *bad-object*. This normal splitting behavior at this stage of ego development protects the infant from being overwhelmed by his own conflicting emotions. The infant has not had the opportunity to establish a memory trace of the good-self or good-object, and the bad-self or bad-object feelings are experienced separately from the good. Children will normally be able to separate and individuate, and they will integrate opposite affects, if they can take autonomous steps away from the mother while still experiencing her support in a type of emotional "refueling." Mahler[4] describes this in her rapprochement subphase of the separation-individuation process: the infant may both "shadow" the mother and "dart away," indicating the toddler's wish for both symbiotic reunion with the mother/object and a fear of reengulfment by her. If the mother does not provide warm support for the toddler at this phase in the efforts to separate or if the mother becomes overly clinging and demanding, the toddler may develop tremendous rage and aggression toward the mother. Thus, a healthy merging of both negative and positive images of self and object does not occur, and splitting is maintained in a destructive way, with a good-mother/object never having become internalized.

The groundwork has been laid for borderline personality organization, characterized by weak ego development, resulting in a poor sense of self and others. The defense mechanism of splitting is, therefore, an important dynamic to understand when developing a plan of care, since it may give the borderline client the stereotyped image of being manipulative. The client views certain staff as *all-good* and others as *all-bad* through the mechanism of projective identification, and this often results in staff tension and conflict. The client is projecting internal conflict over the split affects onto others.

THE THERAPIST-
ADMINISTRATOR SPLIT
AS AN ORGANIZATIONAL
STRUCTURE

Structure is essential in all psychiatric settings. It is especially important in the treatment of borderline clients to prevent the individual from continuing to use the defense mechanisms of splitting and projective identification as a way of dealing with anxiety and conflict. An organizational structure that is effective in managing the defenses used by the borderline client is the separation of the role of therapist from the role of administrator—the T/A split. The administrator is the person who manages the "other twenty-three hours" of the client's day outside the individual psychotherapy hour.

The authors' experience and preference is that the administrator be the skilled and qualified psychiatric nurse. The value of the T/A split for borderline clients is that it provides necessary external limits and opportunities for involvement and self-expression through work with the administrator, while simultaneously providing opportunity for self-exploration and development of adequate internal limits through work with the therapist. This allows the clients to project their split ego onto at least two persons in the environment. It prevents the confusion that might occur when the therapist is both decision maker and confidant. One role often hinders the effectiveness of the other. Although these functions are not neatly divided between the therapist and nurse-administrator, the client generally perceives the therapist as less of an authority figure than the nurse-administrator and perceives the nurse-administrator as less supportive than the therapist. The client may project the split-off good-self/object onto the therapist and the bad-self/object onto the nurse-administrator. It is almost inevitable that the client will try to split the two. The task of the therapist and administrator is to maintain an open line of communication, both to hold a neutral, consistent approach with the client and to refuse to be split off from each other by the client. The authors agree with Woodbury that this starts a "healing process which is eventually internalized within the client's ego with consequent healing of self and object representations."[5]

In establishing a relationship with the borderline client, the nurse-administrator who manages the milieu treatment for a group of clients on the unit will at times be the object of the client's anger. The nurse must be careful not to take the angry attacks personally. This behavior often evokes intense angry and hostile feelings toward the client from nursing staff, so it is important to understand this dynamic and the countertransference feelings involved. The psychiatric nurse-administrator needs to supervise nursing personnel closely to assist them in coping with the hostility, defensiveness, or exhaustion these clients evoke. The nurse who understands the underlying pathology of the client can remain therapeutic and (1) will not counter-attack, (2) will not take the attack personally, and (3) will have energy to sustain the therapeutic relationship.

In the role of nurse-administrator, the nurse encounters the continuous projections of the client. The nurse is the final decision maker and therefore symbolizes the staff member with the most power and control. For instance, though all decisions are discussed in interdisciplinary team meetings, the nurse will make the final decision about an issue and inform the client. If it involves limit setting, such as denial of a pass request, the nurse-administrator may be faced with angry rebuttals. This manifestation of angry behavior seems to constitute the main or the only affect that the borderline client experiences.[6] The nurse may be the target of the client's irritable, argumentative, sarcastic, demanding, or manipulative behavior.[7] The client may make frequent devaluing remarks, expecting to have wishes met, and behave without empathy toward others.[8]

Nurses must be aware that these clients suffer from a continuing conviction that they are unwanted, unloved, unredeemable, and guilty. Borderline clients feel distrustful and threatened in relationships. Being unable to tolerate angry feelings and neutralize their aggression, they act out. Projecting their aggressive impulses onto the environment, in this case onto the nurse-administrator, is a defense against the internal sense of negation and the threat the world imposes on them. Understanding the defense of splitting, whereby the ego is protected from conflict by separation of libidinal/good from aggressive/bad impulses, assists the nurse in maintaining therapeutic neutrality and empathy. The nurse further helps the clients integrate the good-self/object with the bad-self/object. The nurse does this by maintaining neutrality with the clients and a consistent, trusting relationship with the therapist.

NURSING PLANNING AND INTERVENTION IN THE THERAPEUTIC MILIEU

Because the well-developed ego regulates control of impulses, sense of reality, frustration tolerance, and healthy relationships with others, the person with a weak ego has extreme difficulty in all of these areas as they affect life function. Nursing care planning and intervention with the borderline client focuses on helping the individual strengthen ego by:

1. assisting with impulse control

2. presenting reality, especially when client is under stress

3. increasing frustration tolerance level

4. integrating the split or opposite views of self and others

Essential to the above is a unified nursing approach through the application of the nursing process.

Utilizing the therapist–administrator split as an overall organization structure, and applying theory on milieu processes, effective nursing care can be implemented with borderline clients. Five therapeutic activities or processes that occur in a therapeutic milieu, according to Gunderson, are: containment, support, structure, involvement, and validation.[9]

Containment assures the physical well-being of clients. Examples are providing food, shelter, restraining procedures, such as wet packs, seclusion, locked doors, medical care.[10] Containment is stressed with borderline clients in the form of locked doors or wet packs, etc., if the borderline client becomes extremely suicidal or violent. It thus becomes a vehicle to assist the nursing staff in helping the client with impulse control. Containment provides external limits, which over time may become internalized as impulse control, as issues are discussed with both the therapist and nursing staff.

Support refers to conscious efforts to make clients feel less distress and anxiety. Examples of support include escorting clients, giving attention, verbalizations such as direction, reality testing, and education.[11] Clients are assisted in increasing their frustration tolerance and in coping with anxiety by verbalizing feelings rather than acting them out. If the client is not in a state of acute crisis, supportive direction giving and education is useful. If the client is transiently psychotic owing to the stress of entering the hospital, drug or alcohol abuse, and so forth, the nursing staff will present reality, which assists in strengthening this weak aspect of the ego.

Structure is all the aspects of the milieu that provide a predictable organization of time, place, and person. Examples of structure would be hierarchical privilege systems, name tags, use of contracts, regulation of sleeping and eating, and mandatory meetings.[12] The unit structure should provide clear roles for staff, by which clients can then define themselves more clearly. The nursing staff must encourage borderline clients to attend to their schedule of meetings and activities that provides the external boundaries against which clients can test their own internal organizational abilities.[13] This assists the clients in strengthening their sense of identity and contributes to the integration of the split off or opposite views they have of themselves. Within the structure of the therapist-administrator split, the client can see the clearly defined roles, project opposite views onto these two people, and then reintegrate these views into his or her self-identity, as the staff remain neutral and reflect back the behavior. As nursing staff confront discrepancies in behavior, the effect can be an improvement in reality testing and social adjustment. The clients become more aware of their aggressiveness through interactions and involvement in relationships in the milieu. Structure and consistency in relationships with the borderline client enhance the client's capacity to develop more stable relationships and will support increased ego development.

Involvement refers to those processes that cause clients to attend actively to their social environment and to interact within it. Examples would be rounds open to clients, client-led groups, identification of shared goals, mandatory participation in milieu groups, and self-assertiveness experiences.[14] One function of the psychiatric nurse-administrator in planning care for borderline clients is to encourage involvement in one-to-one relationships and in groups, which utilizes clients' egos by expecting that they attend to and interact with their social environment in socially acceptable ways. This process of involvement strengthens the ego and modifies aversive interpersonal patterns. The psychosocial environment of the milieu is an important determinant of clients' functioning and coping ability as well as potentiating the development of healthier patterns of behavior and healthier interpersonal relationships. The nurse-administrator must clinically supervise the staff he or she is responsible for and educate them about impact the client may have on them.

As a group therapy leader, the psychiatric nurse-administrator would encourage the involvement of the clients in the milieu, by having them work on difficulties in interpersonal relationships, in controlling impulses, and in sharing feelings—particularly the feelings of anger they experience so powerfully. In group therapy, the psychiatric nurse would support the individuals' autonomy and function in the milieu, by involving the clients in intrapersonal and interpersonal awareness and by developing relationships on a group level. In group therapy, the clients can share their daily life experiences in the milieu, and a more realistic and integrated view of the world around them can be fostered. Support should be given in group therapy for the person's strengths, based on the beneficial repatterning of maladaptive behaviors. If the reality testing and limit setting are done consistently, the person will begin to feel involved and not abandoned. Thus, the one-to-one relationships and group therapy experience help to strengthen the client's ego by supporting healthy changes in the client.

The borderline client's ego structure is characterized by primitive defenses that keep apart contradictory experiences of the self and others, albeit at the expense of weakening certain aspects of ego function. When a borderline client is regressed, the pathological conflicts of the past are reactivated in the milieu. In the one-to-one relationships with staff, the client may distort the relationship and project aggression onto the staff member. Clinically, this reflects the client's lack of capacity to control aggression. It also intensifies the conceptualization that all relationships are precarious; thus, the repetitive, unhealthy patterns of acting out emerge. The borderline client has a distorted image of relationships and needs reality testing from the staff member to clarify the new and realistic relationships, in contrast to the traumatic one of childhood. These clients often assume one knows what they mean, and staff must persistently clarify communication.

Finally, *validation* refers to those unit activities that affirm a client's individuality. Examples are individualized treatment programming, respect for the right to be alone, frequent exploratory one-to-one talks, and provision of opportunities to fail.[15] This function of a milieu requires an "acceptance of incompetence, regressions, or symptoms as meaningful expressions which need not be terminated or ignored."[16] Thus, the client's ego can be strengthened through a more integrated concept of self.

When a borderline client gives up the option to act on impulses, he or she is still burdened with the internal distress that needs expression. The expression of pathological behaviors needs to be confronted, and the staff should respond to the client as an individual with unique needs and wants. Encouraging staff-patient one-to-one discussions and individualized treatment plans helps the client to cope with a conflict-laden internalized world and fosters the client's uniqueness. It also provides the opportunity for a staff member to give the client realistic feedback regarding this behavior and its effect on relationships. Validation promotes a real-world environment where the client must learn about himself or herself in relation to people, exclusive of distortions. This validation enhances the client's capacity for developing healthier and more stable, consistent relationships. However, this places the client in an even more vulnerable position and there may be a propensity to regress and act out. Nurses must realize that effective treatment with these clients involves risk taking in a relationship. For example, the issue of trust may affect how much responsibility a psychiatric nurse-administrator gives a client. Sometimes it takes months of treatment before the psychiatric nurse-administrator feels able to trust a borderline client significantly. This should not mean giving the client little responsibility and imposing more structure. The nurse-administrator must also be aware that the anxiety staff members feel regarding the potential of a borderline client to act out should not be the determinant in refusing to give the patient more responsibility. Over time, with a neutral, consistent approach as discussed in this article, the borderline client can usually engage in treatment; the client can listen, work with staff, and change behavior. "Validation can help clients develop a greater capacity of closeness and a more consolidated identity."[17]

SUMMARY AND CONCLUSIONS

The repatterning of acting-out behaviors and destructive relationships emerges as the client's ability to verbalize intense feelings of anger, rather than acting them out, is manifested. The increased reality testing in relationships enhances the borderline client's capacity to develop more stable relationships and supports increased ego development. The therapeutic one-to-one relationship and group therapy also increase integration of the all good and all bad self to help control aggressive impulses, and they afford the client the ability to become involved in the milieu and to sublimate acting-out potential. The psychiatric nurse-administrator facilitates the group process and the consistent one-to-one relationship between staff and client for repatterning behavior.

The authors have presented an overview of the current conceptualization of the borderline client. A brief description of the underlying psychodynamics was given, and an organizational structure referred to as the therapist-administrator (T/A) split was discussed. This structure is especially useful in facilitating the nursing management of milieu activities in work with borderline clients.

Notes

1. Kernberg, Otto. "Borderline Personality Organization," *Journal of the American Psychoanalytic Association*, 1967, 15(3). pp. 641–643.

2. *Diagnostic and Statistical Manual of Mental Disorders*, 3rd ed. Washington, D.C.: American Psychiatric Association, 1982, pp. 322, 323.

3. Kernberg, Otto F. "The Structural Diagnosis of Borderline Personality Disorder, In *Borderline Personality Disorders*, edited by Peter Hartocollis. New York: International Universities Press, 1977. pp. 87–121.

4. Mahler, Margaret. *On Human Symbiosis and the Vicissitudes of Individuation*, New York, International Universities Press, Inc. 1968, pp. 17, 28.

5. Woodbury, Michael. "Object Relations in the Psychiatric Hospital," *International Journal of Psychoanalysis*, 1967, 48(1). p. 86.

6. Gunderson, J., and Singer, M. T. "Defining Borderline Patients: An Overview," *American Journal of Psychiatry*, January 1975, 132(1). p. 3.

7. & 8. Perry, J. C., and Klerman, G. "The Borderline Patient: A Comparative Analysis of Four Sets of Diagnostic Criteria," *Archives of General Psychiatry*, February 1978, 35(2). p. 148.

9., 10., 11., 12. & 14. Gunderson, John. "Defining the Therapeutic Processes in Psychiatric Milieus," *Psychiatry*, November, 1978, 41(4). pp. 329–331.

13. Gunderson, John. "Functions of Milieu Therapy," unpublished paper. Amsterdam, Holland: 1978.

15., 16. & 17. Gunderson, John. "Defining the Therapeutic Processes in Psychiatric Milieus," *Psychiatry*, November, 1978, pp. 331–332.

References

Adler, Gerald. "The Myth of Alliance with Borderline Patients," *American Journal of Psychiatry*, May, 1979.
——— "Hospital Treatment of Borderline Patients," *American Journal of P;sychiatry*, January, 1973.
Brown, Lawrence. "The Therapeutic Milieu in the Treatment of Patients with Borderline Personality Disorder," *Bulletin of Menninger Clinic*, September, 1981.
Carser, Diane. "The Defense Mechanism of Splitting: Developmental Origins, Effects on Staff, Recommendations for Nursing Care," *Journal of Psychosocial Nursing and Mental Health Services*, March 1979.
Kerr, Norine. "The Destruction of Goodness in Borderline Character Pathology," *Perspectives in Psychiatric Care*, January, 1979.
Mark, Barbara. "Hospital Treatment of Borderline Patients: Toward a Better Understanding of Problematic Issues," *Journal of Psychosocial Nursing and Mental Health Services*, August 1980.
Shapiro, Edward. "The Psychodynamics and Development Psychology of the Borderline Patient," *American Journal of Psychiatry*, November, 1978.

Chapter Eighteen

WAS THIS SUICIDE PREVENTABLE?

Lee Ann Hoff and Marcia Resing

MR. SMITH KILLED HIMSELF only hours after being assessed by several mental health professionals. Judged to be nonsuicidal but in need of hospitalization, he was nevertheless sent home. The mental health facility serving him had no emergency holding service and made no effort to contact his family.

What went wrong? Was this an unnecessary death? What could have been done to prevent this suicide? What is the role of the nurse in preventing unnecessary death?

THE CIRCUMSTANCES

Mr. Smith had sought help two years earlier, when his wife divorced him and obtained custody of their three children. At that time, he was severely depressed and unable to work, but psychotherapy, milieu therapy, and medication enabled him to return to his job. He functioned well until he married for a second time and experienced an increase in job responsibilities. When he reported feelings of paranoia at work, sexual inadequacy, and depression, he was treated with phenothiazines. The phenothiazines, however, caused him to fall asleep at work; and because being awake and alert was vital to his job, the medication resulted in

From "Was This Suicide Preventable?" by Lee Ann Hoff and marcia Resing. Copyright © 1982, American Journal of Nursing Company. Reproduced with permission from *American Journal of Nursing*, July, Vol. 82, No. 7 , pp. 1106–1111.

increased stress. Taking vacation time, he sought psychiatric treatment at the day hospital. Sensing that hospitalization might be necessary, his therapist referred him to the psychiatric evaluation clinic at the main hospital.

[As a graduate student in this evaluation center, one of the authors—Marcia Resing—met Mr. Smith. She describes what happened.]

"Mr. Smith presented as a casually dressed, clean-shaven, attractive man, but he appeared somewhat older than his 36 years. He walked slowly to the interview room, eyes downcast, and shoulders bent. I began by asking his reasons for coming to the evaluation center. He responded slowly, in an expressionless voice. He wasn't sure why he had come and could not state what he needed. It was difficult to get him to relate the events that led to his present difficulties. Throughout the interview his affect remained listless, his eye contact poor. At one point, though, I remember catching his eye and joking with him—and he lifted his head and smiled. I thought to myself: This man has life underneath that mask of depression. I wanted to help liberate that vitality, but how?

"I did a mental status examination and assessed Mr. Smith for suicidal tendencies. I asked him if he felt badly enough about his life to hurt himself. He half-smiled and said no, that he was afraid to really do anything. He said he had tried suicide before by wrecking his car. On another occasion he tried to poison himself by plugging up the car's exhaust system with a hose, but he said that the attempt was unsuccessful because the hose melted.

"After the interview I consulted with another staff member; we decided that Mr. Smith was probably too depressed to act on suicidal impulses. Still, we felt unsure about how to help him.

"I spent the rest of the afternoon consulting with the day-hospital therapist, the administrator of the clinic, and the psychiatric resident, and we agreed that Mr. Smith might need hospitalization. But since the psychiatric resident alone had the authority to admit a client to the inpatient unit, Mr. Smith would have to wait for several more hours to see the resident.

"I felt very uncomfortable with this plan. Mr. Smith had come to us early that morning requesting assistance, and since that time no one had taken direct responsibility for helping him. It appeared that all this agency could offer him was hospitalization, a disposition I was not convinced was proper. I decided, however, that all I could do was document my impressions and hope that this would help the psychiatrist formulate a treatment plan. I wrote, 'no suicidal ideation present.' I left feeling so frustrated that I did not even say good-bye to Mr. Smith.

"Four days later I returned to the clinic and learned that late in the afternoon on the day of the interview, after being seen by the psychiatrist, Mr. Smith had gone home. The next morning he shot himself. The records indicated that the psychiatrist had recommended hospitalization, but because no beds were available, Mr. Smith had been placed on the waiting list. The psychiatrist indicated in the records that Mr. Smith was not suicidal at the time of the interview.

"After hearing this shocking news, I informed my supervisor, cancelled my afternoon appointments, and went home. I was confused, frustrated, angry, and depressed. I did not understand what had gone wrong; I concluded that Mr. Smith's death was totally unnecessary. I wondered whether things might have been different had I told my supervisor about this client on the day I saw him. Still, many professionals had seen Mr. Smith...."

THEORY, ANALYSIS, AND RECOMMENDATIONS

The case of Mr. Smith is tragic. Yet, when we reflect on a suicide, it is important to avoid two common responses—blaming and excusing—and to focus instead on examining what went wrong and what might have prevented the death.

A tenet of crisis theory and suicidology is that the evaluation of a person in emotional distress is incomplete if it does not include direct assessment for suicide risk—a lethality assessment.[1] Most mental health professionals seem to think that a lethality assessment is part of a general psychiatric examination of clients presenting with emotional or mental dysfunction. Evidence for this assumption is revealed during intake conferences by such statements as, "He does not appear to be suicidal," or "I do not believe that she is suicidal." Or the evidence of risk is presented in terms of depression, for example, "He is only mildly depressed," or "She is too seriously depressed to commit suicide." When questioned about the basis for these judgments the worker is often unable to produce facts.

One reason for this indirect approach to lethality assessment may be that some mental health workers deliberately refrain from asking about suicidal ideation out of the mistaken belief that bringing up the subject will put the idea into the client's head. Contrary to this popular myth, the fact is that the motivation to commit suicide is far too complex to be caused by the power of suggestion, particularly when questions are asked by someone intending to help—not harm—the client.

Some health workers believe that persons contemplating suicide won't reveal their plans anyway, so there is no point in asking a direct question. In fact, however, suicidal persons are more likely to conceal their intentions when they sense that the helper is avoiding the subject. By the same token, a worker who is confident and direct will usually convey to suicidal persons that they are talking with someone who can help them control frightening self-destructive tendencies. If the worker doesn't shy away from the issue, the sharing of suicidal plans is a more likely result.

Such data as the client's appearance, the worker's impressions, and the perceived degree of depression are unreliable as indicators of suicidal risk when considered apart from other signs. And direct communication is not only critical to the assessment process; it is a basic step in helping a suicidal person.

Suicide researchers propose that in considering signs that help predict suicide we must identify those signs that characterize people who actually kill themselves, and differentiate them from signs that are also present in the larger group of suicide attempters, as well as in the population at large.[2,3,4] Even though health and mental health professionals have historically used depression as a major criterion for predicting suicide risk, studies of completed suicides show that depression *alone* is not an accurate predictor. A considerable number of people suffer from varying degrees of depression and may or may not be suicidal.

In assessing suicide risk, then, which signs are the most reliable? Some authorities suggest that workers should identify not only particular signs, but also the *patterning* of signs.[4,5] In this context, assessing risk for suicide is aided by an understanding of two concepts central to the process of self-destruction—ambivalence and communication.

Ambivalence.   People who kill themselves have invariably gone through a process of weighing the relative advantages of life and death, even though the process may not seem to outsiders to have been thorough or objective. In fact, a suicidal person's ambivalent state of mind (simultaneously desiring life and death) forms the very foundation for the possibility of intervention. Contrary to the popular belief that once a person has decided to commit suicide, there's nothing we can do to stop him or her, so long as a person has not in fact committed suicide, one can safely assume that he or she is still open to considering other responses to life's stresses and problems. Thus, the outcome of suicide is not inevitable.

Communication.   People who engage in self-destructive behavior are sending cries for help to those around them. Some examples are: "I'm angry at my mother....She'll really be sorry when I'm dead." "I can't take any more problems without some relief."

Unlike most people, who usually try to get what they need or want by simply asking for it, self-destructive people typically have a history of failed communication. They are either unable to express their needs directly, or their needs are insatiable and therefore impossible to fulfill. Failing to communicate their needs by ordinary means, self-destructive persons learn that self-injury is a powerful method of telling those around them that they are hurting and probably desperate. For some, the message is, "I really want to die....life is no longer worth living." Others are less certain: "I don't really want to die....I just want someone to understand how miserable I am and that if things don't change I will, in fact, kill myself."

Thus, the helping person faces a double challenge: to discover the degree of ambivalence in the self-destructive person and to determine the essential message the person is trying to communicate.

There are numerous signs that can be used to predict whether or not a person is a high suicide risk:

Suicide Plan.   Studies reveal that the majority of persons who die by suicide have deliberately planned to do so by an available "high-lethal" method—a gun, sleeping pills, carbon monoxide poisoning. The risk of death is further increased if the attempter has full knowledge that the method is lethal and if no possibility of rescue is included in the plan.

History of Suicide Attempts.   Among those who kill themselves, significant numbers have a history of other suicide attempts. Those who have made previous attempts with high-lethal methods or who have changed the method of self-injury from low- to high-lethal are at greater risk than those with a history of low-lethal attempts.

Resources and Communication with Significant Others.   Internal resources include emotional strength, problem-solving ability, and other personality factors that help in coping with difficulties and stress. External social resources consist of a network of persons on whom one can rely during times of stress and crisis.

Therefore, if a person has a *history of high-lethal suicide attempts, a specific plan for suicide, an available high-lethal method, and lacks both personal and social resources*, his or her immediate and long-range risk for probable suicide is very high.

There are other demographic and personal factors that increase risk: For example, the general ratio of male to female suicides in America is approximately 3 to 1. The rate among young urban black males between ages 25 and 40 is twice that for white males the same age.[6]

Suicide risk is higher among those who have suffered a recent *loss*, whether through marital separation, death, or divorce. Other significant losses include job termination, a decline in social status, or financial disaster.

The presence of *physical illness, drug, or alcohol problems* also increases suicide risk. People who are suicidal are often physically isolated; such *isolation* exacerbates feelings of being cut off, socially and psychologically, from significant others. In cases of extreme isolation, hospitalization can be a life-saving measure if other high-risk signs are also present. Suicide risk can, however, be increased by hospitalization—well intended though it may be—if hospitalization results in the patient's feeling even more cut off from significant others.

How can we apply these indicators of suicidal danger to specific people like Mr. Smith, who are giving covert and overt signals of distress? First, it should be remembered that *all* self-destructive behavior is serious, indicating either a cry for help or a message of intent to die. Secondly, since self-destructive behavior is serious, the challenge lies in distinguishing self-destructive behavior that is an indication of intent to die from that which is a cry for help. A person who takes ten tranquilizers knowing death is not likely, but who hopes thereby to bring about some change to make life more bearable, is a low risk for suicide in the immediate sense, but may be a high risk in the future, depending on what happens as a result of the current attempt.

In Mr. Smith's case, hindsight tells us that he was in fact a high risk for suicide. We have seen how Mr. Smith was assessed in the psychiatric evaluation clinic. His denial was accompanied by a half-smile, the meaning of which was not pursued. Was Mr. Smith's half-smile related to the suicidal plan he was considering but which no one asked him about? And was he perhaps testing the interviewer to determine whether she could handle his scary ideas without panic or censure? We do not know. But we do know that these possibilities were not explored by direct, detailed questioning, and that Mr. Smith was judged to be nonsuicidal without data regarding his current plans.

Clearly, if the assessment team had judged Mr. Smith to be an immediate high risk for suicide, their response would have been different. However, many health and mental health workers apparently do not have up-to-date knowledge or training in the theory and techniques of lethality assessment. The standard assessment procedure in psychiatric practice— the mental status examination—reveals data about a client's cognition and judgment. This assessment technique, however, is *not* sufficient to determine suicidal danger.[7]

The American Association of Suicidology (AAS)—the national standard-setting body for suicide prevention and crisis services— recommends that health and mental health workers receive a minimum of 40 hours of training in crisis intervention and suicide prevention.[8] The nurse who interviewed Mr. Smith was in her second quarter of a master's program in psychiatric nursing and, at the time of the suicide, had not yet received the mere six hours of crisis content planned for her program. Because nurses, like police, pastors, and teachers, are front-line personnel in suicide prevention and crisis work, they frequently are the first contact for desperate people who use self-injury or suicide as solutions to critical life events.

One of the lessons to be learned from this tragic case is the great importance of assessment based on more than guesswork or vague generalizations. While there was an attempt to assess Mr. Smith for danger of suicide, what was lacking was the knowledge that a history of high-lethal suicide attempts is very significant. Because Mr. Smith had tried to kill himself by a car crash and with carbon monoxide poisoning a year earlier, he should have been asked in detail about his current plans for suicide.

Not only is such direct questioning a most valuable tool for assessment, but it can also be an essential link between life and death. It establishes direct communication between the suicidal person and a caring human being, and this can help to counteract the sense of isolation and despair the client is feeling.

Effective communication with potentially suicidal people does not require extensive training in psychotherapy or counseling, but can be carried out in the ordinary course of gathering information and expressing concern for a person who appears upset or depressed.[9] (See the sample interview and discussion of how Mr. Smith's case might have been handled.)

While recognizing that crisis intervention is not a panacea, we hope that this analysis and sharing of our experience will be helpful in preventing unnecessary deaths as well as in preventing unnecessary pain for health and mental health workers. A suicide is always a painful message, but we believe that the guilt, scapegoating, and/or frustration so common to survivors can be minimized for workers with up-to-date knowledge and experience in assessing and helping people at risk for suicide.

HOW IT MIGHT HAVE BEEN

The following interview excerpt illustrates some recommended techniques for assessing lethality and establishing the basis of a service plan for a suicidal person. It is not a complete assessment interview, rather it focuses on critical lethality assessment techniques.

Principles and Techniques	Interview
— problem identification	*Nurse:* Hello Mr. Smith, I'm Lois Haney. Can you tell me what's troubling you? *Mr. Smith:* Well, it seems like everything is going wrong.
— reflection	*Nurse:* Everything's going wrong? *Mr. Smith:* It sure is.
— focusing	*Nurse:* What seems to be troubling you most?
— identifying hazardous event	*Mr. Smith:* It's hard to say, because everything seems all mixed together in a big mess.

— empathy — focusing	*Nurse:* You really sound frustrated...Why don't you start with what's been happening in just the last couple of days. *Mr. Smith:* Well, I've been off work on account of falling asleep on the job.... I've been trying to get things worked out with my wife (we just got married a few weeks ago), and my medication is bugging me....I'm not sure I should be taking it anymore. Nothing seem to be working out right.
— empathy	*Nurse:* That's a lot of things to put up with. How long has this been going on?
— determining extent and boundary of problem	*Mr. Smith:* Oh, maybe the last 4 or 5 weeks or so. That's why I took some time off work.
— summarizing — identifying precipitating factor	*Nurse:* I see....so there's a problem with your wife, and you've got questions about your medicine, and you're having trouble staying awake at work. I think we need to talk about these things some more, but before we do, can you tell me what made you come in today, since these things have been going on for awhile? *Mr. Smith:* We'll, I'm supposed to go back to work tomorrow and I just can't face it.
— empathy	*Nurse:* You sound like you don't know which way to turn...really frustrated. *Mr. Smith:* Yes, I am. I just don't know how I can stand it anymore.
— clarification	*Nurse:* You mean you sort of feel like giving up? *Mr. Smith:* I sure do.
— reflection — empathy — assessing for suicidal ideation and possible plan	*Nurse:* Sounds to me like you're pretty desperate. Are you so discouraged that you've maybe thought about killing yourself? *Mr. Smith:* Well, yes, I've thought about it

	but I don't think I could go through with it.
— exploring ambivalence — direct questioning — determining suicidal method	*Nurse:* So you're thinking about suicide but aren't sure...What have you thought about doing? *Mr. Smith:* I guess something better than last time.
— clarification	*Nurse:* Last time? *Mr. Smith:* That's right...when I tried to do it before.
— determining history of suicide attempts	*Nurse:* You mean you've tried to kill yourself before? *Mr. Smith:* Yes.
— determining specifics of previous attempts (time, method, outcome)	*Nurse:* When was that? *Mr. Smith:* Oh...not long ago, just about a year....I think it was April. *Nurse:* What did you do to yourself then? *Mr. Smith:* I tried to wreck my car by driving off the road. *Nurse:* What happened? *Mr. Smith:* I went off the road, but I didn't really get hurt. *Nurse:* When was that? *Mr. Smith:* A year ago, after my wife left me.
— determining history of communication patterns	*Nurse:* When that happened did you talk with anyone about your suicide attempt? *Mr. Smith:* No, I felt too foolish to talk to anyone about it.
— determining further history of suicide attempts	*Nurse:* have you made other attempts to end your life besides that one? *Mr. Smith:* I tried to block the exhaust of my car once with a hose, but it melted. I did that about the same time last year ....That was the only other time.
— identifying ambivalence	*Nurse:* So you've tried twice before to kill yourself, and now you feel as badly as

	you did then...but you're not sure you could go through with it. *Mr. Smith:* (nods yes)
— determining method of current plan	*Nurse:* You mentioned that if you decide you want to end your life now you would choose a different method than before. *Mr. Smith:* I have guns at home.
— determining specificity of current plan — assessing for danger to others	*Nurse:* Are you thinking about shooting yourself or anyone else? *Mr. Smith:* Only myself.
— empathy	*Nurse:* It sounds like you're feeling very desperate. *Mr. Smith:* I guess I am.
— identifying social resources — establishing links to social network	*Nurse:* Is there someone at home now who can be with you? *Mr. Smith:* My wife. *Nurse:* I'm concerned about your returning home when you're feeling this way. I think you need to have some help right now. I would like to call your wife and have her come in so we can talk together. *Mr. Smith:* I guess it's OK.

At this point, the interview and assessment process might proceed in several directions. Mrs. Smith needs to be assessed as a potential social resource for Mr. Smith's protection from self-destruction. If it is found that, for the time being at least, she is part of the problem rather than a resource for crisis resolution, other resources such as hospitalization should be explored.

Let's assume, however, that the following additional data have been obtained from Mr. and Mrs. Smith: Mrs. Smith is upset about the possibility of Mr. Smith's not returning to work the next day. She is also concerned about his problem of impotence and has only vague knowledge of his previous suicide attempts. She agrees to remove the guns from the house and then come in to see the counselor with her husband. (Removal of lethal weapons is a crucial suicide prevention technique that should be carried out as soon as possible.) Both Mr. and Mrs. Smith are afraid that even though the guns are removed, if they have an argument he might try some other means of attempting suicide.

From the above interview data, then, what is Mr. Smith's risk for suicide, and how can possible suicide best be prevented? First, the data suggest that Mr. Smith is a high risk for suicide because he has a *specific plan, an available high-lethal method, a history of previous high-lethal suicide attempts, and is unable to communicate his desperate suicidal feelings to his significant others.*

Planning, then, should be based on this assessment of suicide risk, with Mr. and Mrs. Smith actively involved in the planning process. Also, in crisis situations it is acceptable for the helper to assume a more active role in the helping process than would be appropriate in, say, psychotherapy. For example, the worker can suggest to Mr. and Mrs. Smith that the guns should be removed from the home. Once a self-destructive person like Mr. Smith trusts that the worker is willing and able to help protect him from his self-destructive impulses, he will feel more secure and will welcome such a safety measure as removal of the guns. Thus, he would probably agree to the worker's suggestion that his wife remove the guns before coming to the clinic.

A service plan for Mr. Smith might have included the following:

Crisis Intervention. 1. Have wife remove guns from home. 2. Arrange interview with Mrs. Smith individually and with her husband. 3. Arrange for Mr. Smith to stay in the hospital 24-hour emergency holding unit. This will provide immediate protection against suicide while further evaluation of Mr. Smith's home and marital situation, his medication regimen, and possible need for hospitalization are done. We recognize that such 24-hour emergency holding units are not a routine part of many emergency psychiatric programs. However, this does not detract from their need and usefulness, particularly if mental health and crisis workers subscribe to the philosophy that the majority of crises can be successfully managed in the community and that psychiatric hospitalization can as easily be the source of still another crisis as it can be the solution to the crisis initially presented.[1, 10-14] 4. Make appointment for Mr. and Mrs. Smith to be seen in crisis counseling sessions daily or every other day until the acute suicidal urges have subsided and other immediate problems have been resolved.

Follow-up Service. 1. Mrs. Smith should have ongoing individual and/or group therapy for his depression. 2. His medication regimen should be reevaluated on a regular basis. 3. Family/marital therapy may be indicated as the recent marriage was an identified stressor in Mr. Smith's current crisis.

Since Mr. Smith, in fact, killed himself, crisis intervention and follow-up efforts should have been focused on his wife and other survivors of the suicide.

While there are no absolutes in the challenging business of

lethality assessment, suicide prevention, and crisis work, in certain cases suicide is definitely preventable. We think that Mr. Smith's was one such case.

References

1. Hoff, L. A. *People in Crisis*. Menlo Park, Calif., Addison-Wesley Publishing Co., 1978, Chap. 5.

2. Breed, Warren. Five components of a basic syndrome. *Life-Threatening Behav.* 2:3–18, Spring 1972.

3. Beck, A. T., and others, eds. *The Prediction of Suicide*. Bowie, Md., Charles Press, 1974, p. 194.

4. Brown, T. R., and Sheran, T. J. Suicide prediction: a review. *Life-Threatening Behav.* 2:67–98, Summer 1972.

5. Farberow, Norman, ed. *Suicide in Different Cultures*. Baltimore, University Park Press, 1975.

6. Hoff, *op. cit.*, pp. 122–130.

7. *Ibid.*, pp. 293–327.

8. Hoff, L. A., and others, eds. *Certification Standard Manual for Suicide Prevention and Crisis Intervention Programs*. 2nd ed. Denver, American Association of Suicidology, 1981.

9. McGee, R. K. *Crisis Intervention in the Community*. Baltimore, University Park Press, 1974.

10. Langsley, D. G., and Kaplan, D. M. *Treatment of Families in Crisis*. New York, Grune & Stratton, 1968.

11. Polak, P. R., and Kirby, M. W. The crisis of admission. *Soc. Psychiatry* 2 (4): 150–157, 1967.

12. _____ . Social systems intervention. *Arch. Gen. Psychiatry* 25:110–117, Aug. 1971.

13. _____ . A model to replace psychiatric hospitals. *J. Nerv. Ment. Dis.* 162:13–22, Jan. 1976.

14. Harsell, Norris. *The Person in Distress*. New York, Human Services Press, 1976.

Chapter Nineteen

LIMIT SETTING AS A THERAPEUTIC TOOL

Glee Gamble Lyon

THE SETTING IS A day room of a state mental hospital. A cute, young, dark-haired student nurse is sitting talking with a tall, slender, nineteen-year-old boy with hippie style hair and long sideburns.

P: *I'm uncomfortable. I think I'll take my clothes off.*

SN: *How will that make you comfortable, John?*

P: *I'll feel free. I can talk better when I feel free.*

SN: *I don't understand. How does taking your clothes off make you feel free to talk?*

P: *I don't know—I guess it's my hang-up.*

SN: *John, what do you think will happen if you take off your clothes?*

P: *They always put me in the short hall.*

SN: *Do you think you'll feel free to talk in there?*

(The patient does not answer, but walks off. The student nurse remains seated in the day room. Shortly the patient returns with no clothes on.)

P: *There, now I can talk. Am I embarrassing you?*

SN: *Yes, you are. I'm afraid I don't understand how this helps you to talk.*

From "Limit Setting as a Therapeutic Tool," by Glee Gamble Lyon, *Journal of Psychiatric Nursing and Mental Health Services*, November/December, 1970, pp. 17–24. Reprinted by permission of SLACK, Inc., Medical Publishers, Thorofare, NJ.

(At this point an attendant intervenes and puts John in his own room in the short hall. The student nurse returns a little later—the patient is in his room with his clothes still off.)

SN: *John I'm leaving now, and I won't be back until Monday, but I'd like to talk with you again.*

P: OK.

SN: *But I cannot talk to you unless you keep your clothes on, OK?*

P: OK, *that's fine.*

This student, like many new people entering the field of mental health, was attempting to show her acceptance of the patient, as well as her very nonjudgmental attitude. The first two principles stressed were: *accept the patient as he is,* and *focus on the patient's feelings.* New personnel in a psychiatric setting often find what appears to be a very permissive atmosphere. However, this acceptance and permissiveness needs to be limited. *That the patient feels the way he does is accepted, that he has a right to feel that way is accepted, but limits are established beyond which acting out his feelings is not allowed.*

Often a patient "asks" for limits, or tests out his unclear understanding of what is expected and accepted behavior. In the above example John really wanted external help in controllling his behavior. The next week he was with the same student nurse:

P: *I think I'll take my clothes off.*
SN: *No, John, you'll have to leave your clothes on, or I can't stay and talk with you.*

P: *Oh, OK.*
(His anxiety decreases and he spends a half hour talking with the student nurse.)

WHY THERE IS A NEED FOR LIMITS

The need for limits is closely related to the feelings of security and trust. Everyone has the basic need to feel secure, to have a sense of assurance and predictability about himself and his environment. When this feeling does not exist, much of his behavior is motivated by the need for security.

The feelings of security are learned. In the process of growing up, children try to find security by attempting to control and direct parental authority, and in so doing go through many periods of anxiety.[1] If the parents are themselves secure, able to respond to the child's behavior with consistency and predictability, and able to encourage the child to be independent in his behavior according to his capabilities and judgment, the child accepts the restrictions, and through this guidance learns to control his own behavior. Each time the child gains mastery over one more area of his life he receives not only parental approval, but (more importantly) the increased feelings of security and of self-worth in knowing that he can handle himself and his behavior in a growing number of situations.[2]

However, if the parents are constantly anxious and unpredictable, the child is faced with the impossible situation of trying to find security in a desperate struggle where the rules are constantly changing. The child reacts by giving up the struggle and spends the rest of his life acting out roles that he thinks will gain approval, while constantly carrying a burden of anxious, angry, and frustrated feelings.[3]

The person who comes to the mental hospital is usually experiencing insecurity. He is often overwhelmed by the amount of anxiety with which he has to deal, overpowered to the point that he cannot function adequately in his daily living. In order to relieve the anxiety the patient does something; he often feels compelled to do something without understanding why he is doing it—it is his way of trying to deal with the lack of security, his attempt to gain mastery over himself and his environment. It is intended to relieve his anxiety, but often this acting out behavior brings further loss of control, loss of self esteem and more anxiety.

The hospital setting and the nurse-patient relationship must both offer the patient a structure that is secure, consistent, and that communicates what is expected behavior. Within this structure, the patient may experience what he may not have had earlier, an atmosphere that will allow freedom to try out and learn new ways of behaving. Limit setting is one aspect of the nurse-patient relationship which helps the patient to reduce his anxiety, enabling him to reestablish himself and to function on a more acceptable level. This new level of functioning will bring new responses (approval instead of disapproval) from those around him. He can then use these different responses to change his concept of himself, to learn new behaviors, to manage his own life, and to experience success in areas in which he was not successful before.

TYPES OF BEHAVIOR
NEEDING LIMITS

Limits are established for the broad categories of acting out behavior and manipulative behavior. *Acting out* is behavior in which the patient is responding to a present situation as if it were a past situation, seeking gratification of unconscious impulses or desires.[4] Acting out might include behavior which is potentially harmful to the patient or to others, and behavior which in a particular situation is socially unacceptable, such as nudity or sexual misconduct. *Manipulative behavior* is a process by which one person influences another to function according to his needs without regard for the other person's needs.[5] This behavior might include gift giving, flattery, or asking for special favors.

DEFINITION AND PURPOSE OF LIMIT SETTING

Limit setting is a process through which someone in authority determines temporary and artificial ego boundaries for another person. Determining for the patient the boundaries of acceptable behavior provides protection for the patient and others, provides security, decreases the patient's anxiety, and provides a reality contact between the person and his environment. The limit forms a framework within which the person is freer to function more adequately, to learn new behaviors, and is thus able to develop his self identity and to raise his self esteem.

STEPS AND TECHNIQUES IN SETTING LIMITS

Identify the Need for the Limit.   In any situation the need for limits must be considered within the context of the particular situation and patient. The nurse's use of rational authority in setting limits is based on her knowledge and understanding of the dynamics of the patient's behavior. The more capable the nurse is in understanding and interpreting the meaning of the patient's behavior, the more likely she will be able to establish both realistic and meaningful limits for the patient. For example, a nurse who interpreted a patient's slow, systematic way of getting dressed as a way of manipulating her, and preventing her from moving on to her other duties, tried to set limits on the patient's "unnecessary" and time-consuming actions, which resulted in an increase in the patient's anxiety. Another nurse, aware that this was the patient's compulsive ritual and his way to give structure and security to his environment, not only found no need to

184

try to stop the behavior but was able to remain with the patient very patiently and to facilitate a relaxed atmosphere in which the patient could carry out his ritual and, therefore, reduce his anxiety.

In every situation the nurse needs to ask herself, "Why do limits need to be set? What is the patient trying to say with his behavior at this time? And what about this person's personality structure and resulting behavior makes it necessary to take over his ego function temporarily? And furthermore, does this limit lead to growth for the person?"[6]

In answering the above questions about the patient in relation to limit setting, the nurse must also ask and seek answers about herself. She needs to look at her own feelings about limits, about the particular patient and his behavior. She needs to ask herself, "Is the limit for my own comfort or is it because it meets some need of the patient? Is what's being done really limit setting or is it punishment?"[7]

Just as too hasty a judgment and setting of limits might be a serious misuse of rational authority, the nurse's failure to identify the need and to set limits can also deprive the patient of needed guidance and learning experiences. Sometimes in the process of building a relationship, the nurse is afraid that she will spoil a good relationship if she sets limits. She does not set limits for fear the patient will interpret the limit as her rejection of him, or she is afraid that the patient in return might reject her. Or the nurse may rationalize that the patient has suffered enough and she does not want to add any further hardship or hurt by setting limits on the patient's behavior. The nurse's own feelings and attitudes toward authority and limits need to be explored so that they do not interfere with her ability to evaluate the situation, recognize the need, and be able to establish effective limits.

Communicate Expected Behavior.   In many situations before a limit is definitely stated, the nurse communicates expected behavior in the particular situation to the patient, which gives the patient a structure within which he can operate. This might be done through a nonverbal motion such as indicating "no" with a shake of the head, or the nurse's motioning for the patient to leave a room. In effect, in communicating expected behavior the nurse forewarns the patient that a limit will be set if the expected behavior is not followed. For example, "It is time for you to take your medicine," or "Make your bed," or "This is a time for you to talk about yourself," communicate to the patient what is expected of him at a given time.

State the Limit.   After the need for the limits has been identified and, if indicating the expected behavior did not precipitate the necessary behavior, the nurse needs to inform the patient exactly what the limit is. The limit is stated clearly as a statement of fact and is not presented as advice, bribery, or punishment. It tells the patient specifically what he is to do, or specifically what he must not do in the situation.

When stating what is unacceptable behavior and putting a limit on it, the nurse needs to also offer a substitute—a behavior that is acceptable. For example, a patient who was continuously asking a student about her personal life was told: "We are not to talk about me and my life outside the hospital. We can talk about what you did today....tell me what you did in the OT metal shop." Or, after stating the limit, the nurse can offer the patient a choice of alternative behaviors: "You cannot hit Mr. W. You can tell me how you feel about Mr. W., or you can go run in the gym."

The best limit is total, not partial, so that the boundaries are very clear. A patient was banging a board loudly on the table. The staff member said, "You are not to make so much noise; you can bang a little, but don't make too much noise." The patient was left without any clear criterion with which to judge the boundaries so he continued to bang, becoming increasingly louder until he found out what was meant by "too much noise."

The limit should be stated firmly with the nurse's conviction and belief in the value of the limit reflected in her voice, which increases the patient's security in knowing the limit is meant and will be carried out. If she is not sure about the limit, or what to do in the situation, the nurse should not do anything until she has further thought through the situation and her own feelings. If the nurse is ambivalent toward the limit, her uncertainty might challenge the patient to argue against the limit, or to test it.

There is some disagreement about whether to warn the patient of the consequences, or of what he can expect if the limit is tested or if he continues the inappropriate behavior. Often the statements of consequences act as threats—or invitations—to repeat the behavior, as "If you do it once more... ," the patient tends not to hear the "if you" and hears only "do it once more" and sometimes interprets it as "she expects me to do it once more." The warning of the consequences can serve as a challenge and "to do it once more" to retain his self esteem and show himself not as a weakling, or someone who is afraid.[8]

In other situations, the explanation of consequences is of therapeutic value, for it presents the patient with responsibility for the effects or results of his behavior. Within the limit-setting situation the patient is encouraged to look at his own behavior and the resulting consequences, and to then make a choice or decision about his behavior. For example, a patient was told, "You are expected to go to school each day; if you don't you will be restricted from the next hospital extracurricular activity." In understanding the expected behavior and the resulting effect, the patient was given the opportunity to govern his own behavior, to learn how to postpone immediate pleasure for future gratification, and thus to act more responsibly.

Help the Patient Understand the Reason for the Limit.   To increase the therapeutic and learning value of the situation the person needs to understand the limit. The nurse tells the patient as clearly, simply, and concretely as possible the reason for the limit. The amount of explanation varies according to the situation and to the patient's need and ability to understand. For example, a patient who refused her medicine and was to receive an injection was told: "The Doctor ordered this medicine, he thinks it will help you feel better." Even if the person is unable to accept the limit at first, he will be less likely to misinterpret the nurse's motives if a brief explanation is given.

Enforce the Limit.   To be effective, the limit must be one that can be realistically enforced or put into effect if the patient tests it. If there is no way to enforce the limit, then there is no point in setting the limit in the first place. A patient was told that she was to clean her room. After several attempts to make the patient clean her room, including locking her in her room with the needed supplies, the patient was told if she did not clean her room she would not eat. By this time the patient had accepted the challenge and remained more stubborn than the staff until the staff, unable to enforce the limit beyond several missed meals, allowed the patient to eat without the room being cleaned. The limit and the consequences of not following it were not enforceable; thus the limit was useless.

To be effective the limit must be realistic and reasonable; in addition, the consequences should be related to the limit. In the last example, an effective limit would be: "You are to clean your room. Until it is clean, you are restricted to your room." This limit is not only enforceable, but it presents the patient with a choice, to clean her room and be able to join in the other ward activities, or to not clean her room and suffer the consequences of wallowing in the messiness of her room, deprived of any activities going on outside of her room.

Limit setting has a cause and effect relationship; if the limit is not followed then another action will be initiated by the staff member. For example: a patient was told to get off the top of a table; when he did not, the limit was enforced by the necessary staff members physically removing him from the top of the table. When it is necessary to enforce the limit, it is done quickly and with a sense of conviction and sureness on the part of staff. If the patient has exceeded the limit or not followed the restriction, this is not the time to be drawn into long discussions of the fairness of the limit—or even to give further explanation. When a patient exceeds a limit, it causes him anxiety; if the nurse talks too much or is hesitant to act to enforce the limit, it conveys to the patient some uncertainty and weakness at a time when he needs most to know that his environment will provide security and that he can lean on the others for support and strength.

Help the Patient Verbalize His Feelings about the Limit.   To prevent the patient from accepting limits docilely and without questioning, as though he had nothing to say and no control over what is happening to him, the nurse or staff member needs to help the person express his feelings about the limit. When the staff member encourages the patient to say what he feels, acceptance is conveyed to the person. This also helps to involve the person more in the total limit-setting process, helping the patient to better evaluate reality and to judge rational controls. If the patient is unable to express how he feels about the restriction, the staff member can verbalize to the patient what she believes he is feeling, such as "I wonder if you were angry with me this morning when I told you not to leave the ward."

Often it is not appropriate to help the patient verbalize feelings right at the time that the limit is being set. However, after the limit has been enforced and the patient is less anxious, the patient should be given the opportunity to better understand the limit and to verbalize feelings. This might be within an hour or maybe not even until the next day; however, the important thing is that the nurse does approach the patient to discuss the total limit-setting situation, giving him the opportunity to integrate it into his total life experiences.

Evaluate the Limit.   Effective limits should make the patient more secure, for he knows what others expect of him, what behaviors he can and cannot do, and what others will do in relation to him. The setting of a limit often communicates that the nurse does care and is interested, that she will stop a behavior which would later make the patient feel ashamed or embarrassed. For example, when a patient entered the day room hall exposed, the nurse told her to button her blouse. The patient would not, and the nurse did it for the patient although the latter vehemently protested. The next day the patient apologized for her behavior and thanked the nurse. As in this situation, although a limit is needed, it does not mean the patient will readily accept the restriction.

The patient's initial behavioral response cannot always be used to evaluate the effectiveness of a limit. The patient may need to question rational authorities' interest and conviction in himself and in the limit by testing to see if the staff person really means what he says and can be relied upon to follow through and actually supply the boundaries indicated by the limit. The patient needs to know that he can count on the boundaries, and his continued—or even increased—acting-out behavior is calculated to test the boundary for its strength and reliability before accepting rational controls. If the patient interprets a limit as someone in authority trying to control him, and to leave him powerless, his behavior will also probably be in the direction opposite that of the limit. He might resort to even greater acting out or regressive behavior in an attempt to decrease the overwhelming feeling of powerlessness and anxiety. Knowing a patient's previous experience with authority figures and limits often helps in understanding the patient's behavior. However, in many situations it is difficult to evaluate whether the limit itself is not appropriate or whether the behavior is just the initial reaction to the new experience of rational control. If the limit is reevaluated and then continued with consistency, the patient's behavior over a longer period of time should serve as a measurement of the effectiveness of the limit.

The evaluation of the limit needs to be continuous; limits are not established for an indefinite period of time. As the limit is gradually internalized and used by the patient in the management of his own behavior, staff must relinquish their own external controls and return the responsibility for control to the patient.

These then are the basic steps involved in setting limits. Because each patient in each situation is different, limit setting needs to be flexible within this basic framework. Each limit-setting situation will vary in terms of how many of these actual steps are necessary and the order and emphasis placed on each step. In addition to using the principles and techniques already indicated in each step, one aspect that must prevail over the total limit-setting situation is consistency.

Consistency.   Consistency is necessary in order for the limit-setting process to be effective. This consistency must be present in the individual authority figure. When a staff member states the limit, she must then be consistent in her attitude and actions, communicating the same thing nonverbally that her words are communicating. She must be consistent over a period of time. If she has put a limit on a particular behavior, she must enforce it each time; not overlook it because she is tired or because it is easier than causing a "scene" when there are visitors on the ward.

There must also be consistency among all the staff members who have contact with the person. It is necessary for the staff to both understand and accept the particular limit. If there is not consistency on the part of all the staff members, the patient will usually respond with increased anxiety and behavior which is more "out of control." A ward setting where inconsistency thrives can easily result in the patient playing one part of the staff against the other with a breakdown in staff working relationships and the patient's growing distrust of the staff's ability to use rational authority to help him control his behavior.

TWO EXAMPLES OF
LIMIT SETTING

The types of situations within a nurse-patient relationship requiring limit setting are innumerable. However, two types of situations which seem to be particularly difficult are those in which the patient tries to deal with his feelings about the nurse and their relationship through inappropriate behavior which has a sexual connotation or through a gift-giving behavior.

Within a nurse-patient relationship, the patient often has difficulty expressing his feelings for the nurse, and his attempt to communicate positive feelings often results in inappropriate behavior. This is particularly true in a situation where a nurse works with a patient of the opposite sex.

P: *Is it OK if I sit here? I mean I wouldn't want to take you away from Gary* (another patient). *I mean, after all, he loves you, and I love you too, but you're too good to love. I mean I love you like a nurse.*

(The patient is talking very fast and moving his hand over the nurse's hand, which is in her lap.)

SN: (Picking up his hand and moving it away) *Eric, I don't want you to hold my hand. It makes me uncomfortable to have people touch me—and this is not the behavior a nurse and patient should show.*

P: (Pause; then he touches the student nurse's knee)

SN: *I told you I don't want to be touched.*

P: (Pulls hand back very fast) *Oh, that's right—you're too good to be touched. I wouldn't want to touch you. I'm sorry. I won't touch you again, but that doesn't mean I can't look at you.*

(The patient becomes increasingly restless and very shortly gets up and leaves.)

In this situation, although the nurse set a limit on the patient's behavior and the behavior stopped, the patient's anxiety did not decrease and he had to leave the situation.

A patient's behavior, in this case putting his hands on the student nurse, in other situations trying to kiss the nurse, is his way of communicating his caring for and liking the person who is working with him. Although the behavior is not appropriate, only to limit the behavior blocks the patient's attempt to communicate his feelings—and leaves his anxiety increasing with no outlet. The nurse must assume, if he knew a healthier way to express his feelings, he would have used it. So in addition to limiting the inappropriate behavior, she needs to either help him communicate verbally or to seek validation of her understanding of what he is trying to communicate. She also needs to tell what is appropriate behavior. For example:

N: *You can't hold me or kiss me, but I think you want to show me you care; I'm glad you like me, but I wish you would tell me—how you feel.*

The nurse accepts the patient's positive feelings toward her, but not his mode of communicating; and helps him learn a healthier way to deal with his feelings.

Gift giving is another behavior through which a patient may try to communicate; it may be to show appreciation, to seek closeness, to gain favor, to attempt to manipulate the relationship of that of a friend or servant, or to bribe for some future favor. By accepting the gift, the nurse communicates that she understands the meaning of the patient's gift giving and that there is no need for the patient to verbalize the meaning. In this way she may be approving and reinforcing a patient's problematic or pathological behavior.[9] Sometimes the nurse accepts the gift to meet her own needs to be liked or appreciated.

Gift giving requires limit setting; yet, if the nurse rejects the gift, the patient and the nurse often feel that the patient himself is being rejected. The nurse's intervention must reject the gift and set limits on that form of communicating while accepting the patient and providing a more healthy way to communicate feelings.

P: (Handing the nurse a bottle of hand lotion) *Here, I have something for you.*

N: *Oh, Mrs. P, I can't accept this but I'd like to sit here and talk with you.*

Although she rejected the gift, she did not reject the patient but stayed to talk over the situation with the patient. After they were seated, Mrs. P. put away the hand lotion and brought out a tube of lipstick.

P: *Here—you'd like this better anyway.*

N: *No, Mrs. P., but you seem to want to give me something.*

P: *Yes—you're a nice girl—here.* Looking in her purse)

N: *I wonder how you feel when I say I don't want you give me anything.*

P: *I guess you don't want my gifts.* (Looking very rejected, returns to looking in her purse)

N: *No, I don't want to accept your gifts and I won't be giving you any gifts—but we both can share lots of things—our feelings and ideas when we spend time and talk.*

P: *I guess I'd like that.* (Smiling, closes purse)

After the nurse indicated another way of accepting and sharing with the patient—spending time and talking—and put limits on gift giving in their relationship, only once more did she attempt to give; this time to share food. However, the gift giving did continue between this patient and other people. In many of these situations the nurse had an opportunity to help the patient look at her behavior, express her feelings, and explore the desire ("I want other people to like me and to do things for me") behind the behavior. The patient and nurse were then able to do some problem-solving and help the patient to learn some new ways to meet her need for acceptance.

In any limit-setting situation, controlling inappropriate behavior is only one of the goals and only the beginning of the therapeutic value. The very process involved in setting limits provides many opportunities for the nurse to help the patient meet his other basic needs—the need for physical safety, for security, for acceptance, for self esteem; and to develop the abilities to assess, to evaluate, and to problem solve, as well as the ability to change. Once the patient gains control over his behavior he is able to make use of other therapeutic processes that can further influence his path toward growth and health.

References

1. Holmes, Marguerite J., and Werner, Jean A., *Psychiatric Nursing in a Therapeutic Community* (New York: The Macmillan Company, 1966), p. 44.

2. Borel, Jack C., "Security as a Motivation of Human Behavior," *Archives of General Psychiatry* 10:107, February, 1964.

3. Borel, pp. 106–107.

4. Edwin, Lawrence Abt., and Weissman, Stuart L. (editors), *Acting Out, Theoretical and Clinical Aspects* (New York: Grune and Stratton, Inc., 1965), pp. 3, 40–41.

5. Kumler, Fern R., "An Interpersonal Interpretation of Manipulation," *Some Clinical Approaches to Psychiatric Nursing*, Burd, Shirley and Marshall, Margaret A. (editors) (New York: The Macmillan Company, 1963), p. 116.

6. Holmes, p. 51.

7. Holmes, p. 50.

8. Ginott, Haim G., *Between Parent and Child* (New York: The Macmillan Company, 1965), p. 53.

9. Clark, Janice, "The Patient's Gift," *Some Clinical Approaches to Psychiatric Nursing*, Burd, Shirley and Marshall, Margaret A. (editors) pp. 91–92.

Bibliography

Cohen, Raquel and Grinspoon, Lester, "Limit Setting as a Corrective Ego Experience," *Archives of General Psychiatry,* 8:74–79, January, 1963.

Wolf, Nancy Anderson, "Setting Reasonable Limits on Behavior," *The American Journal of Nursing,* 62:104–106, March, 1962.

Chapter Twenty

TEACHING PATIENTS SELF CARE: A CRITICAL ASPECT OF PSYCHIATRIC DISCHARGE PLANNING

Kathleen Coen Buckwalter and Karlene M. Kerfoot

ABSTRACT

THIS ARTICLE ADDRESSES TECHNIQUES that can be incorporated into both inpatient and outpatient programs in psychiatric-mental health nursing to decrease chances of rehospitalization. The authors write from their clinical experience in these settings and from research by the first author that has examined discharge planning techniques and outcome measures.

From "Teaching Patients Self Care: A Critical Aspect of Psychiatric Discharge Planning," by Kathleen Coen Buckwalter and Karlene M. Kerfoot, *Journal of Psychiatric Nursing and Mental Health Services*, May, 1982, Vol. 20, No. 5, pp. 15–20. Reprinted by permission of SLACK, Inc., Medical Publishers, Thorofare, NJ.

INTRODUCTION

The key to helping patients successfully manage after psychiatric discharge is self care—the art and science of helping patients to understand their illness, cope with the medical regimen, and prevent relapse by recognizing symptoms if and when they recur. The most successful kind of teaching in psychiatric-mental health nursing is that which allows patients to take charge of their illness and become partners in the treatment process.

The dimensions of self care perhaps have been defined best by Dorothea Orem (1971) as "The practice of activities that individuals personally initiate and perform on their own behalf in maintaining life, health, and well-being." Teaching and anticipatory guidance are important aspects of self-care assistance that are emphasized in this article. The theoretical implications of self care have been substantiated in research conducted by the first author (Buckwalter, 1980), which demonstrated that inclusion of the patient's family in a predischarge planning program (Figure) positively influenced social and community adjustment variables, satisfaction and stress levels, and compliance with medication regimens and aftercare appointments.

Recidivism rates are indicative of the ultimate failure of self-care teaching. Although deinstitutionalization has brought about an impressive decline in the number of psychiatric inpatients, this has been countered by the fact that there also has been an increasing readmission rate to state and county mental hospitals every year from the 1950s to the 1970s. Moon and Patton (1965) reported that readmission rates for 1960 to 1963 increased 12% over 1948 to 1955 rates. Friedman, Von Mering, and Hinks (1966) noted that high discharge rates and modern treatment methods were accompanied by readmission rates of up to 64%. While some episodes of relapse cannot be prevented, many can be handled on an outpatient basis if effective patient teaching has taken place. Readmission to the hospital often is unnecessary and most often is precipitated by the inability of patients and family members to cope with a crisis in an outpatient setting.

Relapse statistics are related to several factors. If treatment is initiated as soon as signs and symptoms worsen, outpatient management rather than rehospitalization is more likely. This form of treatment is successful only if patients are knowledgeable about their illnesses, and have support groups that understand their conditions. The family's knowledge of the illness and their support for medical treatment is an essential aspect of outpatient management. It is often much easier for families to return the patient to the hospital than to cope with the illness, but ultimately the patient suffers because of renewed stigma associated with rehospitalization and the development of a "failure identity" (Glasser, 1972).

Knowing how to handle the crisis of recurrent illness is essential to managing the relapse, and the manner in which family and patient handle stress is indicative of the methods they will use to cope with recurrent illness. Finally, medication compliance is an important factor in determining length of community tenure. This entails not only patient knowledge of medications, their proper dosage, and potential therapeutic and adverse side effects, but also awareness and support on the part of family and significant others in the patient's home setting.

This article addresses techniques that can be incorporated into both inpatient and outpatient programs in psychiatric-mental health nursing to decrease chances of rehospitalization. The authors write from their clinical experiences in these settings and from research by Buckwalter (1980) that has examined discharge planning techniques and outcome measures.

UNDERSTANDING THE DIAGNOSIS

Psychiatric nomenclature often is confusing to patients and sometimes is considered nothing more than just a label. However, if patients can understand what their diagnosis means and how to cope with their particular symptoms, the chances of adaptive living in the community are enhanced. One of the primary aims of discharge teaching, therefore, is a full explanation of the psychiatric diagnosis that includes both understanding of the symptoms and the implications of the psychosocial and biochemical aspects.

Many nurses, because they do not understand fully the neurophysiological and biochemical basis of psychiatric disorders, are unable to explain the physiological components of the diagnosis to patients. We have found that patients' compliance with the treatment regimen is enhanced if they can see the illness in more concrete physiological terms. We explain to them the basic concepts of neurotransmitters and how a psychiatric illness such as depression or mania can change the way these neurotransmitters function. We use a diagram to illustrate the way in which neurotransmitters work between synapses and use pictures of neurons available in the drug and medical literature. We also explain how the patient's particular drug is thought to act on the synapse and how medication therapy can cause changes in symptomatology.

We find it useful to compare psychiatric illness with a physical illness. Many patients have some knowledge of a common disease such as diabetes and easily can relate the biochemical imbalances of a psychiatric illness to the blood sugar imbalances of diabetes. Using the analogy of medication and insulin, patients can understand that psychiatric medication can restore some of their former functioning through biochemical means. Therefore, the patient does not view medications as merely tranquilizers but sees them as altering neurotransmitter function. If patients understand the biochemical basis for their symptoms, they often feel less stigmatized and are more accepting of a psychiatric diagnosis.

Another aspect of understanding one's illness is an appreciation of the fact that psychiatric illness is not static. Rather, it can be cyclical and possibly can recur. For example, when dealing with someone experiencing a depression, we try to determine the natural history of the disorder. Some patients will note seasonal variations and only become depressed in the fall or spring. If such a pattern can be established, then preventive measures can be instituted more effectively. With other patients, depression tends to recur in a cycle of several months or years, or in response to specific stressors such as the loss of significant others through divorce, separation, or death. Many patients believe that if they have one episode of depression they will have no more. If a relapse occurs, they feel defeated and believe they have done something "wrong" to precipitate the recurrence. It is helpful for patients to understand that in some people depressions occur in self-limiting cycles, and it is therefore best to prepare them for the possibility of a recurrence so they might accept it with fewer feelings of failure. We find that patients who feel good about themselves and their postdischarge progress, and believe they have some measure of control over their illness, are more likely to return for treatment with the onset of the first signs and symptoms of relapse.

Our experience suggests that certain patients benefit from conceptualizing their illness in terms of "coping" rather than "curing." Patients get discouraged when they cannot, in spite of concerted efforts, become totally symptom free. Psychiatry is not at the point where it can promise cures for every diagnosis. The outcome measure then becomes not the absence of symptoms, but how well patients cope with symptoms when they recur. Since nurses cannot promise patients that they will remain symptom free after discharge, it is helpful to teach patients the techniques of anticipatory guidance to help them cope with the initial signs of recurrent illness.

We feel it is essential to work with the families of psychiatric patients. This may sound trite, but one of the most significant aspects determining the success or failure of teaching psychiatric patients is the awareness, support, and knowledge of the family members. Our definition of "family" in this context includes significant others such as roommates, friends, or any other person with whom the patient has any type of enduring relationship.

Families commonly feel a great deal of guilt and responsibility when one of their members becomes psychiatrically ill. A discussion of guilt and concerns is imperative in order to work effectively with the family. This enables the family to work with the patient in a more realistic manner. It has been useful to point out to patients that the family often spots trouble before they do. We help the patient understand that in so doing the family is not being overly suspicious, placing less faith in them, or criticizing them unduly. When a family member suspects that symptoms are becoming worse, we encourage the patient and the family to schedule an outpatient appointment immediately, so that a nurse-therapist can make a decision regarding imminent relapse and begin appropriate interventions if necessary. We conceptualize the family and patient acting as a team, with the therapist functioning in a "coaching" role to help patients and their family members to function within this framework.

Bibliotherapy can be an effective patient teaching strategy. There are books on the market now for lay people that do a good job of explaining affective disorders. We also use articles from popular periodicals, news magazines, and pharmaceutical pamphlets that explain medications and illnesses in a relatively simple and yet accurate manner. Another advantage of using lay literature is that it effectively explains psychiatric illness in understandable terms and thus helps lessen the stigma. These articles usually have a positive focus and emphasize the commonality of the problem. Local mental health associations supply many excellent pamphlets as well.

Another effective technique is the assignment of homework that requires both the patient and family to read instructive material between appointments. The following appointment then is used to clarify any misconceptions they may have. We incorporate techniques of learning such as return demonstration and explanation into our patient teaching and encourage feedback so that we can evaluate if learning has taken place. If the patient is unable to read because of emotional problems, illiteracy, or blurry vision secondary to medication, we record pertinent information on tape. If this is not appropriate, we devote therapy time to explaining written material.

Yet another approach is to note that famous people have had similar psychiatric problems and have been able to cope with their mental illnesses. For example, when explaining depression, we point out that Abraham Lincoln and Winston Churchill suffered depressive episodes and considered suicide, or give examples of people in show business who have handled depression or mania successfully. When patients understand that many productive and admired individuals have coped with similar problems, they often feel more confident in handling their own situation.

STRESSORS

The prehospitalization phase often is accompanied by a series of stressors. The nature of these stressors can be discovered by taking a thorough history of events leading up to the crisis. One problem with this approach is that patients tend to look for external causes of illness when in fact there may be none. However, for many patients, there is a clear history of stressors such as childbirth, a new job, or a change in marital status, that can precede a relapse for certain individuals.

When a clear history of stressors has been elicited, the therapist can continue to teach prevention of future relapses and techniques to lessen the severity of recurrence within an anticipatory guidance framework. Patients are taught to be "tuned into" potential stressors in their lives. If they have a great deal of unavoidable stress in one area, they are instructed to try and relieve stress in other areas. Changes in signs and symptoms may be used as a barometer of the phase of the illness to indicate how well or how poorly they are handling stress. Patients are instructed to check with their nurse-therapist for possible medication changes and crisis counseling whenever they are placed in an unusually stressful situation. They are taught to view stress not as an insurmountable problem, but rather as an opportunity to test coping skills. Stress is presented as a challenge to be dealt with rather than something to be feared.

SIGNS AND SYMPTOMS

In order to cope effectively with any psychiatric illness, patients need to know what signs and symptoms are characteristic of their problem and the particular meaning these symptoms have for them. Every patient has a unique pattern of symptoms. Patients need to understand thoroughly that symptoms should not be thought of negatively, but rather seen as indicators for dealing with illness. The patient's individual symptom pattern best can be identified from interviews with the family and patient. For example, the first sign of recurrent depression for some patients is loss of energy. If the family knows this is one of the symptoms to watch for, they will be concerned if the patient becomes inactive at night, falls asleep, and loses interest in outside activities. The patient may interpret this as simple fatigue, but it could signal the beginning of a relapse to family members. If a mental health professional is called in at this point to make a judgment, a further deterioration of the patient's condition may be averted. On the other hand, the family can be reassured that the patient is simply, as he states, over-tired.

The most important point related to changes in signs and symptoms is the consequent initiation of either psychotherapy, medication therapy, or both to abort an impending relapse. In this way, patients develop a real sense of being in charge of their illness and can learn to view symptoms as potentially-helpful, early-warning signs and to seek immediate intervention when appropriate.

RESOCIALIZATION ISSUES

One of the most critical problems patients face when re-entering the community is that of explaining their hospitalization to co-workers and acquaintances. In therapy sessions, we often discuss this issue with patients and encourage them to formulate answers for awkward situations with which they may be confronted after discharge. Role playing can be especially effective with the therapist portraying the role of employer or friend. Patients are asked to relate how they would respond to various situations. Initially, patients may be very uncomfortable with role playing but after several sessions and encouragement to try out many different situations, they usually are able to determine which behavioral and verbal responses are most effective for them.

After discharge, patients may delay rejoining social groups and activities that are important aspects of positive reintegration into the community. There is a fine line between joining too early only to fail and procrastinating so long that the patient becomes phobic of social situations. If patients can explain confidently their absence, they usually are more willing to re-enter social groups at an earlier date.

Following discharge, patients also should be encouraged to continue some of the recreational activities that they participated in while hospitalized as effective ways of managing leisure time and constructively discharging tension.

COMMUNITY SUPPORT

Patients need to learn to call upon community resources they used prior to hospitalization. For example, if a member of the clergy was a mainstay in the patient's life, he or she should be contacted during hospitalization so that appointments can be set up at the time of discharge. One of the roles the minister can play is to help reintegrate the patient into the social and religious life of the church and thus help to rebuild self-confidence. If patients cannot identify any community support groups, the nurse can guide them to such groups. Most communities have self-help organizations such as Recovery, Inc., which consist of former mental patients who provide support and care to people in similar circumstances. Many mental health centers have socialization groups for discharged patients that offer an opportunity for interpersonal contact, support in the community, and an outlet for discussions of problems related to community living. Public health nursing is an excellent source of postdischarge support, and referrals to public health agencies should be a standard part of discharge planning. In order to maintain some patients in the community, services such as

Meals on Wheels, a friendly telephone service, and volunteer visitors also may be considered.

MEDICATION COMPLIANCE

Eighty to 90% of all discharged mental patients are placed on medications. Research related to medication compliance in the aftercare period is somewhat contradictory. Franklin, Kittredge, and Thrasher (1975) found that use of medications, length of time on medication, or dosages after discharge did not relate to readmission, whereas research by Zolick, Levin, and Hubek (1970) and Davis, Dinitz, and Pasamanick (1972) showed hospital returnees had significantly more medication problems than nonreturnees. Siegal and St. Clair (1977) found that only 16 of 86 rehospitalized patients mentioned any medication problems, but research conducted by Sanders, Smith, and Weinman (1967) suggests patients may underestimate medication problems in the aftercare period.

Psychotropic medications provide professionally acceptable reasons for increased staff attention and optimism. The biochemical aspects of psychiatric disorders in many ways have come to be viewed as the key to the solution. However, psychological therapy and retraining are important in helping patients match their behavior to new-found biochemical normalities after hospitalization.

Psychosocial interventions together with medication teaching will ensure optimum treatment. The introduction of psychotropic medications has not "preempted the necessity for developing more effective psychosocial interventions" (Erickson, 1975).

As noted previously, the biochemical aspects of drug treatment are understood poorly by many nurses. Much information about the neurological basis of drug treatment has been available in the past five to ten years but has not been emphasized in the nursing literature. Therefore, many nurses see drug treatment as adjunctive rather than primary treatment. With the explosion of information about the biochemical components of mental disorders and knowledge about neurotransmitters, we have come to understand that drug treatment is, in many cases, of primary importance in the treatment of psychiatric disorders. Medication compliance can be increased if the nurse understands how medications work, knows when to recommend changes in medications, and knows how to teach patients to recognize a need to regulate their own medications after consultation with a professional.

For some patients, it is difficult to remember to take several medications on different time schedules. It is imperative that the nurse examine the scheduling of medications and consult with the physician regarding the most reasonable timetable for administration. Many antidepressant medications can be given at one time in a nightly dose that is more effective than several doses given throughout the day. Patients are more likely to remember to take a single daily dose than multiple doses. Other medication, because it is metabolized in a different manner, will not be amenable to this type of scheduling. It is effective for the patient to learn to pair medication taking with a routine event. For example, patients can remember to take the morning medication if they associate it with a daily morning task such as brushing their teeth. Similarly, if patients have lunch at approximately the same time every day, they can pair medication taking with lunch. If they skip lunch, then medication must be coupled with another routine event. Alternate plans should be made for weekends or periods without an established routine.

It is sometimes difficult for patients to remember if they have taken their medication and an individualized system needs to be developed to ensure that patients will not retake their pills. Pharmacies have many types of plastic drug dispensers available in disc or rectangular form with sections where each day's medication can be placed. Patients are encouraged to purchase these dispensers and carry them in their pockets or purses so that they can see if the medication has been taken by looking at the dispenser. Patients and/or family members also can establish a nightly routine of setting out souffle cups containing the next day's medication. Xeroxed check list forms that the patient can attach to the refrigerator or other conspicuous place detailing the dosage of medication and the time taken are another way of determining if medication has been taken properly.

For the patient who is unreliable and/or suicidal, frequent outpatient appointments are essential, and the patient should be given only enough medication to last for a few days with no refills. Patients never should be given more medication at any one time than their body can handle in case of an overdose. Each dosage of medication may be poured into a paper packet or plastic dispenser and three or four days' worth of medication can be given to the patient. Patients are instructed to return old packets to the nurse, at which time a new series of medications is provided. If the patient should bring in an unused packet, the nurse must avoid accusations that may result in guilt or a sense of failure on the part of the patient. If this happens, the patient will learn to hide mistakes and the nurse will not get an accurate idea of the patient's compliance. Home visits by the nurse-therapist or public health nurse can be enlisted to help with medication compliance by setting up a program in the patient's home. This is most appropriate if it is difficult for a patient to come back to the outpatient treatment center on a frequent basis. This also provides the opportunity to make a home assessment and to uncover any problems that might escape the outpatient nurse-therapist.

In our experience, most patients are compliant with medication regimens when exposed to this kind of teaching. They understand that there is a physiological and biochemical basis for drug usage and that medications are not solely for tranquilization. We thoroughly discuss any side effects that may be expected and teach them how to cope with these. For example, if an employed patient becomes sleepy after a noon dosage and this interferes with job functioning, we discuss with the psychiatrist either lowering or eliminating the noon medication or administering it later in the day. We fully explain to patients that they might feel sleepy for a period of time when on medication therapy, but this will soon abate. If patients know what to expect and realize that side effects are not permanent, they usually are more agreeable to medication therapy.

FIGURE

Standardization Protocol for Depressives and Their Families

Pre-discharge structured planning interview:

Purpose: To provide knowledge, clarification, and support for the patient about to be discharged and for the family. To help the family understand better the meaning of the hospitalization for the patient and to become aware of those problem areas the patient anticipates after discharge.

Introduction: I've asked you to get together with me in an effort to help prepare for (*patient's name*) discharge from the hospital. I'd like to discuss with all of you certain aspects of his/her illness and treatment so that you have a better understanding of what he/she has been through and what to expect after he/she comes home:

Summary of five areas to be covered in patient and family session:

1. Patient's diagnosis; definition of psychiatric illness; type of treatment patient received in hospital, including names and types of medication on which patient will be discharged, their proper administration (correct dosage and times), potential side effects, and need for compliance.

2. Relapse signs and symptoms of recurrent illness and what to do should they reappear at home. Also create an awareness of factors and symptoms that precipitated patient's admission.

3. Resources for both patients and their families (medical, social, and vocational) in the community. Reminder of postdischarge follow-ups scheduled at the local mental health center.

4. Positive support and knowledge, presenting notion that patient can anticipate and avoid some problems that may arise after discharge, i.e., "You are not helpless...you have some power to recognize and control those situations that lead you into illness." Further, just because a family member has been hospitalized for mental problems, all is not hopeless. You may want to explore the notion that having someone in the family hospitalized for psychiatric illness may be a symptom of deeper problems within the family. There may be a biochemical (or genetic) basis for illness, but environmental factors also can bring about fluctuations in mood. There may be a need to reorganize roles and responsibilities within the family once the patient comes home, but family support and belief that the patient can make it are essential for smooth re-entry into the community.

5. Resocialization issues, or potential problems identified by the patient prior to discharge. Patient is encouraged to lead the discussion about those areas in which he or she anticipates problems after discharge, or simply areas of readjustment about which there are concerns.

SUMMARY

This article has dealt with selected issues in patient education that involve teaching patients self care in the mental health delivery system. It has presented several predischarge teaching techniques that have been used in a research study by the first author and other strategies that have been found to be effective in both authors' clinical practice. There are many other areas in need of systematic investigation related to self-care skills. The first author's study is one of very few conducted by psychiatric nurses to document effective self-care treatment techniques (Figure). We hope that other clinicians and researchers will become interested in this area and add to the knowledge base of self care in the field of psychiatric-mental health nursing.

References

Buckwalter, K. C. *Alleviating the discharge crisis: Shared assessment and planning*

with psychiatric patients and their families. Unpublished
manuscript. University of Illinois at the Medical Center,
1980.

Davis, A. E., Dinitiz, S., & Pasamanick, B. The prevention of hospitalization in
schizophrenia: Five years after an experimental program.
American Journal of Orthopsychiatry. April 1972, *42*,
375–388.

Erickson, R. C. Outcome studies in mental hospitals: A review. *Psychological
Bulletin,* July 1975, *82*, 519–540.

Franklin, J. L., Kittredge, L. D., & Thrasher, J. H. A survey of factors related
to mental hospital readmissions. *Hospital and Community
Psychiatry.* November 1975, *26*, 749–751.

Friedman, I., Von Mering, O., & Hinks, E. N. Intermittent patienthood.
Archives of General Psychiatry. April 1966, *14*, 386–392.

Glasser, W. *The identity society.* New York: Harper and Row Publishers, 1972.

Moon, L. E., & Patton, R. E. First admissions and readmissions to New York
State mental hospitals—A statistical evaluation. *Psychiatric
Quarterly,* July 1965, *39*, 476–486.

Orem, D. E. *Nursing: Concepts of practice.* New York: McGraw-Hill, 1971, p.
13.

Sanders, R., Smith, R. S., & Weinman, B. S. *Chronic psychoses and recovery.*
San Francisco: Jossey-Bass, 1967.

Siegal, J. M., & St. Clair, C. Patient problems associated with immediate and
delayed rehospitalization. *Psychiatric Quarterly,* Fall 1977,
49, 204–220.

Zolick, E. S., Levin, I., & Hubek, P. Comprehensive community care and
patient rehospitalization. *Proceedings of the 78th Annual
Convention of the American Psychological Association,* 1970,
pp. 503–504.

Chapter Twenty-One

NONCOMPLIANCE: UNDERSTANDING AND INTERVENING WHEN CLIENTS FAIL TO FOLLOW THE TREATMENT PLAN

Deborah J. Brief, M.A.,
and Josie E. Dorman, M.S.N., R.N.

NONCOMPLIANCE WITH TREATMENT RECOMMENDATIONS is a widespread problem in health care today. Although most clients appear motivated to follow the recommendations of a health professional (Haynes, 1979a), estimates of actual compliance are astonishingly low. For example, Sackett and Snow (1979) have estimated that the average rate of compliance with long-term medication regimens is 54%, and compliance with short-term regimens is only slightly higher— 62%. There is also some evidence that psychiatric clients are less compliant than others (Haynes, 1979b), making it necessary for professionals in this area of health care to be especially concerned with compliance problems.

DEFINING COMPLIANCE

The term *compliance* is generally used to describe the extent to which a client's behavior coincides with the recommendations of a health professional (Haynes, 1979a; Skillern, 1981). Thus, a client who takes medication according to a prescribed schedule or makes lifestyle changes as recommended is considered compliant. The definition of compliance has recently been broadened to include a wider range of client behaviors (Epstein & Cluss, 1982): clients are now viewed as "noncompliant" if they delay seeking care, break appointments, discontinue therapy early, or take inappropriate doses of medication. In the past, clients have primarily been held responsible for poor compliance. However, health professionals have begun to examine their methods of administering treatment, to determine their role in eliciting compliance (Skillern, 1981). Compliance is now more commonly viewed as a collaborative effort between the client and health care provider (Redman, 1976; Villeneuve, 1982).

IMPLEMENTING A PREVENTIVE OR REMEDIAL STRATEGY

Some clients experience more difficulties in adhering to therapeutic regimens than others and, therefore, might be identified as *high risks* to develop compliance problems. It is important to recognize which clients fall into this category, because noncompliance is not always immediately detectable. By providing these clients with more attention in the early stages of treatment, noncompliance and its effects may be prevented. However, in most cases, it will be necessary to develop a strategy to remediate noncompliant behavior once it has been observed.

The development of an appropriate strategy to increase compliance depends on an accurate assessment of the factors that give rise to the noncompliance (Dunbar, Marshall, & Hovell, 1979; Shelton & Levy, 1981). There are a number of questions that nurses can use to guide their assessment of these factors and to plan appropriate preventive or remedial intervention strategies.

1. *Does the client appear to have a physiological deficit that would interfere with carrying out the prescribed treatment regimen?* Physiological deficits, such as decreased auditory or visual capacity, may interfere with compliance and should be identified by a standard examination procedure and treated if their contribution to noncompliance is expected. The hearing-impaired client who withdraws socially and evidences signs of depression cannot be expected to become more interested in socializing until the hearing defect is corrected. Similarly, a client who beings to stay at home because of failing vision may not be interested in complying with treatment recommendations involving increased outdoor activity until the visual impairment is corrected.

Memory and concentration difficulties may also interfere with the client's ability to follow a recommended treatment regimen. In some cases, the client may recognize and report the onset of these types of difficulties. More often it is the family members who are able to provide significant information about the onset of memory difficulties and the degree to which they appear to interfere with the individual's functioning (e.g., does the client forget to perform routine activities?). If these types of deficits are suspected and appear to interfere with compliance, the client should be referred to a qualified professional, such as a clinical neuropsychologist, for a complete evaluation. It is important to recognize that some psychiatric clients may exhibit memory or concentration difficulties upon admission to the hospital or at the time of a follow-up appointment but that these difficulties may decrease with appropriate treatment. Thus, it may be necessary to assess whether these deficits are present on more than one occasion before the client is referred for additional evaluation.

If at all possible, the ultimate goal of an intervention should be aimed at increasing the client's responsibility for compliant behavior. Some clients may need short-term help because they are not capable of assuming responsibility when treatment is started. However, if a client does have a deficit that cannot be corrected and that will continue to interfere with compliance, then the clinic staff may need to assume responsibility for the client's compliance during the early stages of treatment, and the family may need to assume responsibility for compliance on a long-term basis. For the client on neuroleptic medication, a long-acting form (e.g., prolixin) that can be injected once every two weeks may be appropriate in some cases (Haynes, 1979b).

2. *Does the client have false beliefs about the illness or efficacy of treatment?* Historically, nurses have played an important role in transmitting information to clients about the seriousness of their illness and the rationale for recommended treatments (Hogue, 1979). This continues to be an especially important role for nurses, because they are frequently perceived as less threatening than physicians and may have more contact with clients than the physicians. There are several types of erroneous beliefs that psychiatric clients may have and that nurses may need to challenge in order to improve compliance.

Many clients believe that symptoms are reliable indicators of the severity of illness and that the absence of symptoms implies that they have been "cured." As a result, clients may regulate their medication according to the presence or severity of symptoms and discontinue medication when symptoms subside (Leventhal, 1982). Schizophrenic clients who are prescribed a neuroleptic drug during an acute psychotic episode may stop taking medication once the acute symptomatology subsides because they feel better. However, the client may have been instructed to continue to take the medication prophylactically, in order to prevent relapse. In this situation, the nurse must inform the client that psychotropic medication can *control* symptoms, but cannot *cure* the underlying disorder and that a recurrence of symptoms is likely if the medication is not taken as prescribed.

Clients frequently have unrealistic expectations about the ability of medication to produce changes in their lives (Cohen & Amdur, 1981; Hogue, 1979). Depressed, socially anxious clients may expect antidepressant medication to produce an elevation in mood and improve their social lives. It is probable that the antidepressant medication is necessary to elevate the clients' moods, so that they will be motivated to improve their lives by learning new social or independent living skills, by increasing levels of activity, or by entering situations previously avoided. A frequent consequence of this type of belief is that clients will be noncompliant with recommendations for lifestyle changes and will become disappointed in the medical treatment. Similar behavior may result if clients believe that they lack the responsibility or ability to change their lifestyles (Finnerty, 1980; Redman, 1976). Educating clients about the limitations of pharmacological therapy is essential in these circumstances.

3. *Is the client experiencing drug-induced side effects that make compliance difficult?* Side effects of psychotropic medication have been found to contribute to noncompliance in two ways. First, in many cases and particularly with neuroleptic drugs, side effects will persist as long as the client is taking the drug. Under these circumstances the client may be able to decide whether it is preferable to risk the illness or to experience drug-induced side effects. It appears helpful in this regard for clients to be informed, prior to the medication being started, what the expected side effects are and how long the will last (Cohen & Amdur, 1981). There are several ways in which side effects can be minimized for the client who has decided that it is preferable to take medication as it is prescribed (Cohen & Amdur, 1981). These ways (which of course require the physician's collaboration) are as follows: (a) decrease the dose during the relapse prevention stage; (b) use alternative drugs, with fewer side effects if possible, during the prophylactic stage (e.g., thioridazine instead of chlorpromazine); (c) use supplementary medication to decrease side effects (e.g., antiparkinsonian drugs with neuroleptics); and (d) have the patient take all or the largest dose of medication at bedtime. Forming a group of clients to discuss their medication and methods of coping with side effects has been reported to help some clients (Cohen & Amdur, 1981).

Second, side effects contribute to compliance problems when they precede the therapeutic effects. Neuroleptic drugs may produce involuntary movements, rapid weight gain, and sedation almost immediately after being started, yet it generally takes two or three weeks for a positive, therapeutic benefit to be observed. Similarly, the therapeutic effects of an antidepressant may not be detectable until ten days after it is first administered, yet sedative effects are almost immediate. Under these circumstances, clients need to know the exact nature of the relationship between the time of treatment onset and expected therapeutic benefit.

4. *Is the client on a regimen that makes compliance difficult?* Research has shown that the more complex and demanding the plan of medical care is, the more likely it is that the client will not be compliant (Blackwell, 1979; Epstein & Cluss, 1982; Haynes, 1979b; Raskin, 1980; Redman, 1976; Villeneuve, 1982). Complexity can be broken down into several elements, including the number of different medications, dose of medication, and frequency with which medication must be taken. Of these elements, the number of different medications seems to have the greatest impact on compliance. Thus, clients who are required to take more than one type of medication (e.g., a benzodiazepine and an antidepressant in the treatment of an anxiety disorder) will experience more compliance problems than clients treated with a single type of medication (Blackwell, 1979; Hulka, 1979). An effort should be made, therefore, to simplify medication schedules early in the treatment program as much as possible.

5. *Does the client lack the necessary knowledge to carry out a prescribed regimen?* A client may appear to be noncompliant because of a lack of understanding of what is required (Shelton & Levy, 1981). Clients on medical regimens frequently make scheduling errors due to a misinterpretation of the instructions. Nurses can be particularly helpful, if the client lacks this knowledge, by providing the client with both verbal and written instructions containing specific details about the medication (Haynes, 1979c; Hecht, 1974). These instructions might include the name of the drug, the recommended schedule (i.e., number of times/day), the color of the medication (if more than one is prescribed), and the possible side effects of each drug. Clients who most frequently make scheduling errors are those who have no knowledge of the drug's function or of the drug's name (Hulka, 1979). Therefore, educating the client about these matters can increase compliance (Latiolas & Berry, 1969).

Confusion of this type can also occur with recommendations for lifestyle changes. For example, a depressed client who is told to increase her activity level by exercising may not know what type of exercise to do, how often to exercise, or where to find exercise classes.

When presenting information to a client about a medication or lifestyle-change regimen, it is important to use terms that the client will understand and to assess periodically whether the client comprehends your instructions. In some cases it may be necessary to test for language comprehension, such as when English is not the client's first language.

6. *Does the client lack the necessary skills to carry out a prescribed regimen?* The client may have the appropriate knowledge about the regimen but still not be able to perform the appropriate behavior, because of a lack of necessary skills (Shelton & Levy, 1981). This frequently occurs when lifestyle changes are needed. A schizophrenic client may not know how to increase social contacts because of a lack of social skills. Similarly, a depressed or anxious client may not know how to improve the quality of interactions with others, because of a lack of skills necessary to elicit positive reactions from others. If the client cannot demonstrate the skills, but knows what is required, then skill training may be necessary.

7. *Is there something about the client's social support system or daily routine that is interfering with compliance?* Whenever possible, it is important to collaborate with family members to help the client to comply (Hogue, 1979). First, it may be important to determine whether the client is being rewarded for being ill. Is a depressed client, for example, receiving a lot of attention from family members for staying in bed all day, crying, or verbalizing low self-esteem? If this is the case, then the family may need to be instructed to ignore these behaviors and to reinforce nondepressed behaviors, such as getting up in the morning, grooming appropriately, and exercising regularly. Second, when a client returns home after a long hospitalization, the family may want to become involved in helping the client by taking over the nurse's role of reinforcing compliance (e.g., with medication schedules, going to work on time, or scheduling pleasurable activities on the weekends).

For clients who require long-term programs, the importance of extended supervision by nurses and/or the involvement of family members in treatment appears to increase dramatically (Glanz, 1980; Haynes, 1979c). However, the crucial element to maintaining compliance with long-term treatments may be transferring the responsibility of managing all aspects of treatment to the client.

It is also desirable to try to fit a client's regimen into the daily routine, once the client has moved home (Hecht, 1974). This means that the nurse may need to take some time to establish each client's individual schedule. Often there is something about the client's daily routine that may be used as a *reminder* or a *cue*, such as taking the medication every night before going to bed and before work in the morning. The medication might be placed in the medicine cabinet on the shelf with the toothbrush or on the night table beside the bed. Artificial cues, such as medication buzzers, calendars, and pill dispensers are also useful but are most effective on a short-term basis (Haynes, 1979c). If therapy is long-term it is more desirable for the client to incorporate the behavior into the daily routine.

SUMMARY

It has become clear that health professionals cannot expect clients to be compliant by simply providing them with information about what is required with a treatment regimen. In fact, health professionals can expect a compliance rate of only about 50%, if traditional methods of administering treatment are employed (Haynes, 1979a). Although it is important to analyze each case individually, there are some general principles that are now recognized as important, in order to prevent noncompliance or improve compliance when problems occur. It is important that each client

1. be free of physiological deficits which would interfere with compliance

2. have appropriate beliefs and knowledge about the illness and treatment

3. understand the type and time course of possible side effects of treatment

4. be on the least complex regimen possible

5. have the necessary skills to be compliant

6. and have a social support system or daily routine that enhances compliance.

The information provided here may serve as a guide to practicing nurses to facilitate behavioral changes in clients who must adjust their lives to control psychiatric illness.

References

Blackwell, B. The drug regimen and treatment compliance. In R. B. Haynes, D. W. Taylor & P. L. Sackett, (Eds.), *Compliance in Health Care* (pp. 144–156). Baltimore: Johns Hopkins Press, 1979.

Cohen, M. and Amdur, M. Medication group for psychiatric patients. *American Journal of Nursing*, 1981, 81, 343–345.

Dunbar, J. M., Marshall, G. D., and Hovell, M. F. Behavioral strategies for improving compliance. In R. B. Haynes, D. W. Taylor & P. L. Sackett, (Eds.), *Compliance in Health Care* (pp. 174–190). Baltimore: Johns Hopkins Press, 1979.

Epstein, L. and Cluss, P. A. A behavioral medicine and perspective on adherence to long-term medical regimens. *Journal of Consulting and Clinical Psychology*, 1982, 50 (6), 950–971.

Finnerty, F. A. Hypertension—specially trained personnel can improve compliance. *Consultant*, 1980, 20, 226–228.

Glanz, K. Compliance with dietary regimens: Its magnitude, measurement and determinants. *Preventative Medicine*, 1980, 9, 787-804.

Haynes, R. B. Introduction. In R. B. Haynes, D. W. Taylor & P. L. Sackett, (Eds.), *Compliance in Health Care* (pp. 1-7). Baltimore: Johns Hopkins Press, 1979a.

———Determinants of compliance: The disease and mechanics of treatment. In R. B. Haynes, D. W. Taylor & P. L. Sackett, (Eds.), *Compliance in Health Care* (pp. 49-62). Baltimore: Johns Hopkins Press, 1979b.

———Strategies to improve compliance with referrals, appointments and prescribed medical regimens. In R. B. Haynes, D. W. Taylor & P. L. Sackett, (Eds.), *Compliance in Health Care* (pp. 121-143). Baltimore: Johns Hopkins Press, 1979c.

Hecht, A. B. Improving medication compliance by teaching outpatients. *Nursing Forum*, 1974, *13* (2), 113-129.

Hogue, C. C. Nursing compliance. In R. B. Haynes, D. W. Taylor & P. L. Sackett, (Eds.), *Compliance in Health Care* (pp. 247-259). Baltimore: Johns Hopkins Press, 1979.

Hulka, B. Patient-clinician interactions and compliance. In R. B. Haynes, D. W. Taylor & P. L. Sackett, (Eds.), *Compliance in Health Care* (pp. 63-77). Baltimore: Johns Hopkins Press, 1979.

Latioilas, C. J. and Berry, C. C. Misuse of prescription medications by outpatients. *Drug Intelligence & Clinical Pharmacy*, 1969, *3*, 270-277.

Leventhal, H. Wrongheaded ideas about illness. *Psychology Today*, 1982, *16*, 48-55.

Raskin, D. E. Patients who don't follow instruction. *Consultant*, 1980, *20*, 226-228.

Redman, B. K. *The Process of Patient Teaching* (3rd edition). St. Louis: C. V. Mosby Company, 1976.

Sackett, D. and Snow, J. C. The magnitude of compliance and noncompliance. In R. B. Haynes, D. W. Taylor & P. L. Sackett, (Eds.), *Compliance in Health Care* (pp. 11-22). Baltimore: Johns Hopkins Press, 1979.

Shelton, J. L. and Levy, P. L. Enhancing compliance with behavioral assignments. In *Behavioral Assignments and Treatment Compliance* (37-89). Champaign, IL: Research Press, 1981.

Skillern, P. G. Noncompliance: 8 steps for improving patient cooperation. *Consultant*, 1981, July, 206-211.

Villeneuve, M. E. The patient compliance puzzle. . . nursing practice in relation to insulin administration. *Nursing Management*, 1982, *13* (5), 54-56.

Part Four

INTERVENTIONS WITH GROUPS AND FAMILIES AND THE THERAPEUTIC MILIEU

In most settings, nurses are involved in formal and informal groups on a daily basis. With knowledge of group dynamics and with some experience in analyzing group behavior, nurses can make valuable contributions in leadership roles. Diabetic and newborn care classes, ward and therapeutic community meetings, activity groups, floor staff conferences, and psychotherapy groups are only some examples of the kinds of groups nurses organize and lead.

Swanson's article provides several checklists that are helpful to both new and experienced group leaders. Specific suggestions are offered in response to questions about the value of group activities for psychiatric clients, goals for group achievement, selection of the group members, and choice of effective leadership styles. Swanson follows with a checklist the leader can use for self-appraisal and as a guide for evaluating group and leader performance at various stages of group development.

In her article, Slimmer provides brief examples of group interventions derived from three theoretical models: the focal-conflict model, the communication model, and the group dynamics model. Her work is a good example of how nurses can use theory to guide them in decisions about how to manage the problem behaviors encountered in their work with groups.

"How Can an Alcoholic Change in 28 Days?" According to Yearwood and Hess, the group process has an extremely important role in helping alcoholics begin to accept responsibility for their behavior. They discuss a number of ways in which the group process influences the patient to change self-defeating behavior patterns. It should be noted that the psychoanalytic theory of the etiology of alcoholism described in the article is no longer as popular as it once was.

Like group therapy, family therapy is a relatively new form of treatment in mental health settings. Family therapy is not treatment of an individual with the family present; it involves assessing and treating the family system itself as a client. Working with the complex communication patterns of a family system requires specialized techniques and training; for this reason, undergraduate students and others without advanced training are not expected to assume the role of family therapist. However, knowledge of the goals and methods of family therapy may facilitate referrals, and at times family therapy techniques may be incorporated into the practice of students and other practitioners.

The article by Harris and Fregly describes Harris's experience, while in a graduate program, with family crisis intervention. Harris worked with a family of two parents, thirteen children, and two grandchildren over a period of five months, during which time the family underwent four major crises. The authors describe in considerable detail how the nurse helped the family cope with each crisis and emerge strengthened by the experience.

Nursing students and practitioners can help, in an important way, with the identification and treatment of battered women. These clients can be extremely difficult, not only because of their helplessness and ambivalence but also because of the emotions they arouse in the care provider. Nurses in all settings need to know the specific responses that are most likely to help the abused woman take advantage of the treatment resources available. Iyer describes exactly what nurses can say and do when confronted with a battered woman.

Too often, practitioners are quick to blame families for aggravating or even causing the mental health problems of clients. Lamb and Oliphant offer an excellent discussion of the problems families face when a member has chronic psychiatric problems. They believe that relatives (and ultimately the client) can be helped a great deal by sensible, practical advice from mental health professionals; numerous examples and suggestions are included in their article.

Chapter Twenty-Two

A CHECKLIST FOR GROUP LEADERS

Mary G. Swanson

WORKING WITH GROUPS OF patients has become one of the most frequently used approaches in psychiatric nursing, particularly in large federal and state mental hospitals. In some of these hospitals the goal now seems to be to have every patient, every nurse, and every psychiatric aide participate in some kind of patient group every week or even every day. In many hospitals the more experienced and better-prepared nurses serve as co-therapists or even group leaders in group therapy, as leaders of remotivation groups, and as organizers or leaders of special hobby or interest groups. They are also often expected to participate in the training and supervision of psychiatric aides who lead remotivation or hobby groups.

Many nurses, when they accept employment in large mental hospitals, find that group work is included in their assignments, lack preparation for this responsibility. True, most graduate programs in psychiatric nursing now provide training for work with groups of patients, especially in formal therapy groups. In most basic nursing programs, however, little or nothing is taught about group techniques; the psychiatric nursing courses are focused almost entirely on teaching the students to function effectively in a one-to-one relationship with patients. Thus, the area of group work with psychiatric patients is one in which many graduate nurses find they need some additional reading, observing, and training after arriving in their job settings.

From "A Check List for Group Leaders," by Mary G. Swanson, *Perspectives in Psychiatric Care*, 1969, Vol. 7, No. 3, pp. 120–126. Reprinted by permission.

VALUES OF GROUP WORK

Several reasons account for the increasing use of group work in psychiatric hospitals. At first glance the main reason might seem to be economy in the use of staff, which in large hospitals is almost never numerically adequate to provide a one-to-one relationship for every patient who could benefit from it. However, economy is not the only reason; there are therapeutic values for a patient in group interaction which supplement the benefits he can derive from even a very satisfactory one-to-one relationship. Some of these values are:

> *Socialization; increased self-confidence and enjoyment in interacting with groups of people.*
>
> *Moving out of the dependent and self-centered role of patient and regaining the feeling of interacting with a group and becoming more aware of and responsive to the feelings and ideas of other people.*
>
> *Increased sense of well-being. This goal is sometimes the only realistic one for group work with chronic patients with considerable organic brain damage or with fairly advanced senility. It is a legitimate goal: when a patient cannot be "cured" it is still worthwhile to make him as happy and comfortable as possible.*
>
> *Practice in problem solving as a member of a group. Such activity helps the patient to recognize and take into account the opinions and suggestions of others and to develop an increased flexibility in sometimes working to influence other people and sometimes changing his own opinion in response to what he learns by listening to them.*
>
> *Clearer realization of how one's personality and actions appear to others. For a patient to persist in denial when a group of his peers express an opinion about him and his problems is harder than for him to insist that his therapist does not like him or understand him.*
>
> *The impact of group pressure in the direction of conformity rather than toward deviant or unhealthy behavior.*
>
> *The development of psychological insight into one's unconscious feelings. The responses of group members to a patient's disclosures can facilitate the development of insight. Also, many patients gain some insights by realizing their similarities to some of the other patients who are describing their situations and feelings.*
>
> *Diminution of the feeling that many psychiatric patients have of being alone and unique in their suffering from emotional problems.*

*Increased hope that one may improve, derived from the
observation of other patients who are improving during therapy.*

*An opportunity to practice an alternative method of handling
anxiety, anger, or despair for the patient whose usual response to
such emotions has been to withdraw and regress rather than seek out
other people to help him cope with these emotions more successfully.*

*A stimulus to the practice of clearer communication with
others derived from the patient's realization that others cannot
understand his present mode of communication or that he is not
receiving communication from others adequately.*

*Formation of relationships with other patients which often
result in more interaction among patients on the ward between group
meetings and less sitting and staring into space during hours when
activities are not scheduled.*

*Increased feeling of community with others and the consequent
lessening of the anxiety and anger that accompany feelings of being
shut out and ignored by other people.*

This last-mentioned benefit is supported by some evidence that simply
being required to function as a group member is therapeutic, even if the
group does not discuss psychiatric problems. One study which seems to
demonstrate this is the experiment by Anker and Walsh[1] in which
matched groups of long-term schizophrenic patients were assigned either to
group therapy or to produce plays for the entertainment of the hospital
population. The plays were not psychodrama, but were selected by the
patients from books of plays. The group therapy was in charge of a
trained therapist, but the drama group had no staff help except for a
recreation leader who was told to help the patients obtain materials for
scenery, costumes, and so on but to furnish no other leadership.
Observations and tests of the two groups over a one-year period indicated
that the drama group had made the greater improvement.

One can only speculate about why the activity group members
improved more than the patients in the therapy group. One possibility is
that if destructive or deteriorating personality changes can take place
without a patient's conscious knowledge of the process, reconstructive
changes can also take place unconsciously when conditions encourage such
change. Apparently cooperative interaction with peers in and of itself was
enough to produce some constructive changes even without development
of the insight which, in chronic schizophrenic patients, is so difficult to
achieve without arousing the anxiety, despair, and opposition that may
make them regress when talk is directed to their problems, failures, and
traumatic experiences.

The following checklist contains a set of considerations about which
a nurse or other staff member undertaking the leadership of a group of
psychiatric patients would find it profitable to become self-conscious.
Some of the items have been suggested by literature from psychology on

group techniques; others reflect questions that have been asked or problems that have arisen with nursing personnel new to group work. The items fall into two categories: those which pertain to the decisions that should be made before a group is started and those which relate to the abilities needed by the leader.

PRELIMINARY DECISIONS

In planning to initiate a patient group, the leader might well answer the following questions.

What do I most want to help the members of this group to achieve? Among the possible goals are:

Socialization.

Independence and initiative.

Increased sense of well-being.

Learning to cooperate in problem solving.

Productivity from work on a project of mutual benefit.

Insight.

Stimulation of energy and interest.

On what basis shall I choose my patients? Mixture of personalities and diagnostic categories. Many experienced group therapists feel such a mixture is the most beneficial arrangement for the patients.

One special problem, such as drinking, epilepsy, blindness, orientation to the hospital, or preparation for discharge.

Similar diagnosis. This criterion would be a very difficult one to use with groups of withdrawn psychotic patients, but groups of neurotic patients sometimes work well together, as do groups of drug or alcoholic addicts.

Similar ability in verbal expression and abstract thought.

Emotional level.

Sociometric similarity—that is, putting patients who like working together in the same group. This can be done by getting patients to indicate preferences in individual interviews before the group is established.

The patient's choice that results from permitting each patient to choose one of several available interest groups.

How large will my group be? Why this size? How is the size I select related to group goals? If the group goal is to apply pressure outside the group, a large group is effective (as with a political party or a labor union). If the group goals include the full functioning of every member, a small group (five to fifteen) is better.

What type of leadership shall I try to maintain? Why?

Democratic. Such leadership results in more friendliness, group mindedness, motivation, and originality.

Authoritarian. More work is done, but more discontent, hostility, and dependency may develop. Nonetheless this type of leadership may be better in some kinds of group therapy, especially short-term therapy in which the aim is suppression of sensitive material and the patients' acceptance of practical arrangements for living, in contrast to long-term therapy aimed at the patients' development of insight into their unconscious feelings.

Laissez-faire. The quality and quantity of work may be less, but this approach may be best for some chronic patients who need to be placed in a position of setting up their own organization.[2,3]

CHECKLIST FOR SELF-APPRAISAL

How do I appraise myself as a leader according to the following criteria? In which areas would I like to improve?

Am I successful in reducing the patients' anxiety about participating in this group?

Do I let the patients become acquainted with me before the group begins?

Do I relate to patients with warmth, supportiveness, and nonthreatening humor during the orientation phase?

Do I arrange for comfortable surroundings and refreshments if appropriate?

Do I exhibit a matter-of-fact, businesslike attitude if the group includes many patients who tend to be suspicious of direct friendliness?

Do I reward participation or otherwise promote progress toward group goals? Do I use verbal conditioning, smiling, nodding, and so on, or more direct praise or statement of approval?

Have I established expectations among the patients that participation is the group norm? This is most easily done while the patients are new in the group. The most frequent error of new group leaders is to make a long preliminary speech at the first session.

Am I successful in drawing out persons so that all members participate? The leader achieves this goal by:

Accepting contributions.

Making reluctant individuals feel their ideas are wanted and needed.

Preventing talkative individuals from dominating without rejecting them.

Keeping discussion and activity moving forward.

Accepting the feelings and attitudes of all participants as valid points for consideration.

Protecting individuals whom other group members might attack verbally.

Accepting conflict or disagreement in the group as therapeutic if it is expressed with reasonable appropriateness.

Do I "wait out" pauses? Usually the group "takes over" more after the first few pauses.

Do I hear the ideas and feelings expressed and restate them accurately in shorter, more pointed, clearer form? In this way the leader shows he is paying attention, understands what is said, and accepts the views of the person who expresses them. This kind of acceptance does not always mean agreement, but in demonstrating it the leader shows that he respects the right of every member to contribute.

Am I sensitive to nonverbal communication from group members? For example, silence can connote concentration, hostility, or lack of interest, and it is important for the group leader to know which of these attitudes is being reflected. She also should be able to identify restlessness and other feelings reflected in nonverbal communication.

Do I ask questions which stimulate problem-solving behavior? Among such questions are those which clarify situations that have been unclearly described, those which inquire about the emotions surrounding a situation, and those which promote investigation of alternative solutions. The questions should be difficult enough to keep the patients interested. Good questions direct exploration along fruitful lines as well as prevent the persistence of thinking in areas where failure has repeatedly been experienced. Questions which the group members see as threatening rather than helpful should be avoided.

How much did I learn about each patient before the group started?

How well am I keeping up contact with the patients between group sessions and learning about them outside of the group? Knowing group members well enhances the leader's ability to ask questions of the appropriate member if the occasion arises. Also, if patients already know and trust the leader, they are more likely to feel secure in answering questions. Knowing the patients also enables the group leader to promote group cohesiveness by pointing out the similarities among some group members or to promote interaction by pointing out differences in viewpoint or in experiences among them.

Do I summarize as the need arises? This important skill can be used to:

Move the discussion along.

Indicate progress.

Restate the problem in new form in light of the discussion.

Point up the fact that differences exist in the group and that these differences are part of the problem.

Am I receiving genuine feedback on the verbal level? If not, why are patients not telling me what they think and how they feel?

Do I maintain standards that are high enough to keep the group interested and to prevent fake questions and the selection of tasks that are too easy or too difficult? Do I keep the group moving toward new problems and activities as they tire of old ones and thus promote a sense of momentum?
Am I varying techniques and formats for meetings in order to keep interest up? Some possibilities are:

Pictures and equipment, relevant to topics being discussed. It is desirable for these materials to be collected with the help of a patient or a patient committee.

Role playing.

Goal-directed fantasy, a technique which involves helping the patients to talk about things they would like to do as part of the motivation program.[4]

Psychodrama.

Didactic sessions characterized by lectures which give patients information that is new to them followed by discussion.

Film followed by discussion.

Outings.

"Guest leaders"—that is, volunteers or other staff members expert in some topics of interest to the group.

Group tasks selected and approved by the group.

Group recreational activities selected by the group.

Do I display ingenuity in arranging for the group to do its own work? The leader should not perform any task, however small, that a patient or a committee of patients could do. Even such a small job as arranging the chairs in a circle for the meeting should be left to the group members if they can accomplish it. Is my attitude that of getting the group to learn to solve problems with me, or do I tell them what to do?

Am I alert to every opportunity to give the group as much real power to make choices as possible? Patient groups usually prove to be more conservative than staff when they are permitted to make choices and may often be trusted to make appropriate decisions about matters that affect them. Some psychiatric hospitals now permit patient groups to have considerable choice in setting schedules for their unit, making and enforcing many of their own rules, and setting up most of their own recreational programs. The effective group leader limits himself to supplying essential facts and clarifying the areas of choice without suggesting the decision. For example, if the group has decided to have a party, the leader might have to tell them what the amount of money and the times available are, but should let the group decide how to spend the time and money as long as the decisions are within permissible limits.

Do I turn activity and responsibility over to the group as soon as possible and keep turning it back to them as needed? In many psychiatric patient groups the turning of responsibility back to the group has to be repeated frequently.

Am I using group deviants wisely? The quantity of interaction increases when a deviant is in the group, and recognition and discussion of differences of opinion make a group more active. However, in some cases the leader should intervene to prevent a deviant from being subjected to a harmful degree of scapegoating. Among psychiatric patients, scapegoating seems to occur most often when there is strong external pressure on the group or when an especially odd or deviant patient arouses fears in the other patients that they may resemble him. When strong pressure for scapegoating appears in a group, direct suppression is not always the most effective way of stopping it; the leader should also look for and deal with feelings of individual worthlessness among patients, fear of revelation of weakness, and fear of similarity to the scapegoat.

Am I contributing to group cohesiveness? Cohesiveness is highest when goals are strongly desired and agreed on and when the means for achieving them and the norms are agreed on. The leader can facilitate cohesiveness by encouraging the group to make its own choices, to talk out and resolve differences, and to review and alter goals as needed. The leader of a group of psychiatric patients can usually work best by helping the patients do the work of facilitating progress toward their own goals, but if there is an influential group member who tries to persuade the group to adopt unhealthy goals, the leader must sometimes exert her influence to help the group maintain goals that will be therapeutic for the members. This threat to therapeutic goals is most likely to occur in a group of adolescent patients or in one with several adult sociopaths.

What am I doing to develop leadership among the patients?

Rewarding it?

Encouraging the ability of some patients to draw out others?

Encouraging the patients to direct questions and remarks to each other rather than to me?

Sitting back quietly whenever possible?

Am I encouraging shared or circulating leadership among the patients instead of merely replacing a "staff leader" with a "patient leader"?

Am I bringing in new members or removing present members from time to time when therapeutic considerations indicate this?

Am I bringing new members into the group at the best time for them? Research has shown that many people seem much more attracted to interaction in groups when their anxiety is high because of changes in or uncertainty about their own situations. This finding would seem to indicate that the best time to move many patients into a group is when they have just been brought into the hospital or moved to a new setting within the hospital or when changes in staff or in hospital procedures have increased their anxiety.

Is the group actually moving toward goals? How can I facilitate this progress more? Most group progress occurs when the group has chosen goals and agreed on methods of reaching them. If it is not possible for the patients to choose all of their goals, maximum progress will occur if they see the goals as important to them and agree on ways to reach them. Progress is also facilitated if the group leader keeps the group aware of gains they are making, and keeps further goals visible to them.

Am I flexible enough to revise goals as patients progress or other circumstances change?

Probably no group leader will ever reach the point where she can honestly respond "Yes, I always succeed in doing this" to every question on this list. But the group leader who, as she periodically checks her performance against the list, finds that her answers are progressing from "sometimes" to "often" to "usually" will not only experience the rewards that come from observing improvement in patients, but also the satisfaction that occurs when one realizes one's own growth and one's increasing effectiveness in working with patients.

References

1. Anker, J. M., and Walsh, R. P.: "Group Psychotherapy, A Special Activity Program and Group Structure in the Treatment of Chronic Schizophrenia," *Journal of Consulting Psychiatry*, 1961, 25:476–481.

2. White, R., and Lippitt, R.: "Leader Behavior and Member Reaction in Three 'Social Climates'." In D. Cartwright and A. Zander (eds.) *Group Dynamics*, Evanston, Ill.: Row Peterson, 1953, Ch. 40.

3. Mullan, H., and Rosenbaum, M.: *Group Psychotherapy*, New York: Free Press of Glencoe, 1968.

4. McClelland, D. C.: "Toward a Theory of Motive Acquisition," *American Psychologist*, 1965, 20:321–333.

Bibliography

Armstrong, S. W. and Rouslin, S.: *Group Psychotherapy in Nursing Practice*, New York: Macmillan Co., 1963.

Goldstein, A. P., Heller, K., and Sechrest, L. B.: *Psychotherapy and the Psychology of Behavior Change*, New York: John Wiley and Sons, 1966.

Lewin, K., Lippitt, R., and White, R.: "Patterns of Aggressive Behavior in Experimentally Created 'Social Climates,'" *Journal of Social Psychology*, 1939, 10:271–299.

Maier, N.: *Psychology in Industry*, Boston: Houghton Mifflin Co., 1965.

Chapter Twenty-Three

USE OF THE NURSING PROCESS TO FACILITATE GROUP THERAPY

Lynda W. Slimmer

REGARDLESS OF A PSYCHIATRIC client's diagnosis, his primary problems include ineffective problem-solving ability, faulty reality testing, and difficulty with interpersonal relationships. The intended use of group therapy in psychiatric-mental health treatment settings is to offer the client needed ego support and a safe environment in which he can practice problem solving, reality testing, and relating with others. However, often the intended purpose of the group is not fully realized because the group leader does not examine the group process and plan her subsequent interventions according to what is happening in the group. I have found that I am most effective as a group therapist and that my clients benefit most from the group experience if I apply the steps of the nursing process to my leadership behaviors. After each group session, I assess what occurred in the group; compile and/or update a titled, numbered problem list for the group; plan what interventions to employ at the next session; and evaluate the effectiveness of the interventions that I have just employed at the previous session.

Therapists have long used theoretical models to explain or predict

From "Use of the Nursing Process to Facilitate Group Therapy," by Lynda W. Slimmer, *Journal of Psychiatric Nursing and Mental Health Services*, February 1978, Volume 16, pp. 42–44. Reprinted by permission of SLACK, Inc., Medical Publishers, Thorofare, NJ.

group phenomena. However, too often the use of the model is an intellectual exercise and the knowledge gained is not actually used by the therapist to enhance the group experience. Although there are many group theoretical models, I have found three of them most useful as group assessment guides: the focal-conflict model, the communication model, and the group dynamics model.

The focal-conflict model is based on the premise that everything that occurs in a group is caused by an underlying, here and now concern shared by all group members. This concern or focal conflict has two components: a wish or disturbing motive and a fear or reactive motive.[1] The disturbing motive usually concerns something the clients would like to do, but that is difficult for them because of their problem in relating with others; for example, they may wish to openly reveal their feelings to the group. The reactive motive usually concerns a fear or reservation that they have about actually carrying out what they would like to do because of negative experiences they have had in the past; for example, they fear that if they openly reveal their feelings to the group, the other group members may ridicule them as others have in the past. The conflict between the wish and the fear causes anxiety within the group. The group works to decrease this anxiety by finding a solution that will reduce the fear while allowing them to satisfy the wish as much as possible. Thus, the overt behavior seen in the group is a result of the group members' unconscious efforts to work out solutions to focal conflicts. An example of such a solution is shown in Figure 1.

FIGURE 1

Disturbing Motive (wish)
wish to show anger toward therapist for not selecting discussion topic.

Reactive Motive (fear)
fear that therapist will abandon them or be angry with them if they do not comply with her request to select own discussion topic.

Solution
(decreased fear and partially fulfilled wish)
discuss how chaotic the hospital library is because the librarian will not help you find material to read that is of interest (Group selected own topic, but displaced its anger toward the therapist onto the librarian.)

After employing the focal-conflict model to assess what is occurring in a group, I make a nursing diagnosis or compile a problem list for the group that comes directly from information I now have concerning the group's focal conflict. The problems usually concern feelings that group members have that contribute to the fear or unhealthy coping mechanisms they use to decrease the fear. Using the above example of a group's focal conflict, the problem list would include: 1. Mistrust of leader, 2. Displacement of anger.

The goal of the leader who uses the focal-conflict model is to facilitate the group members' ability to satisfy their wish. The leader can accomplish this goal through the use of interventions which resolve the identified problems. If displacement of anger is a problem, then the leader assists group members to recognize the real source of their anger, allows them to role play being angry, and serves as a role model by consistently expressing her true feelings in a therapeutic manner. When using the focal-conflict model, evaluating the effectiveness of interventions can easily be done by determining if identified problems have been resolved and a specific group wish has been fulfilled.

The communication model is based on five propositions:

1. Communication is inevitable; one cannot not communicate.

2. Communication is a multilevel phenomenon; messages may impart content information and/or describe the relationship the sender wants to have with the receiver.

3. Messages connote and denote; the message sent is not necessarily the message received.

4. Communication has overt and covert elements; the sender is aware of and can control his overt communication, but he is not aware of and has little control of his covert communication such as body language and tone of voice.

5. Dysfunctional communication results if the sender cannot assume the responsibility for interpersonal interaction; if a person feels unable to handle the feelings that he has or the responses of others to his feelings, he will avoid directly communicating these feelings.[2]

When using the communication model to assess what occurs in a group, I look at who talked and who did not talk; I examine what content information was given in the group and how various members communicated to the group their desired relationship with the group; I determine whether messages sent were messages received; I determine whether the covert communication of members was consistent with the overt communication; and I describe any dysfunctional communication observed. From this assessment, a problem list can be compiled, such as the following:

1. Two non-participating members.

2. Group members choose to attend to information content only and ignore statements about relationships.

3. Negative feedback sent is not received.

4. Double-bind messages being sent.

5. Members intellectualize and do not reveal gut feelings.

The goal of the leader who uses the communication model is to facilitate group members' ability to communicate effectively. The leader can accomplish this goal through the use of interventions which resolve the identified problems. For example, if non-participating members are a problem, the leader points out to such members that their lack of active participation is actually communicating something to the group and assists them to verbalize what they are feeling. The leader may simply acknowledge the non-verbal message (Paul, your body is very tense.); she may acknowledge the non-verbal message with understanding (Paul, your body is very tense. This conversation is making you angry.); or she may acknowledge the non-verbal message without understanding (Paul, your body is very tense, but I'm not sure I know what that means.). Each of the above interventions lets the group member know that someone care enough to try to understand what he is thinking or feeling and provides him with an opportunity to verbally respond. The leader can best assist the group to learn effective communicating by being a model communicator. When using the communication model, evaluation of intervention effectiveness can be done by determining if identified problems have been resolved and behavioral criteria for healthy communication are being met.

The group dynamics model is based on three propositions:

1. Groups are in a constant state of flux; the interactional patterns and emotional tone is dynamic, not static.

2. Group movement has stages usually related to the group's level of cohesion.

3. Groups may develop in a healthy or an unhealthy manner; healthy development allows effective decision making to occur;[2] healthy development necessitates an effective leadership style, appropriate structure, effective role fulfillment, adequate norms, and cohesion.

When using the group dynamics model to assess what occurs in a group, first, I examine sociograms that were made during the group session to determine the interactional pattern of the group. Second, I write a content process recording for each session so I have a record of how decision making was done; in addition, I describe in the process recording the body language of each member as he participates and the overall emotional atmosphere of the group as it changes. Third, I assess five primary group properties: (1) Is the structure of the group formal or informal? (2) Who plays what role in the group? (3) What norms govern the group? (4) What is the level of cohesion? (5) What is the leadership style?

From this assessment, I can determine what interactional problems the group is experiencing. Such a problem list might include:

1. Lack of cohesion.

2. Autocratic leadership.

3. Group norm does not allow anger to be vented openly.

4. Each member directs all communication to leader.

5. Group anxiety level high.

The goal of the leader who uses the group dynamics model is to facilitate the group's ability to develop in a healthy manner.[2] This healthy development can occur if interventions are directed toward resolving the identified problems. If a problem is lack of cohesion, the leader can increase cohesion by assisting members to discover similarities among themselves (hobbies), selecting topics for discussion that focus on common concerns, and helping members identify common difficulties in coping. When using this model, the evaluation of intervention effectiveness is done by determining if identified problems have been resolved and effective decision making occurs in the group.

After one becomes skilled in using one of the specific theoretical models to assess what occurs in a group, she may choose to employ a more eclectic approach to group assessment. She may select parts from several models that she is most comfortable using and devise her own group assessment tool. For example, when I use the focal-conflict model, I also assess the group properties (roles, structure, cohesion, leadership style, norms) because I feel such an assessment tells me more about how the group members may choose to resolve the conflict.

The most important guidelines to remember when using the nursing process to facilitate group therapy are: (1) identified problems must relate to whatever model is being used as an assessment guide; (2) problems must relate to the group as a whole, and not be a member's individual problem; and (3) interventions must be directed toward specific problems.

The schematic representation shown in Figure 2 might be used to organize the therapeutic plan for a group.

FIGURE 2

Therapeutic Model Used as Assessment Guide: Communication

Problem (title and number)	Intervention	Rationale (for intervention)	Criteria for Evaluation
1. Non-participating members	Acknowledge non-verbal messages without understanding.	Lets member know that someone cares enough to try to understand what he is thinking or feeling. Provides member with opportunity to verbally respond.	Member states what he is thinking or feeling.

232

References

1. Whitaker, D., Lieberman, M. *Psychotherapy Through the Group Process.* New York, Atherton Press, 1970, Ch. 2.

2. Marram, G. *The Group Approach in Nursing Practice.* St. Louis, C. V. Mosby Co., 1973, pp. 103–112.

Chapter Twenty-Four

HOW CAN AN ALCOHOLIC CHANGE IN 28 DAYS?

Alma C. Yearwood and Susanne K. Hess

ON HIS FIRST DAY in the therapy group, Gene radiated hostility. He sat with his arms folded over his chest. His eyes, narrowed in a defiant glare, seemed to dare anyone to come close.

As with most alcoholic patients, he had started treatment under duress. For him, it was fear of an enlarged liver that his doctor had told him was caused by his drinking. His wife had threatened to leave him and his job was in jeopardy, but Gene was unable to relate these facts to his drinking. Instead, he blamed such external pressures as these for his problems and saw no reason to change his own actions. The task of the group was clear—to help him make the transition from external blame to internal motivation for change.

The patient group Gene joined was one of several that meet daily at the Smithers Rehabilitation Unit, part of the Smithers Alcoholism Treatment and Training Center of Roosevelt Hospital, New York City. The rehabilitation unit, located in a renovated mansion, has a 51-bed capacity (32 male, 19 female). The patient population is socially and economically mixed. The patients are 16 years of age or older, ambulatory, able to participate in an English-speaking therapeutic community and, in addition to their alcoholism, may have a problem with

From "How Can an Alcoholic Change in 28 Days?" by Alma C. Yearwood and Susanne K. Hess. Copyright © 1979, American Journal of Nursing Company. Reproduced with permission from *American Journal of Nursing*, August, Vol. 78, No. 8, pp. 1436–1438.

other mood-altering chemicals. Their stay is a minimum of 28 days (although no one is kept against his or her will). In addition, patients must be free of psychoactive drugs (including tranquilizers and antidepressants, and so forth) while at the rehabilitation unit. Alcohol detoxification can be managed during the first five days at Smithers if the physical dependency is minimal and if the patient is sufficiently lucid to understand the commitment he is making to treatment.

Gene is a prototype of the alcoholic who exists in a world with a population of one—himself. The alcoholic is inner-directed and totally self-absorbed. He or she has a low frustration tolerance—inability to deal with stress, no reciprocal relationships, and a lack of self-reliance. To say definitely whether or not these psychodynamics occur before addiction is beyond the scope of this paper. Rather, we will focus on some of the personality issues that unfold within a short-term group such as ours, and what *beginnings* of change can occur.

Alcoholism is a form of behavior that one might look at from different dynamic points of view. According to one psychoanalytic theory, excessive dependency needs in later life are often the consequence of early inadequate mothering. The early lack of gratification is later experienced by the alcoholic as an emptiness that must be filled from outside. Since all energies are focused on suppressing the deprivation, there are no emotional forces left to tolerate tension, endure frustration, or establish meaningful interpersonal relationships.

Optimally, the mother provides a "benign environment" in which the child can grow and develop coping mechanisms. D. W. Winnicott speaks of the "benign environment" as the optimal surroundings in which an infant can gradually internalize the mother's strong ego and develop the capacity to be in touch with his own internal experience.[1] Not having this secure atmosphere, the alcoholic finds, in alcohol, an illusory and fantasied substitute for the missed state of oneness with the mother.

Lester Farber finds that intrinsic to the addictive personality is the assumption that life cannot be lived without drugs. Chemicals or alcohol are used in an attempt to compensate for or ease the feelings of overwhelming emptiness brought about by early inadequate mothering.[2] As the disease progresses, this escape becomes the crux of the alcoholic's existence as external and internal discomfort has to be masked. Each time discomfort is masked and not experienced, the capacity for effective coping is diminished.

At the Smithers Rehabilitation Unit, the primary task of the therapy group is to provide the "benign" environment in which the alcoholic can become aware of his internal experience and risk new ways of behaving. The group provides ego strength that the patient can borrow, in a sense supplying the experience missing from childhood.

Within 24 hours after admission, each patient is assigned to an ongoing group consisting of 10 members and 2 cotherapists. On the first day, a contract is established with the group, for recovery is dependent upon the patients' ability to identify with each other. This therapeutic dynamic of group identification is the foundation upon which the group work rests. For example, despite Gene's defensive posture, sitting within the group and listening to other members tell how they, too, blamed others for their drinking began the process of group identification for him.

Listening to another member relate her panic when rushed to the hospital hemorrhaging from esophageal varices provided a point of identification for Gene. The therapist was able to use Gene's fear of liver disease to begin to confront his defense strategy of rationalization. Defense strategies continue in the recovering alcoholic and need to be confronted in treatment. They include rationalization of use, projection of blame, and denial, which allow the alcoholic to continue drinking in the face of disastrous consequences because a favorable view of reality is maintained. As one patient explained to Gene, "I could live life as it's supposed to be rather than as it is."

It is unrealistic to expect that there always will be a permanent characterological change in patients in a short-term group. However, the beginning of change can be effected. In order to facilitate change, the therapist needs to know some of the curative factors provided by the group experience.[3] For example, as his denial is confronted, the alcoholic is faced with the reality of his drunken behavior and its consequences. In expressing shame and embarrassment, patients relate feelings of isolation and uniqueness. One of the goals of the group is to alleviate this empty, lonely feeling through the discovery that we are all human and, therefore, more similar than different.

A curative factor in the ongoing group process is imparting information. By explaining that blackouts (periods of temporary amnesia), persistent remorse, resentments, and indefinable fears are some of the symptoms of chemical dependency, anxiety may be alleviated in patients who often feel that they have "gone mad."

For recovery to be enduring, interpersonal learning must occur. Our personality is almost entirely the product of interaction with significant others. The group, therefore, helps a patient learn how others perceive and experience him in contrast to how he perceives and experiences himself. Hopefully change can occur by encouraging the patient to recognize, to integrate, and to give free expression to previously denied parts of himself. The therapist can encourage such interpersonal learning by giving assignments; for example, revealing three previously undisclosed secrets in the group atmosphere of acceptance assists integration of a disowned part of the self. In fact, what often happens is that the patient becomes aware of the universality of the human experience.

After a period of time in the group, Gene was asked to give three self-descriptive adjectives. The group, in turn, gave three descriptive adjectives of him. Gene described himself as "shy, insecure, and unable to express myself." The group said he was "proud, angry, and arrogant." The therapist helped him explore the discrepancy between the two perceptions. Gene learned that while he thought his questioning others was helpful, others felt they were being interrogated. Thus, the group provides external reality testing that gradually can become internalized.

The therapist, at all times, must be aware of the patient's particular way of interacting within the group that mirrors his disordered interpersonal relations. For example, Gene's condescending judgmentalism not only isolated him from his children at home, but soon began to isolate him from his peers. The other patients were encouraged to talk, rather than act to isolate him, while Gene was encouraged to voice his experience of being isolated, the role he played in it, and whether or not he wanted to change it.

At all times, the use of alcohol is explored in terms of easing the anxieties of living and relating to others. It is important to acquaint the patient with the way he has been using alcohol to minimize or avoid anxiety. The group provides a forum for exploring painful past drunken behavior in the here-and-now while exploring more effective ways of coping in the future without the use of a chemical.

The therapist helps the patient accept responsibility for his behavior. For example, Gene, who believed that alcohol made him more outgoing and more productive, minimized the difficulties he would have being abstinent after discharge. The group confronted the romantic ideas he had about his drinking times, for instance, that he had been productive when, in fact, his employer had been instrumental in his coming to treatment.

Gene was asked to fantasize an abstinent day hour by hour. He was unable to do this. The anxiety he experienced by having to face his customary drinking times without a drink was shared by the group who then helped define what resources he had for coping. With each new experience of frustration, stress, anxiety—all of the previously denied emotions—an adaptive spiral of coping is set into motion. Although it was uncomfortable for Gene, he was able to accept the group's confrontation of his behavior, which was the beginning of a more realistic self-appraisal.

Termination from the group is as important as the introduction to the group. The patient is helped to reexamine the original goals he set for himself, what he has accomplished, and what is left undone.

Optimally, the patient has begun to internalize some of the acceptance and understanding from the group, which will enable him to carry the new behavior learned. There is the hope that the beginning of self-reliance has been accomplished in this short time and that further support through AA and other treatment modalities will be sought.

Since his discharge, Gene has continued to examine his way of relating to others, which has helped him to become a more tolerant and caring family member. As his recovery progresses, his increasing awareness of chemical-free competence has enabled him to be a more productive employee. His profitable group experience serves as a foundation on which he continues to build.

References

1. Winnicott, D. W. *The Maturational Processes and the Facilitating Environment.* New York, International Universities Press, 1965.

2. Farber, L. H. Our kindly family physician, chief crazy horse. In *Lying, Despair, Jealousy, Envy, Sex, Suicide, Drugs and the Good Life.* New York, Basic Books, 1976, pp. 106–119.

3. Yalom, I. D. *The Theory and Practice of Group Psychotherapy.* 2nd ed. New York, Basic Books, 1975.

Chapter Twenty-Five

INTERVENTION AND INVESTMENT IN COMMUNITY MENTAL HEALTH—A FAMILY IN CRISIS

Faye Gary Harris and Marilyn S. Fregly

WHILE STUDYING FOR A master's degree in psychiatric nursing, I worked for five months with a family of seventeen members who during this period underwent four major crises. My method of therapy was based upon the preventive psychiatry model of Gerald Caplan and the crisis theory of Erich Lindemann.

THE HIGGINS FAMILY

The Higgins family, consisting of the parents, thirteen children, and two grandchildren, live on the west side of Chicago in a rapidly changing suburb. The drab, overcrowded buildings with broken windows, rickety staircases, and dank odors symbolize the basic discouragement the

From "Intervention and Investment in Community Mental Health — A Family in Crisis," by Faye Gary Harris and Marilyn S. Fregly, *Nursing Clinics of North America*, December, 1971, Vol. 6, No. 4, pp. 769–784. Reprinted by permission.

inhabitants feel toward their lives. The same incohesive structure is found in the family unit, huddled in a thrown-together style, each member "doing his own thing" without much awareness of the consequences of his individual actions on the others.

My introduction to the family occurred when the principal of the grade school where I conducted group therapy with emotionally disturbed students referred Mrs. Higgins to me. She had come for help in dealing with her 10-year-old son who attended the school. Our first meetings were at the school, but because of baby-sitting problems we agreed to meet in her home. In the home we were surrounded and frequently interrupted by her many children. The conditions were not exactly ideal for a satisfactory interchange, so we often used the telephone in the evenings as a means of holding a one-to-one conversation.

Mrs. Higgins is a 35-year-old black mother of thirteen children and has two grandchildren. The children range in age from two months to 24 years. Though living under deplorable conditions, she keeps herself and her children clean. She also seeks self-improvement for them and herself. She related with some enthusiasm her experiences in the adult education program held at night at the community school, her parts in plays there, and how she tutors her younger children with their homework, as well as preparing them for school in the morning.

Her interest in her children showed on our first meeting in the principal's office, a familiar place for her but a relatively strange one to me. She knew the physical structure of the building and was pleased to show me around—to the ladies' lounge, to her children's classroom, and to the rooms of teachers she knew. She assumed a leadership role and I enjoyed following her.

However, she was not completely at ease at the school or with me. She never removed her coat and scarf. She always said, "No, thank you. I will keep it on because I cannot stay too long this time," yet she stayed at least an hour each time. When she indicated that it was time to go, I tried to end the session by planning for the next one. "We will see each other next week same time and same station." Also, I wrote her name and the time of the next session in a notebook and put an asterisk by it with a comment, "I will be here waiting for you; see you next week." She liked the special attention and the feeling of importance that I tried to create. I tried to convey the message that on a particular day, at a particular time, my only concern was to see her—everything else was secondary.

Her concern about her "importance" and her "impression on me" was apparent at our fourth session, the first held in her home. I arrived early in the midst of her cleaning. She was apologetic for not having the house in order. I told her, "I understand about the house not being tidy. I am a member of a large family too." We both chuckled as she moved various articles from a chair to give me a seat. Yet almost by an unconscious time mechanism, she communicated that my visit here, too, was to last for one hour. "My, it is almost time for Judy to go to school, and I have not even started to get her ready. I got to fix lunch for my children." She also communicated this nonverbally: her hand twisting, looking out the window, turning the TV on and adjusting it many times, and making frequent comments to her children about their behavior. As I left, I wrote her name in my notebook, the time I would return, and the big asterisk. I hoped to convey the same message of significance and importance.

After a few more visits in her home, I learned each of her children's names and something about them in order to fix their names and individualities in my memory. Whenever family members were present, which was usually the case, I always chatted with them before starting the session.

Because chores had such a high priority, Mrs. Higgins' kitchen became the focal spot for our conversations. While we talked, she prepared lunch, ironed, and tended the children. She impressed me as a warm person who was overwhelmed by her family and its many problems. But when she came to talk about these problems, she became defensive and talked as if she were an outsider looking in.

I discovered at the end of the first home visit that Mr. Higgins had been sent out of the house, not to return until 12 noon, after I had left. For this reason, I decided that I should always call before coming to the house. I found out why when I met Mr. Higgins.

THE UNSEEN
OTHER FORCE

Mrs. Higgins' restless behavior and her side remarks about Mr. Higgins led me to wonder about her fear of him and her fear of his disapproval of my being there.

I met Mr. Higgins on my fifth visit. He looked me up and down, from head to foot. I stood up to acknowledge his presence, extended my hand, and he shook it. Mrs. Higgins fell silent when he entered. He took the aggressive leadership role, and seemed hostile. "What you here for, and how long you be here?" I responded: "I am here because I want to help you with some of the problems you are having. I think I can be of some help, and I hope you will allow me to try. I will leave at any time you suggest, but I am hoping you will allow me to stay in your home so that we can work together."

He fired more questions at me: "Where are you from? About how old are you? Who told you about us? Who do you work for?" I answered each question truthfully and fully. After I had responded to his barrage of questions, he voluntarily began to talk about himself. By the end of the session, he had relaxed and was less defensive. He invited me to come again and we shook hands when I left. Having met him, I felt I could win his trust and confidence as well as continue coming back to the home. He was concerned about the family name, about what the neighbors would think if they learned he was not "man" enough to handle his own family. I assured him his family would not be discussed with anyone but my colleagues.

Mr. Higgins always asked about my little blue book (of process notes). I told him the notes were recorded and shared with my teacher. I offered to share the notes with him or any member of the family who chose to read them. They never read them, but occasionally he would ask, "How the notes coming?"

He was also suspicious of his wife's telephone conversations with me. One morning I called to say I would be late because of bad weather and Mr. Higgins, who answered the phone, advised me to stay home. I did not go.

One reason for the lack of trust on the part of both parents was my age. Mrs. Higgins had difficulty in perceiving me as a person with ability to be therapeutically helpful because she had a daughter as old as I. Her daughter was not helpful to her; therefore, she associated youth with immaturity, lack of knowledge, and understanding.

It took about five weeks and ten visits to establish myself in their confidence as a decent and genuine human being as well as a competent member of the therapy team.

FOUR CRISES

During my five months' work with the family, four crises developed, any one of which could have destroyed the already tenuous family unit and produced new problems for the "uninvolved" members.

The first crisis involved Bill, the seventh child, a hefty 10-year-old who prided himself on being "the toughest kid in the neighborhood." Bill was already being seen by another member of the health team.

The center of another crisis was Judy, the fourth child, a shy 15-year-old whose assets were seen in her interest in cooking and in tending to the younger children. She became an unwed mother during the period of intervention.

Mary, the fifth child, an obedient but hostile 14-year-old, was described as "fast and selfish" with no interest in home responsibilities. The onset of menses produced another problem as Mary threatened to have sexual relations with her boy friend, which started a power struggle between her mother as to who was to set the limits for night hours.

The fourth crisis involved Mrs. Higgins herself when she sought and accepted employment. Her step toward economic independence threatened the weak ego structure of her unemployed husband as well as the traditional family role pattern.

Crisis One

Bill had broken into the school building during the weekend with a group of boys who lived in the neighborhood. He had been taken, with the others, to the district police station for questioning. Bill did not mention the incident to his parents, but another neighborhood boy did. The parents completely denied the neighbor boy's statement and said nothing to Bill.

The principal told Mrs. Higgins about the incident when she came to school to keep her appointment with me the following week. During our session Mrs. Higgins cried, then we sat in silence for a long time. When Mrs. Higgins did speak, she expressed guilt and a feeling of failure. "Maybe I could have helped my little boy more than I did." The guilt was explored to some extent by allowing Mrs. Higgins to talk about her feelings concerning Bill. She tried to place blame on her husband as the cause of all the family's misfortunes and failures: "My husband could help too. I have everything to do. Jim will not cooperate." But her attempt to absolve herself was not successful because, as she talked, she grew progressively sadder in expression, her voice became softer, her hand twisting increased, and she shifted positions in her chair many times. When the session ended, we agreed to meet at her home the following week, at which time we would focus on Bill, as we had agreed to during previous sessions.

Mr. Higgins was present when I arrived, and much of my time was spent answering questions he posed concerning myself and my credentials: "Where are you from? Where do you go to school? How long have you been in the city? Is your family here, or do you live alone?" Mr. Higgins showed anger toward and impatience with his son, frequently referring to Bill as being "bull-headed" and "a toughie" who was trying to "get away with everything." He boasted that he punished Bill by beating him with the cord of an electric iron. In fact, he said, "I am the best beater that you have ever seen."

Before the police incident could be completely explored by Mrs. Higgins and me, it was compounded by Bill's attack on a teacher at school. Apparently the teacher had irritated Bill, and he swung at her. Several male teachers were needed to subdue him. The mother was not at home when the principal called, but Mr. Higgins was. He went to the school and returned in a rage, cursing, slamming doors, threatening any available family member, and kicking furniture.

In the meanwhile, the entire family was affected by the parents' attitude toward Bill. Mr. Higgins had instructed Bill to remain quiet in the household. He was to have small portions of food and was not permitted to make the slightest complaint. He was screamed at not only by the parents, but by other brothers and sisters as well. He was laughed at and called names by his brothers and sisters. Both the mother and Bill's therapist agreed in their reporting that Bill was becoming hostile and withdrawn.

During the sessions in the home Mr. Higgins showed his helpless rage toward Bill. He began to compare Bill with Hitler: "He wants to push people around—he wants to have his way." He described to me how he beat Bill. I listened to the outburst of hostility and recognized that the entire household was angry with Bill. Although she was on the verge of tears, the mother was not able to express her feelings, but Mr. Higgins continued loudly and clearly: "That boy is no good. He has caused me nothing but worry and trouble. I am getting tired of him." When the parents were asked about Bill's desirable qualities, Mr. Higgins could recognize none, but Mrs. Higgins mentioned that he was "dutiful" in that he helped to care for the younger children and helped to clean the house.

I helped the parents look at methods they had used in communicating with Bill that might have caused him to become angry and unable to control his aggression. For example, feelings of rejection were being experienced by Bill because of his aggression toward the teacher and fear of some type of punishment by the father and teacher. Everyone in the family could feel free to humiliate him.

Methods of punishment were discussed. I pointed out that the methods used by the father apparently were not the answer. Mr. Higgins said he would try another method, but he assured me that he was "very skilled at beating." He added, "If beating is what he needs, that is what he will get." The three of us concluded that since Bill liked to attend the social center at school, restricting him from doing so might be a more effective method of punishment when punishment was justified. I suggested that identifying the activities that made the parents and the other family members intolerant of Bill might be the most useful method of working with the negative feelings they were experiencing toward him. Finally, I pointed out that Bill's behavior was not necessarily abnormal or odd, but a struggle on his part to be understood. It was apparent that the family was not aware of the struggle Bill was having.

I emphasized that Bill's problems were created by a lack of understanding and communication within the family. Contributing to his problems was his particular phase of growth and development, pre-adolescence. I explained that the pre-adolescent phase is accompanied by emotional and physiological changes, among which are interest in status in peer groups and rebellion through restlessness, hostility, and irritability. Helping Bill successfully complete this phase of development should aid him in becoming more successful in the other phases of growth and development.

Evaluation.   After I assessed the situation, it was clear to me that the crisis was Bill's inability to control basic impulses, aggression and anger, which, in turn, created undesirable behavior that could not be accepted by other family members. In other words, the crisis was a complex problem brought about by Bill's encounter with the police, his aggressive attack on the teacher, and his family's response to his behavior. Bill seemed to be responding to hostility within the family structure by becoming even more aggressive and more hostile. Since all efforts at self-expression were thwarted in the home, Bill took his pent-up frustrations and conflicts with him to the community.

The tension seemed to increase considerably immediately after Bill struck the teacher, and intervention seemed to be most effective at this point. Intervention included:

1. Helping the family members understand how they were contributing to Bill's aggression and hostility.

2. Having the father express reasons for his negative attitude toward Bill.

3. Helping the family understand some of the feelings Bill may be experiencing.

4. Identifying other methods to be used in setting limits.

5. Identifying the activities that made the family intolerant of Bill.

6. Discussing the struggle inherent in the pre-adolescent phase of growth and development.

My effectiveness was dependent on the family's willingness to accept my guidance, support, and clarification. Since they were in a state of crisis, they allowed somewhat tentatively for my intervention.

Crisis Two

While there was an abatement in the intensity of feelings, as well as some success in solving the problems that brought about the first crisis, a second crisis was in process. Mrs. Higgins contacted me by phone over the weekend and said that she had received a certificate of merit for having completed a nurses' aide course. She wanted to display the certificate, but Mr. Higgins refused to let it be shown in the household. She expressed her need and desire for beginning a job as nursing assistant at a general hospital, but said Mr. Higgins disapproved. They had had a violent argument two hours before she called me.

Mrs. Higgins enrolled in a four-week course for nursing assistants and completed it, and Mr. Higgins did not object to her attending school. In fact, he told me that he was attending school for interior designing. Within this framework of confusion, the children could not decide whom to support or not to support.

On my ninth visit to the home, several of the children were in the living room listening to records or watching television. The apartment was noisy. The physical setting reflected the family's depression. The apartment was dark, although it was but 10 a.m.; curtains were drawn, and several of the family members were in pajamas. After Mrs. Higgins came into the living room, the family members lowered the hi-fi and television, but they remained seated. Mr. Higgins, however, began wandering in and out of the living room. In between his pacing, he muttered, "Finishing school is a good and a bad sign." On the next go-around he questioned, "Will she leave us now that she has completed school? Will she think she is better than we are?" Mrs. Higgins talked with me very softly and frequently interrupted our conversation to set limits for Cathy, her youngest child, and Ophelia, her grandchild. Though little verbalization took place, much nonverbal communication went on, and a shifting back and forth within chairs took place. The family members stared at me and talked among themselves, not including Mrs. Higgins or me in the conversation. I feared that the amount of tension and anxiety being experienced by the family, in addition to my verbalization of present problems, would irritate the situation, thus leading to no productive end. I left because the family was too upset to discuss their problems with me. I was feeling uncomfortable also.

The following week, during my tenth meeting in the home, tension and anxiety were still present. Mr. Higgins was home again. He and Mrs. Higgins said that I had helped them, that they could talk with me about the problem within the family without worrying about the neighbors knowing "their business." We began discussing Mr. Higgins' feelings about Mrs. Higgins' coming job. He sounded very jealous of her progress, "She thinks she is better than anyone else. She thinks she is getting too good for me and the children." He stated his concern about the household activities being neglected if Mrs. Higgins should go to work, and emphatically pointed out that she would still be responsible for all household tasks as well as for maintaining her job if *he* decided to *allow* her to work. Mrs. Higgins accepted the job at a nearby hospital one week later.

After I suggested that Mrs. Higgins' duties be shared among other family members so that she could keep her job, the family members began to listen. They wanted to know what I meant, how I thought it would work out: "Who would be doing the work?" We discussed tasks that

could be performed by other members of the household: the older ones
cooking breakfast, Mr. Higgins preparing lunch for younger children,
Judy and Mary getting Cathy ready for kindergarten, and so on. All family
members were to come home immediately after school so that none of the
younger children would be at home alone. Mr. Higgins would not accept
any responsibility in the household, mainly because he insisted that he was
employed. This was refuted by Mrs. Higgins as well as by other family
members. However, he did encourage the other children to "help their
mother out around the home." Mr. Higgins did not object to the
planning, and Mrs. Higgins beamed when he did not object verbally. I
constantly asked him for suggestions and criticism.

When the plans were concluded, Mr. Higgins talked about a social
worker who had visited his home and questioned his role as a father,
challenged him about his unemployment, and told him that his family was
living in deplorable circumstances. As he poured out his feelings of
humiliation, he talked quickly, occasionally stuttering. He also fancied
what he would do if another social worker or anyone else intruded. He
threatened to literally "throw the social worker out of his house" if she
ever came again. I heard all of this as an expression of his feelings of
failure and unworthiness, his need to be recognized as the authority figure
in his family, all brought about by Mrs. Higgins' attempt to make a
decision without consulting him.

After Mrs. Higgins became employed, the family had to accept a
smaller welfare check which meant less total income. I encouraged her in
her attempt to have self-respect and to be self-sufficient even though
necessities were hard to obtain. I told her and the family about a new
food stamp program that would allow Mrs. Higgins to purchase
approximately one hundred dollars worth of food for eighty dollars. Mr.
Higgins volunteered to purchase the food stamps, but Mrs. Higgins was
reluctant to give him the money as she was afraid of his ever-present need
to socialize with his neighborhood drinking friends. However, Mr. Higgins
said he would like to help do things around the house, to help Mrs.
Higgins with some of her duties. He was trying to assume more
responsibility and earn respect within his family and community.

Evaluation.   The crisis identified was the inability of family members to
adjust to a transitional role—a working mother. Mrs. Higgins found it
very difficult to communicate to her family her need for a job and to cope
with the problems resulting from her aggressive steps into a new role as a
nursing assistant in a nearby hospital. Anxiety, tension, fear, and hostility
developed quickly, but family members were unable to express the reasons
for their feelings.

On the ninth visit, I too felt their anxieties and fears, and the threats
to their shaky family structure. This made intervention impossible until
the family had reached that point when their emotional turmoil had
calmed and we could be rational and sensible in dealing with the problem.

Intervention included:

1. Allowing the mother to express fears over the telephone.

2. Postponing active intervention until the family was more amenable to therapeutic help.

3. Allowing Mr. Higgins to verbalize his feelings about Mrs. Higgins' intended employment.

4. Providing Mr. Higgins with an opportunity to express negative feelings about a recent social worker's visit; listening to him express his need for a feeling of worthiness and respect.

5. Discussing with the family members ways of getting household tasks done by reassigning roles to various family members.

6. Providing information about food stamps.

The basic structure of the family was weak and consequently easily affected by any change in traditional roles. The family had rather poor interpersonal relationships: feelings, ideas, information, behavior, and messages were not discussed freely within the family. The family was amenable to help when I intervened and gave direction and support. In this crisis, because of the timing of the intervention, equilibrium was restored temporarily.

Crisis Three

In the midst of the second crisis, I heard a baby crying. When I asked about the weak cry, Mrs. Higgins hedged about their keeping a neighbor's infant. She brought the baby to the living room, and I cuddled her and put her shoes on. No one disagreed with the mother's remark concerning the infant. It turned out that Patricia was not the child of a neighbor but of Judy, the 15-year-old daughter, a fact I learned through conference with my teammates. This shock wave of "upsetness" caused by Judy's becoming a mother out of wedlock became the third crisis that befell the family within this five-month period.

When I made the eleventh home visit, the house was very untidy. Judy was at home with her pajamas on. Mr. Higgins was in the back, and Mrs. Higgins was ironing. We talked first about her new job; she enjoyed being away from home, as well as being a wage earner again. We talked about Bill, who was doing "nicely," and the family members complimented Bill's therapist for his progress. As Mrs. Higgins ironed, I cuddled Patricia and gave her a bottle, I displayed a warmth for the child in such a fashion that the other family members could observe my approach to the infant. I expressed no moral judgment, no ostracism.

Mr. Higgins appeared irritated. He stalked through the dining and living room areas, making frequent demands upon Mrs. Higgins. "It is time for me to eat. Send Ann to the store for a pop." I did not stay long because of the number of duties Mrs. Higgins was commanded to perform. I did not want to make another demand by my presence. Before I left, she assured me that she would call very soon.

During the weekend, Mrs. Higgins called me to tell me that the infant was Judy's baby. A few hours before she called, Mr. Higgins had come into the living room intoxicated and nude. He had begun to humiliate Judy. Mrs. Higgins reported his comments: "No good woman has a baby without a husband. Why aren't you married? You should not be in *my* house with the baby." All of the family members were embarrassed, shocked, and frightened, especially the females, who scurried into their bedrooms. The two older boys subdued the father and put him in a back room for the rest of the night. Mrs. Higgins planned to sleep in a chair in the living room with Judy and the infant in the front bedroom for security. Above the noise in the background, I learned that the family had begun to reject Judy because she had had a baby out of wedlock. In fact, they had become hostile toward her. Mrs. Higgins pleaded with me to come as soon as I could find the time.

Two days later, I went to the home. Again, the baby was crying. I cuddled the infant while Mr. and Mrs. Higgins, Judy, and Aaron slowly settled in the living room. Aaron, their second son, is mentally retarded. Everyone was quiet. The family apparently had wanted to keep Judy's pregnancy a secret because of Mr. Higgins' attitude. He was very concerned about what his friends would think. Mrs. Higgins said she was finding it difficult to talk about illegitimate pregnancies because her oldest child, Carmen, was born out of wedlock. Mrs. Higgins was experiencing an awakening of old conflicts, guilt, shame, and failure. Mrs. Higgins also said that Carmen, at the age of 19, had given birth to an illegitimate child who lived in the home at present.

My approach was to encourage the family to talk about how they felt concerning Judy and the infant. Mr. Higgins said he felt as though he had failed; he was ashamed and was feeling guilty. Then he fell silent. I broke the silence when I asked how they thought Judy was feeling. No one commented. She looked very remorseful, hands folded in lap and head bowed. I asked Judy about *her* reaction to having a baby and seeing the family become so disorganized and irritated. Judy responded, "I am tired from washing and ironing. I cannot go out of the house. My friends are having fun without me. My face is fat and big. The baby is so tiny—I am not sure if I can care for it. I have not seen my boy friend in a long time. I feel that I have disgraced my family."

The family members present said they were not aware of how Judy felt concerning her baby. They seemed to have overlooked the fact that Judy was experiencing mixed feelings about the infant, too. Mr. and Mrs. Higgins thought Judy enjoyed being a mother, especially since she was always so "dutiful" around the home with her younger sisters and brothers. I pointed out that Mr. Higgins' behavior may have caused Judy to "dislike herself," and pointed out that his attitude could have played a part in influencing the other family members to respond to Judy in a hostile, detached manner.

The next step was to try to get the family to help Judy through the crisis, as well as to restore the equilibrium within the family. Mr. Higgins began to soften a bit and asked for suggestions as to how things could be "quieted." I guided the members of the family who were present in identifying the constructive methods to resolve the crisis.

Some suggestions elicited were the following:

1. Responsibility for the care of the baby should be shared by the members of the family.

2. The family, along with Judy, should keep the infant at different times so that Judy could return to school.

3. Judy should continue to live in the home.

4. No derogatory behavior toward Judy should be permitted.

5. Talks about feelings of disappointment, shame, failure, and guilt should be carried on within the family structure.

6. Judy, the father of the child, and Mr. and Mrs. Higgins should be permitted to talk about marriage.

7. The infant should be accepted by other members of the family.

8. Judy should be permitted to participate in the core of family life as she had previously done.

I emphasized that Judy was experiencing mixed feelings concerning the baby, and that she needed their help more than ever before. At this comment, Judy's face seemed to light up. Mr. Higgins very loudly and clearly said that the family had his support. Mrs. Higgins challenged him, "He never does anything." I added that maybe he was trying to assume more responsibility and be a better father; why not give him a chance to improve?

I stayed a long time at the home, approximately three hours. Feeling that the session had been most profitable, I left with the satisfaction of having been helpful.

Evaluation.   The crisis (a family member, Judy, becoming a parent out of wedlock) was identified. The family viewed Judy's behavior as "disgraceful" and had begun to take steps to punish her within the family setting. As a consequence, Judy withdrew, and experienced feelings of shame, failure, unworthiness, and ugliness.

Had there been better interpersonal communication, the family might have been better equipped to deal more effectively with the birth of Judy's infant. The family was obsessively concerned about their reputation, their "image," their "impression on others." This was their reason for keeping the pregnancy a secret. They denied the parentage of the child, and decided to reject both the mother and child.

In this value judgment, I decided to focus upon Mr. Higgins as the law giver and injustice collector. Even though the family members were fond of Judy, they responded to his plans to "put her out," and, by her absence, thus restore the equilibrium to solve his status problem.

He seemed to have no understanding of any standard but his own— no feeling for the emotional trauma that Judy was experiencing—and thus no basis for reevaluating his actions to integrate or compromise for the sake of family unity.

Intervention included:

1. Displaying my acceptance of the child by cuddling her and feeding her.

2. Listening to the mother talk about frightening incidents over the telephone.

3. Being receptive to the family's expressions of failure, shame, guilt, and hostility.

4. Encouraging Mr. Higgins to look at his behavior and the responses it provoked within the family.

5. Encouraging Judy to express her feelings about giving birth to the infant.

6. Encouraging the family to be more accepting of and helpful to Judy through crisis and to permit her to live within the home, as well as to participate in family life.

7. Helping the family put their family love for Judy and her baby in a higher priority than the opinion of the neighbors.

Crisis Four

After the third crisis, I was not able to contact Mrs. Higgins for about three weeks. I called several times and was told by the child who answered the phone that Mrs. Higgins "was busy" or "not at home." I always left a message saying I had called, but she did not return the calls. No home visits were made because I could not contact any of the older family members.

After my many thwarted attempts to see the family again, Mrs. Higgins phoned me one afternoon. We talked about Bill, Judy, and her new job. Everything was working out nicely. She asked to see me again and we agreed to meet in her home the following week. When I arrived at the home, I talked for the first time with Mary, the 14-year-old daughter. She was pouting because her mother would not allow her at attend a two-week meeting for teen-age girls being cosponsored by a local university, and a YWCA. Mary was dressed like many adolescents—socks, slim skirt, and pony tail. Mrs. Higgins described her as "fast and fresh."

After Mary had left the room, Mrs. Higgins assembled her ironing equipment. Having finished several menial tasks, she settled down and began to talk about a "problem that may develop," namely, Mary's difficulty in adjusting to the beginning of adolescence. Mrs. Higgins said that Mary had threatened to "have a sexual affair" with her steady boy friend. She had told Mrs. Higgins about her "deep love" for her boy friend, which caused Mrs. Higgins to tell Mary about birth control methods. Although she cautioned her about becoming involved sexually before marriage, she added that Mary should use some form of contraceptive if she "just *must* become involved." She related that at some time earlier the boy had visited with Mary in the home, but the visits were embarrassing. Mr. Higgins argued with the boy friend or anyone available, used profane language, and disrupted the entire household. The house was crowded and noisy with the younger children. Privacy was impossible. Because of all this, Mary decided not to invite her date home again. Instead, she would go *out* with him.

I perceived this story as another potential crisis and planned to intervene before the entire household became upset. At the time of our discussion, other family members were not aware of the struggle that Mary and her mother were involved in. I, therefore, wanted to act quickly to forestall as much conflict as possible within the family, and, at the same time, give Mrs. Higgins and Mary freedom to solve their problems.

During this visit, Mrs. Higgins focused on sex education. She had told her other daughters the same thing she was telling Mary. To the boys, when they became of age (approximately thirteen), she said, "Be careful and always protect the girl." Mrs. Higgins thought this was extensive enough, valid and proper. To defend herself from criticism, she added, "That is what I was told."

Our session then focused upon the double message she was giving Mary. The two older girls had responded to the covert message, "Don't, but if you *do*, use a contraceptive." Yet she hoped Mary would not have a baby out of wedlock. Consequently, we decided that Mrs. Higgins should go into greater detail about the physiologic changes that accompany growing up, as well as healthier ways of relating to members of the opposite sex. Curfews should be set for Mary, and she should be expected to obey them. Family members should be told beforehand when Mary's guest would be coming into the home in order to allow for some privacy. I pointed out that Mary would need help in channeling her sexual behavior in socially acceptable ways. Her interests in dancing, dating, and "speaking a private language" were merely a phase in growth and development used as a means to explore and master her environment.

I stressed Mary's need to be able to talk about her problems. Mrs. Higgins agreed to make herself available to Mary whenever she indicated that she would like to talk. Her need for privacy should be respected by all the family. At the time of our discussion, she was keeping her "private things" in a suitcase under her bed.

Getting back to Mary's attending the two-week meeting for teenagers, Mrs. Higgins' reason for not allowing her to participate was that Mary did not have proper clothing. I suggested that she could take what she had, and launder it frequently. This suggestion was not accepted because of Mrs. Higgins' fear of embarrassment. I was not able to convince her that the meeting would no doubt prove to be helpful and educational for Mary.

Evaluation.   The crisis identified was a power struggle between mother and daughter over the daughter's method of adjusting to the adolescent phase of growth and development. The crisis was aborted because the mother identified the situation and sought help early. When I came to the home, chaos had not spread throughout the entire household as it had in previous crises. The problem was still limited to Mary and her mother.

Mary found this phase of growth and development especially difficult because of the type of sex education she received from her mother. Initially, Mary's behavior was viewed by the mother as "fast," "selfish," and "fresh," and not as an attempt to grow up. The fear that Mary provoked within Mrs. Higgins was familiar, a fact that possibly motivated her to call me again. Having had two other daughters with babies out of wedlock was an appropriate reason for Mrs. Higgins to seek help when another daughter began to reach this period of development.

I intervened before the tension was at a peak, and when intervening, I tried to let Mrs. Higgins handle the problem. I wanted to give her guidance and support while she worked through the problem. Mary did not participate in the session, but I felt that Mrs. Higgins was the dominant force in the family and that helping her would be the best way to reach all of the family members. Intervention included:

1. Helping Mrs. Higgins understand Mary's struggle with the adolescent phase of growth and development.

2. Encouraging Mrs. Higgins to reexamine her methods of teaching sex education.

3. Assisting with devising methods of manipulating the environment when Mary had company.

4. Encouraging Mrs. Higgins to help other family members to understand Mary's need for privacy.

CONCLUSION

Termination after five months had been prepared for at the outset of my work with the Higgins family, because the date was determined by my plan to leave the area after completing the master's program. The thirty sessions had meant a great deal to me, not only because the Higgins home was less tense and family members seemed strengthened from having weathered these crises, but also because they had allowed me to be allied with them in their struggle with these crises.

References

Books

Ackerman, Nathan: The Psychodynamics of Family Life. New York, Basic Books, 1958.

Bellak, Leopold, Ed.: Community Psychiatry and Community Mental Health. New York, Grune and Stratton, 1964.

Berlo, D. K.: The Process of Communication. New York, Holt, Rinehart and Winston, 1960.

Caplan, Gerald: An Approach to Community Mental Health. New York, Grune and Stratton, 1961.

Caplan, Gerald, Ed.: Emotional Problems of Early Childhood. New York, Basic Books, 1955.

Caplan, Gerald: Principles of Preventive Psychiatry. New York, Basic Books, 1964.

Josselyn, Irene: Psychosocial Development of Children. New York, Family Service Association of America, 1948.

Kotinsky, Ruth, and Witmer, Helen E.: Community Programs for Mental Health. Cambridge, The Commonwealth Fund, Harvard University Press, 1955.

Lindemann, Erich: Symptomology and Management of Acute Grief. In Parad, H. J., Ed.: Crisis Intervention: Selected Readings. New York, Family Service Association of America, 1965.

Orlando, Ida Jean: The Dynamic Nurse-Patient Relationship. New York, G. P. Putnam's Sons, 1961.

Parad, H. J., and Caplan, Gerald: A Framework for Studying Families in Crisis. In Parad, H. J., Ed.: Crisis Intervention: Selected Readings. New York, Family Service Association of America, 1965.

Articles

Backscheider, Joan E.: The influence of sociocultural factors on the mentally ill patient. Perspect. Psychiatric Care, 3:12–16, #3, 1965.

Connolly, Mary Grace: Mental health and use of community resources J. Psychiat. Nursing, 1:5–8, Jan., 1963.

Eller, Florence: A psychiatric nurse's experience in community nursing. Perspect. Psychiat. Care, 3:14–18, #6, 1965.

Harris, Faye G.: A psychiatric nursing experience with a troubled child in the community. Perspect. Psychiat. Care, 5:92–97, #2, 1967.

Harris, Faye G.: Psychiatric and Mental Health Nursing. Failure at Four. In ANA Regional Clinical Conferences (1969). New York, Appleton-Century-Crofts, 1970, pp. 259–265.

Harrison, Mary: Lindemann's crisis theory and Dabrowski's positive disintegration theory—a comparative analysis. Perspect. Psychiat. Care, 3:8–13, #6, 1965.

Mereness, Dorothy: The potential significant role of the nurse in community mental health services. Perspect. Psychiat. Care, 1:34–37, #3, 1963.

Norris, Catherine: The trend toward community mental health centers. Perspect. Psychiat. Care, 1:36–40, #1, Jan., 1963.

Chapter Twenty-Six

THE BATTERED WIFE

Patricia W. Iyer

BATTERED WIVES ONCE FELT so ashamed and helpless that they hid their bruises behind their own doors. But the battering is no longer the wife's burdensome secret. The wife who's punched, kicked, slapped, or in some way brutally mistreated now knows she's not alone. One estimate says that in the United States this year, some four million wives will be physically abused by their husbands. (The term "husband" is used loosely to cover the man who shares a home with the woman; it also includes the man who's divorced or separated from the woman but will sometimes return to physically assault her.)

Not only is the battered wife learning that other women are coping with "her" problem—she's also learning about organizations and people who can help. More often now she's daring to walk away from the man who abused her, and she shows up in the emergency department (ED) of her hospital, in the doctor's office, and in the mental health clinics. If she has access to the appropriate information, she'll use the hot lines, task forces, and temporary safe shelters set up for her chiefly by feminists.

WHEN YOU MEET THE BATTERED WOMAN

You're sympathetic and you *want* to help the battered woman. But you're puzzled: Why would a woman stay with such a man? *You* wouldn't.

From "The Battered Wife," by Patricia W. Iyer, *Nursing 80*, July, Vol. 10, No. 7, pp. 53–55. Reprinted by permission.

Only when you understand the forces that hold her will you see her difficulty in extricating herself. She stays, as we've learned from recent studies:

Because she's ambivalent. Her situation is not as clear-cut in her mind as it can be in yours. In spite of the abuse, she has ties of loyalty—and even affection. She *did* marry him; he is her husband—and she doesn't find it easy to step away. She hopes he'll change. In self-protection, some wives will "forget" the abuse—until it happens again; some will even defend the husband as "a good man—except when he's drinking."

Because she has no financial resources of her own. The battered wife is often incapable of leaving because she has almost no money, no skills with which to earn her living—and no opportunity in the marriage to acquire either. (The possibility of working, or learning to work, is further reduced if she has young children.) Her husband will often close down the avenues for her escape by making *sure* she has no money, no means of transportation, and no friends. Note that the economically powerless wife isn't confined to lower income groups. The battering occurs at *all* income and social levels; and the husband who abuses his wife is likely to exercise deliberate control over all family money—whether there's alot or a little.

Because she's protecting her children. She has no means of supporting them if she leaves *with* them. But she's afraid to go *without* them—lest the husband maltreat them or demand custody of the children in the courts. (The husband's also been known to physically abuse or threaten to abuse the wife's mother and other members of her family.)

Because she's isolated. The battered wife's shut off from the outside world. She feels guilty, feels she somehow provoked her husband's attack and is at fault in the marriage. In her guilt and confusion, she's ashamed to reveal the problem to friends or family who might help her. The lower her self-confidence and self-image, the more aggressive her husband becomes—and the more powerless, the more fearful she becomes. In time, her feelings of helplessness prevent her from attempting to break the spiraling cycle of violence.

Because recourse to the law may make her situation worse rather than better. The threat of further violence from the husband is more powerful than legal action. Police have often failed to protect the wife when called upon and have even discouraged her from filing a complaint against her husband. These "forces" of the law sometimes tend to look upon domestic violence as a family squabble in which outsiders should not interfere—and therefore do not provide her with adequate protection against the battering. The police—and sometimes judges and lawyers as well—feel their actions are pointless, since most women drop the charges against the husband anyhow.

Because she fears her husband's reprisal.   Husbands have followed wives, dragged them home, and continued to abuse them.

Because while the laws say a man may not strike his wife, public opinion is not so sure.   According to a recent Harris poll, 20% of all Americans approve of hitting a spouse under certain circumstances; and among the college educated, the approval rises to 25%.

Because of her background of abuse.   Statistically, the woman who comes from a background of domestic violence is more likely to remain in her own abusive situation than the woman whose background did not include domestic violence. The latter is more likely to leave and seek a resolution of the problem.

WHERE NURSING BEGINS

When the battered wife shows up in your clinic or office, your first job is to identify her. As much as she needs your help, she rarely admits the true source of her injuries at first. She'll tell you she "bumped into a door" or "fell down the stairs." But you can suspect abuse:

- if the bruises are in the wrong place for the accident she's described

- if the injuries have healed somewhat, indicating that the woman hesitated to seek help immediately

- if signs of earlier injuries are apparent, or if this woman has appeared before with a similar "fall" or "bump"

But the real giveaway is the battered wife's attitude and behavior: She's timid and evasive. She avoids looking at you directly—because she's not telling the truth. You sense that she's frightened and ashamed. Her composure seems as fragile as her story. Sadly, in the press of other emergencies and duties, the battered wife is only too easy for you to miss.

But once you're certain you're facing a battered wife, keep the following guidelines in mind:

Try to wait until the woman is willing to tell you she's been abused. But once you're convinced that she's hiding the truth, ask her outright if another person has done this to her. She may *need* to be asked before she can open up. Be gentle about it—but firm. Get the facts out in the open— if you can. *Not* asking may *seem* sensitive and thoughtful, but ultimately this kind of "sensitivity" protects the husband and helps perpetuate the situation.

Don't berate the absent husband. Don't chide her for "allowing" herself to be hurt: She already feels guilty, depressed, helpless. In fact, do not be judgmental in any way. Your expression of sympathy should be confined to her bruises and her physical needs rather than to her life situation.

Let her know that you recognize her feelings—whatever they are— and accept her right to feel as she does.

Take the woman aside and treat her injuries in private.

Appear unhurried and interested. Take the time to listen.

Allow her to express her anger. But be prepared: What surfaces at first may be anger at *you* or the hospital staff. This will seem strange and unfair to you. But she cannot yet feel free to express the *real* anger: the huge anger she feels toward the man who's maltreated her.

You're going to feel a bit like you're walking a tightrope. Yes, the situation undoubtedly calls for your utmost tact and skill. If and when the woman *does* tell you she's been abused, she's likely to cry—and pour out the whole story. At this point, she's ready for some TLC. Ask if she'd like to rest for a few hours—or perhaps the night—in a vacant room. (Sometimes she'll clearly be reluctant to leave the ED.) Find her a small tray of food—even if it's only hot tea and saltines.

But if in spite of her needs, the woman is unable to level with you, suggest that she return in about 48 hours to let you have another look at her injuries. She'll be calmer then—and better able to be open about the facts. Your seeing her again is good nursing and may become another chance for establishing rapport.

Tell the doctor who's slated to see her that you suspect battering. Sometimes a woman's able to tell her story only once—and prefers to tell it to a doctor.

OFFERING PRACTICAL HELP

The battered wife needs your practical as well as your emotional help. Offer the services of your hospital social worker or mental health professional. But above all, be sure *you* know what resources your community can offer her: hot line, task force for battered wives, women's crisis center, legal counseling, pastoral counseling, or public assistance.

Keep the telephone numbers handy. Some task forces will send one of
their people to the ED to support and counsel the woman in crisis; some
will provide an advocate to accompany the woman to the courts, to legal
aid, or to social service interviews. These services are far more than token:
If the woman in her distraught state is left to fight her way through
organizational red tape alone, she'll become quickly frustrated and
defeated.

In the past 5 years, women's centers have been springing up across
the country. These centers offer a variety of services, including temporary
safe shelter for the battered woman. In the safe shelter, the woman's
whereabouts are kept secret; here she has a brief respite—time to recover
a bit and think through her situation. The shelter also offers counseling
and helps the woman find housing and employment, as well as financial
and legal assistance. Unfortunately, the need for shelters far outruns the
supply. At present there are an estimated 200 to 300 shelters existing
around the country.

For further information on the existing women's centers and safe
shelters in your community, call your local or regional chapter of the
National Organization for Women (NOW), or the women's commission
(if there is one) in your state or local government.

AFTER YOUR
INTERVENTION

But after you've cared for the battered wife, after you've referred her to
others who may help, what then?

The harsh reality is that whichever way she turns, she's not likely to
find a fairy-tale ending. Therefore, the warmth and humanity you—and
others along the way—offer may become her only emotional sustenance
and reason for hope. When you care for her, be especially understanding;
her spirit is as battered as her body.

Further Reading

Hendrix, M., LaGodna, G., and Bohen, C.: The Battererd Wife, AMERICAN
JOURNAL OF NURSING. 78:650, April 1978.

Parker, B., and Schumacher, D.: *The Battered Wife Syndrome and Violence in the Nuclear Family of Origin: A Controlled Pilot Study,* AMERICAN JOURNAL OF PUBLIC HEALTH. 67(8):760, August 1977.

Petro, J., Quann, P., and Graham, W.: *Wife Abuse, the Diagnosis and its Implications,* JOURNAL OF THE AMERICAN MEDICAL ASSOCIATION. 240:240, 1978.

Resnik, M.: WIFE BEATING: COUNSELOR TRAINING MANUAL, #1. Ann Arbor, Mich. National Organization for Women, 1976.

Rounsaville, B.: *Battered Wives: Barriers to Identification and Treatment,* AMERICAN JOURNAL OF ORTHOPSYCHIATRY. 48(3):487, July 1978.

Chapter Twenty-Seven

SCHIZOPHRENIA THROUGH THE EYES OF FAMILIES

H. Richard Lamb and Eve Oliphant

IN THIS ERA OF deinstitutionalization, families have become the real primary care agents for a large proportion of schizophrenics released from mental hospitals. For example, a recent study found that more than 50 percent of the long-term severely disabled patients in San Mateo County, California, were living with their relatives.[1] Yet until recently this seemingly obvious development went almost unnoticed by mental health professionals. Only now is attention beginning to be turned to the problems of dealing with chronic schizophrenics at home.

Relatives must learn to live with unpredictable, socially embarrassing behavior and even occasional violence. They must come to terms with the patient's social withdrawal, inactivity, and excessive sleeping. The patient's lack of conversation can be a particular hardship for a relative such as a spouse who depends on him for companionship.

If the patient and the relative stay together, they may in time reach an equilibrium that enables the patient to live outside a hospital. But inevitably the situation will severely restrict the family. Often the relative of a schizophrenic cannot even leave the house to go shopping without getting someone to watch him. The relatives may begin to feel not only as if they are jailors but also as if they themselves are in jail.

---

[1]H. R. Lamb and V. Goertzel, "The Long-Term Patient in the Era of Community Treatment," *Archives of General Psychiatry*, Vol. 34, June 1977, pp. 679–692.

From "Schizophrenia Through the Eyes of Families," by H. Richard Lamb and Eve Oliphant, *Hospital and Community Psychiatry*, 1978, Vol. 29, No. 12, pp. 803–806. Reprinted by permission.

Far from recognizing such difficulties, many professionals lay all the blame for the patient's problems at the family's doorstep. Many schools of psychiatric thought hold the patient's family responsible for aggravating and even generating his illness.[2] The professionals do not seem to realize that being the relative of a mentally ill person is traumatic and overwhelming enough. Even before their initial contact with the mental health establishment, the family members are usually guilt-ridden and feel a keen sense of failure for having "produced" a schizophrenic.

Professionals are often not sufficiently aware of such feelings and of the additional impact of a parent's receiving a label such as "schizophrenogenic mother." The concept of the "identified patient," which holds that the entire family is ill and the patient is simply the person who has been labeled the sick one, adds further trauma. To the parents, it means not only that they have driven their child crazy but also that the whole family is crazy.

Moreover, long-term schizophrenics are given low priority in community mental health programs,[3,4] despite the fact that a number of state hospitals have been closed, many thousands of long-term patients have been released into the community, and considerable sums of money have been made available for community mental health. Community programs often use these funds for everything but long-term schizophrenic patients.[5] Such patients are left to find their way into community residential settings of varying types and quality where they are forgotten as completely as they were when they were left on the back wards of state hospitals.

Families have often been appalled at the reluctance of local programs to fund aftercare projects that meet the needs of long-term patients and sheltered vocational workshops that offer them an opportunity to be productive and increase their self-esteem. Families have found that even when their schizophrenic relative is initially accepted for treatment in a community program, he is subsequently rejected by staff who explain, "Our job is not to baby-sit for long-term patients." The problem often has to do with the patient's lack of verbal skills to participate in what is considered a satisfactory way in group and individual therapy. What is

---

[2]S. W. Appleton, "Mistreatment of Patients' Families by Psychiatrists," *American Journal of Psychiatry*, Vol. 131, June 1974, pp. 655–657.

[3]G. Hogarty, "The Plight of Schizophrenics in Modern Treatment Programs," *Hospital & Community Psychiatry*, Vol. 22, July 1971, pp. 197–203.

[4]S. A. Kirk and M. E. Therrien, "Community Mental Health Myths and the Fate of Former Hospitalized Patients," *Psychiatry*, Vol. 38, August 1975, pp. 209–217.

[5]H. R. Lamb and M. B. Edelson, "The Carrot and the Stick: Inducing Local Programs to Serve Long-Term Patients," *Community Mental Health Journal*, Vol. 12, Summer 1976, pp. 137–144.

often lacking is sufficient flexibility in the program and tolerance and patience on the part of staff so that the schizophrenic can remain in the program without being expected to do more than he realistically can.

RELATIVES' GROUPS

Because it has been so difficult for relatives of schizophrenics to deal with these problems and attitudes alone, they began to join together into advocacy and mutual-support groups. Such groups are fast becoming a significant political force. Yet many mental health professionals have not recognized their influence and have failed to realize that they will increasingly be affected and held accountable by these groups. As the members become more powerful and politically sophisticated, professionals will be reminded more and more forcefully when they have been insensitive to the needs of the severely mentally ill and their families.

One of the earliest such organizations, the National Schizophrenia Fellowship, was formed in England in 1972. The fellowship now has 1300 members all over the United Kingdom and Ireland and has been instrumental in the formation of similar organizations in New Zealand, Australia, and West Germany. The group sponsors research on the causes of schizophrenia and works to create a greater understanding of the special problems arising from the illness, to secure the improvement of community care facilities of all kinds, and to encourage patients and their families to help each other and themselves.

The fellowship has also established a liaison with an American counterpart, Parents of Adult Schizophrenics, as part of attempts to form an international organization. Parents of Adult Schizophrenics, based in San Mateo County, California, has a membership there of more than 200 families. In addition, it has spawned eight similar organizations in other California counties, one in Oregon, one in Ohio, and four in the Chicago area. The Chicago groups were formed largely as a result of a radio program and subsequent newspaper article in which one of the authors (EO) was interviewed. Further, other parents' groups have been formed in ten additional California counties as well as in Missouri, Wisconsin, Florida, Georgia, Texas, Louisiana, Washington, and the District of Columbia. Moreover, relatives of patients currently in state hospitals are forming alliances with these groups in the community.

Parents of Adult Schizophrenics began in 1973 when a group of 15 parents who had schizophrenic children over the age of 18 got together to compare notes. They felt they were getting far more than their share of the blame for what happened to their children and that no one in the professional ranks seemed to understand the problems inherent in being the parent of a schizophrenic. They wondered why the parents of a child with leukemia were treated with sympathy and understanding while the parents of a schizophrenic child were treated with scorn and condemnation. They began to wonder if there was not more wrong with the system than with them.

The parents began their advocacy efforts by sending a delegation to community mental health administrators to tell them what they saw as the needs of their sons and daughters. They were not exactly welcomed with open arms. They were informed that if the mental health staff were instructed to run such programs, they would say they were not therapeutic, merely baby-sitting. The parents' suggestions were ignored. They were furious because they believed that gearing a program to the level at which patients can function and grow is not baby-sitting. Besides, they wondered, weren't community mental health programs supposed to be run for patients rather than for the staff?

They did not give up. They realized that if their views and demands were to be taken seriously, they would have to be credible, knowledgeable, vocal, and highly visible. Therefore, they began to use every channel open to them to learn about mental health programs and administration. Many members of the organization now have a better over-all understanding of the mental health system than do some of the professionals who work in it.

They lobbied to have all mental health programs studied and evaluated. They visited local politicians. They went to the newspapers. They had eight to ten people at every meeting of the local mental health advisory board. They discovered the importance of being political.

Having begun with considerable naivete, they have come to recognize how crucial it is to know where the power is, not only in the mental health system but also in the community, and to know what motivates and influences those in power. They have come to realize that having a role in fiscal deliberations and some control over the budget is the key to successful citizen participation.[6]

So far, Parents of Adult Schizophrenics has had considerable success. The members have been influential in getting professionals to change their attitudes toward parents. They have applied pressure and have been successful in getting programs for long-term patients funded and expanded; some of those programs were about to be cut back or dismantled. They have also obtained public money and grants from private foundations to establish a therapeutic housing program for schizophrenics who have not been able to meet the expectations of other community therapeutic housing programs.

---

[6]R. K. Yin et al., Citizen Organizations: Increasing Client Control Over Services, Rand Corporation, Washington, D.C., 1973.

The organization also takes into account the needs of its own members. There is a monthly "woe night" to which any parent is welcome to come and talk about his problems and feelings. The discussions are led by an experienced member of the organization. In some instances, parents have been helped through crises, and emotional breakdowns have been averted.

The organization has helped many of its members feel less isolated. Changes occur in friendships when one family has a schizophrenic child. Friends hesitate to talk about the accomplishments of their own children and do not know whether or not to discuss the illness. The friendship often becomes strained, and the friends begin to see less and less of each other. Within the group, parents find others who have similar problems and with whom they can talk openly. They also begin to re-establish a social life.

Parents' organizations often begin with a concern about the members' own children. Then members gradually begin to want to do something about the over-all problem of community treatment and rehabilitation for the chronic schizophrenic. As a result, there now exist an increasing number of effective citizens' groups devoted to advocacy for the needs and rights of long-term schizophrenics.

It is essential, however, that such organizations maintain their separate identities and not become a part of the mental health establishment. In some instances, when their leaders have been appointed to mental health advisory boards or positions in mental health associations, most of their energy has been directed to that job, leaving the relatives' organizations to falter and collapse. While getting involved in such positions is in one sense a positive development, it nevertheless can deprive the community of an independent, effective advocacy and support group for patients and their relatives.

THE FAMILIES' NEEDS

One of the most important functions relatives' support groups can serve is to pass along to less experienced members the practical tips that can make living with a schizophrenic easier. Relatives do acquire considerable expertise in coping with difficult behaviors, usually through trial and error, since such helpful advice is difficult to obtain from professionals. Frequently mental health professionals totally avoid the issue when asked for advice on the practical management of schizophrenics.[7]

---

[7]C. Creer and J. K. Wing, *Schizophrenia at Home*, National Schizophrenia Fellowship, London, 1974.

When advice is given, it is usually bad. For instance, thinking they are empathizing with the relatives' problems, they advise, "If the patient behaves badly, throw him out and lock the door after him so he cannot get back in." That could be a dangerous course of action for the patient and a difficult one to live with for the relative. Still another common piece of advice is "Forget about him; live your life." That is easy to say but difficult, if not impossible, to do when one feels guilt-ridden about a schizophrenic relative.

There is practical advice that can be extremely helpful. Goals for patients should be realistic; it is important for professionals and relatives to determine together what a patient can achieve. Then, if a relative can maintain objectivity and emotional overinvolvement does not cloud his judgment, he can apply pressure to counteract the patient's social withdrawal. However, the patient must not be pushed to achieve standards beyond his capability, and he must be left with a good deal of control over what he actually does. Many families have learned this lesson through experience over a period of years, but often only at great emotional cost when compared with having help from knowledgeable professionals in setting realistic goals.

Relatives can be helped to see that it is often useless to contradict delusional ideas, but that patients can be told not to talk back to hallucinations in public. They can also be helped to understand that social withdrawal may be a necessary defense for schizophrenics, but that too much withdrawal may lead to a form of institutionalism at home.

A crucial time to deal sensitively with relatives is at the point of the patient's first psychotic break. Professionals need to appreciate the intensity of the guilt and shock relatives feel then. Support and empathy, not condemnation, are essential. Professionals must also be aware of how the patient's illness can strain the marital relationship of the parents.

Relatives must be told that schizophrenia is not purely the result of environmental factors—that there are hereditary factors and almost certainly a biochemical imbalance. Such information reduces their fears that by their actions they will drive other relatives, especially their children, crazy. It also makes them more willing to cooperate with the patient's treatment.

In some instances, assertiveness training may help the relative set limits on the schizophrenic's behavior and deal more effectively with professionals. Of course, some relatives are already too assertive; professionals should tactfully work with them to lessen their assertiveness or to channel it into activities such as advocacy for better services for the schizophrenic relative.

There is a need for adequate treatment and rehabilitative services for the patient so relatives will have help in caring for him. Without these services the family may have all they can do to simply cope with the patient, much less treat and rehabilitate him. A whole range of facilities with all degrees of structure are needed for that large proportion of patients who need out-of-home placement. Otherwise the schizophrenic may be unwilling and the parents too guilt-ridden to effect the separation. One type of schizophrenic patient who probably needs a highly structured program with intense supervision, at times even restriction, is the patient with an alcohol or drug problem or both. Other patients need a less structured, highly nurturing environment. All patients need mental health professionals able to determine who should have what kind of placement.

Many families can manage their schizophrenic relatives well at home if they have access to periodic respite care so that they can take a vacation from the hard work of managing a schizophrenic. Such vacations are also helpful for the siblings, who frequently are neglected in the midst of the family's preoccupation with taking care of the patient.

Part Five

ISSUES, CONTROVERSIES, AND PSYCHIATRIC SOCIAL SYSTEMS

What is "mental illness," and how well are we able to distinguish sanity from insanity, normal from abnormal? What effect does the institutional environment have upon the therapeutic relationship? Can nurses be effective in changing environments? What are the rights of clients in psychiatric settings? What happens to chronic psychiatric clients once they leave the hospital system and return to the community? In this final unit, we have selected articles that look at some of the effects of psychiatric institutions and other social systems upon both nurses and clients.

In the first article Rosenhan describes a study in which "normal" people sought admission to mental hospitals; the results proved both controversial and disturbing. Rosenhan presents a thought provoking discussion of the implications of the study for psychiatric diagnosis, which is followed by an equally significant discussion of the experience of psychiatric hospitalization as recorded and reported by these "pseudopatients." Analyzing the data, Rosenhan attempts to identify sources of the powerlessness and depersonalization that characterized the clients' experience, even in the newest, best-staffed hospitals. Although this article was published in 1973, its conclusions remain significant and should prompt all readers to look more closely and critically at their attitudes toward clients.

Jones advocates that nurses utilize social systems theory and the idea of a therapeutic community to initiate more humane and therapeutic treatment in state mental hospitals. He proposes that the clients' social environment be utilized to help them become more aware of their behavior as seen by others and to facilitate the learning of more appropriate and effective behaviors. Nurses, the care-givers who are in the most daily contact with clients and who have the most knowledge of the clients' activities of daily living, are the significant people to initiate this change. Jones also proposes that an interdisciplinary team approach be utilized in a therapeutic community. One important function of this team is to "process" itself, that is, to focus on how care-givers on the team are working with each other as well as with clients. Initiation of an open social system (such as a therapeutic community where all people, including clients, feel free to comment and plan) may change the usual hospital hierarchy and redistribute the lines of power and decision making.

In the next article, Tuohey suggests that a psychiatric unit's group process, which includes both the communication of the client group to the staff and the staff group's response to this client communication, is a major factor in influencing the emotional climate of the unit. She takes the position that a primary nursing task on a psychiatric unit is to constantly assess the group process of the unit. Based on this ongoing assessment, nurses must then decide when and how to intervene, if necessary, in the group process, in order to maintain an emotional milieu that can be therapeutic for clients and facilitate staff growth and satisfaction. Tuohey presents ways to determine group process, one important factor being to "tune in" on our own feelings for cues to the clients' emotional state. Also presented are phenomena that contribute to a stressful group process.

Hankins-McNary demonstrates how institutional racism, which creates barriers to the full participation of blacks as equals in all areas of psychiatry, influences the client-therapist relationship. She maintains that both black and white therapists are influenced by cultural barriers that have negative effects on their work with black clients and that institutional racism has a negative effect on the attitude of black clients toward their therapists—white or black. Hankins-McNary reviews the origins of some of these attitudes and barriers and suggests ways in which they may be modified. One suggestion is that therapist trainees be given the opportunity in their educational experience to interact therapeutically with clients who are culturally different and be provided with supervision to explore their negative feelings and perceptions.

It is all too easy in providing psychiatric care to assume that we know what is best for our clients and to intervene with our treatment modalities without sufficiently involving the client in the treatment plan. Leichman discusses the legal rights of mentally ill clients, including the right to refuse treatment and the right to be active participants in their treatment. She defines the meaning of rights and identifies sets of ethical principles that are employed in decisions regarding rights. Nurses who provide care that is based on knowledge and respect of clients' rights help to facilitate clients' self-esteem, autonomy, and self-determination.

Krauss looks at the effects of clients being moved from one social system into another. She reviews what happens to chronic psychiatric clients and their families when the clients are deinstitutionalized and discharged into the community. Many clients do not return to their community of origin but cluster in low-income, poor housing areas. Follow-up care often is not utilized. Many clients live isolated lives, experience constant chronic symptomatology, and take large doses of psychotherapeutic drugs. If clients return home to families, the families receive little guidance on how to cope with clients' behaviors and symptoms. Krauss points out that it is the unique educational, professional preparation of psychiatric/mental health nurses that allows them to be the health care givers who can best coordinate and implement the community-based care that chronically ill psychiatric clients require.

"Hour after hour, day after day, health and social service professionals are intimately involved with troubled human beings. What happens to people who work intensely with others, learning their psychological, social or physical problems?" In the last article, Maslach provides some unsettling answers to that question, which is the core of her research on how persons in the healing professions cope with stress. Poverty lawyers, social workers, and others are subject to similar stresses. When the situation becomes overwhelming, they may experience "burnout." In most settings, including psychiatric wards, the time said to be required for this emotional distancing is only two years or less! Is burnout inevitable? Maslach does not think so, and her report indicates some factors that have potential for decreasing this appalling loss of human energy and concern.

Chapter Twenty-Eight

ON BEING SANE IN INSANE PLACES

David L. Rosenhan

IF SANITY AND INSANITY exist, how shall we know them?

The question is neither capricious nor itself insane. However much we may be personally convinced that we can tell the normal from the abnormal, the evidence is simply not compelling. It is commonplace, for example, to read about murder trials wherein eminent psychiatrists for the defense are contradicted by equally eminent psychiatrists for the prosecution on the matter of the defendant's sanity. More generally, there are a great deal of conflicting data on the reliability, utility, and meaning of such terms as "sanity," "insanity," "mental illness," and "schizophrenia" (1). Finally, as early as 1934, Benedict suggested that normality and abnormality are not universal (2). What is viewed as normal in one culture may be seen as quite aberrant in another. Thus, notions of normality and abnormality may not be quite as accurate as people believe they are.

To raise questions regarding normality and abnormality is in no way to question the fact that some behaviors are deviant or odd. Murder is deviant. So, too, are hallucinations. Nor does raising such questions deny the existence of the personal anguish that is often associated with "mental illness." Anxiety and depression exist. Psychological suffering exists. But normality and abnormality, sanity and insanity, and the diagnoses that flow from them may be less substantive than many believe them to be.

At its heart, the question of whether the sane can be distinguished from the insane (and whether degrees of insanity can be distinguished from each other) is a simple matter: do the salient characteristics that lead to diagnoses reside in the patients themselves or in the environments and

From "On Being Sane in Insane Places," by David L. Rosenhan, *Science*, January, 1973, Vol. 179, pp. 250–258. Reprinted by permission.

contexts in which observers find them? From Bleuler, through Kretchmer, through the formulators of the recently revised *Diagnostic and Statistical Manual* of the American Psychiatric Association, the belief has been strong that patients present symptoms, that those symptoms can be categorized, and, implicitly, that the sane are distinguishable from the insane. More recently, however, this belief has been questioned. Based in part on theoretical and anthropological considerations, but also on philosophical, legal, and therapeutic ones, the view has grown that psychological categorization of mental illness is useless at best and downright harmful, misleading, and pejorative at worst. Psychiatric diagnoses, in this view, are in the minds of the observers and are not valid summaries of characteristics displayed by the observed (3–5).

Gains can be made in deciding which of these is more nearly accurate by getting normal people (that is, people who do not have, and have never suffered, symptoms of serious psychiatric disorders) admitted to psychiatric hospitals and then determining whether they were discovered to be sane, and, if so, how. If the sanity of such pseudopatients were always detected, there would be prima facie evidence that a sane individual can be distinguished from the insane context in which he is found. Normality (and presumably abnormality) is distinct enough that it can be recognized wherever it occurs, for it is carried within the person. If, on the other hand, the sanity of the pseudopatients were never discovered, serious difficulties would arise for those who support traditional modes of psychiatric diagnosis. Given that the hospital staff was not incompetent, that the pseudopatient had been behaving as sanely as he had been outside of the hospital, and that it had never been previously suggested that he belonged in a psychiatric hospital, such an unlikely outcome would support the view that psychiatric diagnosis betrays little about the patient but much about the environment in which an observer finds him.

This article describes such an experiment. Eight sane people gained secret admission to 12 different hospitals (6). Their diagnostic experiences constitute the data of the first part of this article; the remainder is devoted to a description of their experiences in psychiatric institutions. Too few psychiatrists and psychologists, even those who have worked in such hospitals, know what the experience is like. They rarely talk about it with former patients, perhaps because they distrust information coming from the previously insane. Those who have worked in psychiatric hospitals are likely to have adapted so thoroughly to the settings that they are insensitive to the impact of that experience. And while there have been occasional reports of researchers who submitted themselves to psychiatric hospitalization (7), these researchers have commonly remained in the hospitals for short periods of time, often with the knowledge of the hospital staff. It is difficult to know the extent to which they were treated like patients or like research colleagues. Nevertheless, their reports about the inside of the psychiatric hospital have been valuable. This article extends those efforts.

PSEUDOPATIENTS AND
THEIR SETTINGS

The eight pseudopatients were a varied group. One was a psychology graduate student in his 20s. The remaining seven were older and "established." Among them were three psychologists, a pediatrician, a psychiatrist, a painter, and a housewife. Three pseudopatients were women, five were men. All of them employed pseudonyms, lest their alleged diagnoses embarrass them later. Those who were in mental health professions alleged another occupation in order to avoid the special attentions that might be accorded by staff, as a matter of courtesy or caution, to ailing colleagues (8). With the exception of myself (I was the first pseudopatient and my presence was known to the hospital administrator and chief psychologist and, so far as I can tell, to them alone), the presence of pseudopatients and the nature of the research program was not known to the hospital staffs (9).

The settings were similarly varied. In order to generalize the findings, admission into a variety of hospitals was sought. The 12 hospitals in the sample were located in five different states on the East and West coasts. Some were old and shabby, some were quite new. Some were research-oriented, others not. Some had good staff-patient ratios, others were quite understaffed. Only one was a strictly private hospital. All of the others were supported by state or federal funds or, in one instance, by university funds.

After calling the hospital for an appointment, the pseudopatient arrived at the admissions office complaining that he had been hearing voices. Asked what the voices said, he replied that they were often unclear, but as far as he could tell they said "empty," "hollow," and "thud." The voices were unfamiliar and were of the same sex as the pseudopatient. The choice of these symptoms was occasioned by their apparent similarity to existential symptoms. Such symptoms are alleged to arise from painful concerns about the perceived meaninglessness of one's life. It is as if the hallucinating person were saying, "My life is empty and hollow." The choice of these symptoms was also determined by the *absence* of a single report of existential psychoses in the literature.

Beyond alleging the symptoms and falsifying name, vocation, and employment, no further alterations of person, history, or circumstances were made. The significant events of the pseudopatient's life history were presented as they had actually occurred. Relationships with parents and siblings, with spouse and children, with people at work and in school, consistent with the aforementioned exceptions, were described as they were or had been. Frustrations and upsets were described along with joys and satisfactions. These facts are important to remember. If anything, they strongly biased the subsequent results in favor of detecting sanity, since none of their histories or current behaviors were seriously pathological in any way.

Immediately upon admission to the psychiatric ward, the pseudopatient ceased simulating *any* symptoms of abnormality. In some cases, there was a brief period of mild nervousness and anxiety, since none of the pseudopatients really believed that they would be admitted so easily. Indeed, their shared fear was that they would be immediately exposed as frauds and greatly embarrassed. Moreover, many of them had never visited a psychiatric ward; even those who had, nevertheless had some genuine fears about what might happen to them. Their nervousness, then, was quite appropriate to the novelty of the hospital setting, and it abated rapidly.

Apart from that short-lived nervousness, the pseudopatient behaved on the ward as he "normally" behaved. The pseudopatient spoke to patients and staff as he might ordinarily. Because there is uncommonly little to do on a psychiatric ward, he attempted to engage others in conversation. When asked by staff how he was feeling, he indicated that he was fine, that he no longer experienced symptoms. He responded to instructions from attendants, to calls for medication (which was not swallowed), and to dining-hall instructions. Beyond such activities as were available to him on the admissions ward, he spent his time writing down his observations about the ward, its patients, and the staff. Initially these notes were written "secretly," but as it soon became clear that no one much cared, they were subsequently written on standard tablets of paper in such public places as the dayroom. No secret was made of these activities.

The pseudopatient, very much as a true psychiatric patient, entered a hospital with no foreknowledge of when he would be discharged. Each was told that he would have to get out by his own devices, essentially by convincing the staff that he was sane. The psychological stresses associated with hospitalization were considerable, and all but one of the pseudopatients desired to be discharged almost immediately after being admitted. They were, therefore, motivated not only to behave sanely, but to be paragons of cooperation. That their behavior was in no way disruptive is confirmed by nursing reports, which have been obtained on most of the patients. These reports uniformly indicate that the patients were "friendly," "cooperative," and "exhibited no abnormal indications."

THE NORMAL ARE NOT DETECTABLY SANE

Despite their public "show" of sanity, the pseudopatients were never detected. Admitted, except in one case, with a diagnosis of schizophrenia

(10), each was discharged with a diagnosis of schizophrenia "in remission." The label "in remission" should in no way be dismissed as a formality, for at no time during any hospitalization had any question been raised about any pseudopatient's simulation. Nor are there any indications in the hospital records that the pseudopatient's status was suspect. Rather, the evidence is strong that, once labeled schizophrenic, the pseudopatient was stuck with that label. If the pseudopatient was to be discharged, he must naturally be "in remission"; but he was not sane, nor, in the institution's view, had he ever been sane.

The uniform failure to recognize sanity cannot be attributed to the quality of the hospitals, for, although there were considerable variations among them, several are considered excellent. Nor can it be alleged that there was simply not enough time to observe the pseudopatients. Length of hospitalization ranged from 7 to 52 days, with an average of 19 days. The pseudopatients were not, in fact, carefully observed, but this failure clearly speaks more to traditions within psychiatric hospitals than to lack of opportunity.

Finally, it cannot be said that the failure to recognize the pseudopatients' sanity was due to the fact that they were not behaving sanely. While there was clearly some tension present in all of them, their daily visitors could detect no serious behavioral consequences—nor, indeed, could other patients. It was quite common for the patients to "detect" the pseudopatients' sanity. During the first three hospitalizations, when accurate counts were kept, 35 of a total of 118 patients on the admissions ward voiced their suspicions, some vigorously. "You're not crazy. You're a journalist, or a professor [referring to the continual note-taking]. You're checking up on the hospital." While most of the patients were reassured by the pseudopatient's insistence that he had been sick before he came in but was fine now, some continued to believe that the pseudopatient was sane throughout his hospitalization (11). The fact that the patients often recognized normality when staff did not raises important questions.

Failure to detect sanity during the course of hospitalization may be due to the fact that physicians operate with a strong bias toward what statisticians call the type 2 error (5). This is to say that physicians are more inclined to call a healthy person sick (a false positive, type 2) than a sick person healthy (a false negative, type 1). The reasons for this are not hard to find: it is clearly more dangerous to misdiagnose illness than health. Better to err on the side of caution, to suspect illness even among the healthy.

But what holds for medicine does not hold equally well for psychiatry. Medical illnesses, while unfortunate, are not commonly pejorative. Psychiatric diagnoses, on the contrary, carry with them personal, legal, and social stigmas (12). It was therefore important to see whether the tendency toward diagnosing the sane insane could be reversed. The following experiment was arranged at a research and teaching hospital whose staff had heard these findings but doubted that such an error could occur in their hospital. The staff was informed that at some time during the following 3 months, one or more pseudopatients would attempt to be admitted into the psychiatric hospital. Each staff member was asked to rate each patient who presented himself at admissions or on the ward according to the likelihood that the patient was a pseudopatient. A 10-point scale was used, with a 1 and 2 reflecting high confidence that the patient was a pseudopatient.

Judgments were obtained on 193 patients who were admitted for psychiatric treatment. All staff who had had sustained contact with or primary responsibility for the patient—attendants, nurses, psychiatrists, physicians, and psychologists—were asked to make judgments. Forty-one patients were alleged, with high confidence, to be pseudopatients by at least one member of the staff. Twenty-three were considered suspect by at least one psychiatrist. Nineteen were suspected by one psychiatrist *and* one other staff member. Actually, no genuine pseudopatient (at least from my group) presented himself during this period.

The experiment is instructive. It indicates that the tendency to designate sane people as insane can be reversed when the stakes (in this case, prestige and diagnostic acumen) are high. But what can be said of the 19 people who were suspected of being "sane" by one psychiatrist and another staff member? Were these people truly "sane," or was it rather the case that in the course of avoiding the type 2 error the staff tended to make more errors of the first sort—calling the crazy "sane"? There is no way of knowing. But one thing is certain: any diagnostic process that lends itself so readily to massive errors of this sort cannot be a very reliable one.

THE STICKINESS OF PSYCHODIAGNOSTIC LABELS

Beyond the tendency to call the healthy sick—a tendency that accounts better for diagnostic behavior on admission than it does for such behavior after a lengthy period of exposure—the data speak to the massive role of labeling in psychiatric assessment. Having once been labeled schizophrenic, there is nothing the pseudopatient can do to overcome the tag. The tag profoundly colors others' perceptions of him and his behavior.

From one viewpoint, these data are hardly surprising, for it has long been known that elements are given meaning by the context in which they occur. Gestalt psychology made this point vigorously, and Asch (*13*) demonstrated that there are "central" personality traits (such as "warm"

278

versus "cold") which are so powerful that they remarkably color the meaning of other information in forming an impression of a given personality (14). "Insane," "schizophrenic," "manic-depressive," and "crazy" are probably among the most powerful of such central traits. Once a person is designated abnormal, all of his other behaviors and characteristics are colored by that label. Indeed, that label is so powerful that many of the pseudopatients' normal behaviors were overlooked entirely or profoundly misinterpreted. Some examples may clarify this issue.

Earlier I indicated that there were no changes in the pseudopatient's personal history and current status beyond those of name, employment, and, where necessary, vocation. Otherwise, a veridical description of personal history and circumstances was offered. Those circumstances were not psychotic. How were they made consonant with the diagnosis of psychosis? Or were those diagnoses modified in such a way as to bring them into accord with the circumstances of the pseudopatient's life, as described by him?

As far as I can determine, diagnoses were in no way affected by the relative health of the circumstances of a pseudopatient's life. Rather, the reverse occurred: the perception of his circumstances was shaped entirely by the diagnosis. A clear example of such translation is found in the case of a pseudopatient who had had a close relationship with his mother but was rather remote from his father during his early childhood. During adolescence and beyond, however, his father became a close friend, while his relationship with his mother cooled. His present relationship with his wife was characteristically close and warm. Apart from occasional angry exchanges, friction was minimal. The children had rarely been spanked. Surely there is nothing especially pathological about such a history. Indeed, many readers may see a similar pattern in their own experiences, with no markedly deleterious consequences. Observe, however, how such a history was translated in the psychopathological context, this from the case summary prepared after the patient was discharged.

> This white 39-year-old male...manifests a long history of
> considerable ambivalence in close relationships, which begins in early
> childhood. A warm relationship with his mother cools during his
> adolescence. A distant relationship to his father is described as
> becoming very intense. Affective stability is absent. His attempts to
> control emotionality with his wife and children are punctuated by
> angry outbursts and, in the case of the children, spankings. And
> while he says that he has several good friends, one senses
> considerable ambivalence embedded in those relationships also....

The facts of the case were unintentionally distorted by the staff to achieve consistency with a popular theory of the dynamics of a schizophrenic reaction (15). Nothing of an ambivalent nature had been described in relations with parents, spouse, or friends. To the extent that ambivalence could be inferred, it was probably not greater than is found in all human relationships. It is true the pseudopatient's relationships with his parents changed over time, but in the ordinary context that would hardly be remarkable—indeed, it might very well be expected. Clearly, the meaning ascribed to his verbalizations (that is, ambivalence, affective instability) was determined by the diagnosis: schizophrenia. An entirely different meaning would have been ascribed if it were known that the man was "normal."

All pseudopatients took extensive notes publicly. Under ordinary circumstances, such behavior would have raised questions in the minds of observers, as, in fact, it did among patients. Indeed, it seemed so certain that the notes would elicit suspicion that elaborate precautions were taken to remove them from the ward each day. But the precautions proved needless. The closest any staff member came to questioning these notes occurred when one pseudopatient asked his physician what kind of medication he was receiving and began to write down the response. "You needn't write it," he was told gently. "If you have trouble remembering, just ask me again."

If no questions were asked of the pseudopatients, how was their writing interpreted? Nursing records for three patients indicate that the writing was seen as an aspect of their pathological behavior. "Patient engages in writing behavior" was the daily nursing comment on one of the pseudopatients who was never questioned about his writing. Given that the patient is in the hospital, he must be psychologically disturbed. And given that he is disturbed, continuous writing must be a behavioral manifestation of that disturbance, perhaps a subset of the compulsive behaviors that are sometimes correlated with schizophrenia.

One tacit characteristic of psychiatric diagnosis is that it locates the sources of aberration within the individual and only rarely within the complex of stimuli that surrounds him. Consequently, behaviors that are stimulated by the environment are very often erroneously attributed to the patient's disorder. For example, one kindly nurse found a pseudopatient pacing the long hospital corridors. "Nervous, Mr. X?" she asked. "No, bored," he said.

The notes kept by pseudopatients are full of patient behaviors that were misinterpreted by well-intentioned staff. Often enough, a patient would go "berserk" because he had, wittingly or unwittingly, been mistreated by, say, an attendant. A nurse coming upon the scene would rarely inquire even cursorily into the environmental stimuli of the patient's behavior. Rather, she assumed that his upset derived from his pathology, not from his present interactions with other staff members. Occasionally, the staff might assume that the patient's family (especially when they had recently visited) or other patients had stimulated the outburst. But never were the staff found to assume that one of themselves or the structure of the hospital had anything to do with a patient's behavior. One psychiatrist pointed to a group of patients who were sitting outside the cafeteria entrance half an hour before lunchtime. To a group of young residents he indicated that such behavior was characteristic of the oral-acquisitive nature of the syndrome. It seemed not to occur to him that there were very few things to anticipate in a psychiatric hospital besides eating.

A psychiatric label has a life and an influence of its own. Once the impression has been formed that the patient is schizophrenic, the expectation is that he will continue to be schizophrenic. When a sufficient amount of time has passed, during which the patient has done nothing bizarre, he is considered to be in remission and available for discharge. But the label endures beyond discharge, with the unconfirmed expectation that he will behave as a schizophrenic again. Such labels, conferred by mental health professionals, are as influential on the patient as they are on his relatives and friends, and it should not surprise anyone that the diagnosis acts on all of them as a self-fulfilling prophecy. Eventually, the patient himself accepts the diagnosis, with all of its surplus meanings and expectations, and behaves accordingly (5).

The inferences to be made from these matters are quite simple. Much as Zigler and Phillips have demonstrated that there is enormous overlap in the symptoms presented by patients who have been variously diagnosed (16), so there is enormous overlap in the behaviors of the sane and the insane. The sane are not "sane" all of the time. We lose our tempers "for no good reason." We are occasionally depressed or anxious, again for no good reason. And we may find it difficult to get along with one or another person—again for no reason that we can specify. Similarly, the insane are not always insane. Indeed, it was the impression of the pseudopatients while living with them that they were sane for long periods of time—that the bizarre behaviors upon which their diagnoses were allegedly predicted constituted only a small fraction of their total behavior. If it makes no sense to label ourselves permanently depressed on the basis of an occasional depression, then it takes better evidence than is presently available to label all patients insane or schizophrenic on the basis of bizarre behaviors or cognitions. It seems more useful, as Mischel (17) has pointed out, to limit our discussions to *behaviors*, the stimuli that provoke them, and their correlates.

It is not known why powerful impressions of personality traits, such as "crazy" or "insane," arise. Conceivably, when the origins of and stimuli that give rise to a behavior are remote or unknown, or when the behavior strikes us as immutable, trait labels regarding the *behavior* arise. When, on the other hand, the origins and stimuli are known and available, discourse is limited to the behavior itself. Thus, I may hallucinate because I am sleeping, or I may hallucinate because I have ingested a peculiar drug. These are termed sleep-induced hallucinations, or dreams, and drug-induced hallucinations, respectively. But when the stimuli to my hallucinations are unknown, that is called craziness, or schizophrenia—as if that inference were somehow as illuminating as the others.

THE EXPERIENCE OF PSYCHIATRIC HOSPITALIZATION

The term "mental illness" is of recent origin. It was coined by people who were humane in their inclinations and who wanted very much to raise the station of (and the public's sympathies toward) the psychologically disturbed from that of witches and "crazies" to one that was akin to the physically ill. And they were at least partially successful, for the treatment of the mentally ill *has* improved considerably over the years. But while treatment has improved, it is doubtful that people really regard the mentally ill in the same way that they view the physically ill. A broken leg is something one recovers from, but mental illness allegedly endures forever (18). A broken leg does not threaten the observer, but a crazy schizophrenic? There is by now a host of evidence that attitudes toward the mentally ill are characterized by fear, hostility, aloofness, suspicion, and dread (19). The mentally ill are society's lepers.

That such attitudes infect the general population is perhaps not surprising, only upsetting. But that they affect the professionals— attendants, nurses, physicians, psychologists, and social workers—who treat and deal with the mentally ill is more disconcerting, both because such attitudes are self-evidently pernicious and because they are unwitting. Most mental health professionals would insist that they are sympathetic toward the mentally ill, that they are neither avoidant nor hostile. But it is more likely that an exquisite ambivalence characterizes their relations with psychiatric patients, such that their avowed impulses are only part of their entire attitude. Negative attitudes are there too and can easily be detected. Such attitudes should not surprise us. They are the natural offspring of the labels patients wear and the places in which they are found.

Consider the structure of the typical psychiatric hospital. Staff and patients are strictly segregated. Staff have their own living space, including their dining facilities, bathrooms, and assembly places. The glassed quarters that contain the professional staff, which the pseudopatients came to call "the cage," sit out on every dayroom. The staff emerge primarily for caretaking purposes—to give medication, to conduct a therapy or group meeting, to instruct or reprimand a patient. Otherwise, staff keep to themselves, almost as if the disorder that afflicts their charges is somehow catching.

So much is patient-staff segregation the rule that, for four public hospitals in which an attempt was made to measure the degree to which staff and patients mingle, it was necessary to use "time out of the staff cage" as the operational measure. While it was not the case that all time spent out of the cage was spent mingling with patients (attendants, for example, would occasionally emerge to watch television in the dayroom), it was the only way in which one could gather reliable data on time for measuring.

The average amount of time spent by attendants outside of the cage was 11.3 percent (range, 3 to 52 percent). This figure does not represent only time spent mingling with patients, but also includes time spent on such chores as folding laundry, supervising patients while they shave, directing ward cleanup, and sending patients to off-ward activities. It was the relatively rare attendant who spent time talking with patients or playing games with them. It proved impossible to obtain a "percent mingling time" for nurses, since the amount of time they spent out of the cage was too brief. Rather, we counted instances of emergence from the cage. On the average, daytime nurses emerged from the cage 11.5 times per shift, including instances when they left the ward entirely (range, 4 to 39 times). Late afternoon and night nurses were even less available, emerging on the average 9.4 times per shift (range 4 to 41 times). Data on early morning nurses, who arrived usually after midnight and departed at 8 a.m., are not available because patients were asleep during most of this period.

Physicians, especially psychiatrists, were even less available. They were rarely seen on the wards. Quite commonly, they would be seen only when they arrived and departed, with the remaining time being spent in their offices or in the cage. On the average, physicians emerged on the ward 6.7 times per day (range, 1 to 17 times). It proved difficult to make an accurate estimate in this regard, since physicians often maintained hours that allowed them to come and go at different times.

The hierarchical organization of the psychiatric hospital has been commented on before (20), but the latent meaning of that kind of organization is worth noting again. Those with the most power have least to do with patients, and those with the least power are most involved with them. Recall, however, that the acquisition of role-appropriate behaviors occurs mainly through the observation of others, with the most powerful having the most influence. Consequently, it is understandable that attendants not only spend more time with patients than do any other members of the staff—that is required by their station in the hierarchy— but also, insofar as they learn from their superiors' behavior, spend as little time with patients as they can. Attendants are seen mainly in the cage, which is where the models, the action, and the power are.

I turn now to a different set of studies, those dealing with staff response to patient-initiated contact. It has long been known that the amount of time a person spends with you can be an index of your significance to him. If he initiates and maintains eye contact, there is reason to believe that he is considering your requests and needs. If he pauses to chat or actually stops and talks, there is added reason to infer that he is individuating you. In four hospitals, the pseudopatient approached the staff member with a request which took the following form: "Pardon me, Mr. [or Dr. or Mrs.] X, could you tell me when I will be eligible for grounds privileges?" (or "...when I will be presented at the staff meeting?" or "...when I am likely to be discharged?"). While the content of the question varied according to the appropriateness of the target and the pseudopatient's (apparent) current needs the form was always a courteous and relevant request for information. Care was taken never to approach a particular member of the staff more than once a day, lest the staff member become suspicious or irritated. In examining these data, remember that the behavior of the pseudopatients was neither bizarre nor disruptive. One could indeed engage in good conversation with them.

The data for these experiments are shown in Table 1, separately for physicians (column 1) and for nurses and attendants (column 2). Minor differences between these four institutions were overwhelmed by the degree to which staff avoided continuing contacts that patients had initiated. By far, their most common response consisted of either a brief response to the question, offered while they were "on the move" and with head averted, or no response at all.

The encounter frequently took the following bizarre form: (pseudopatient) "Pardon me, Dr. X. Could you tell me when I am eligible for grounds privileges?" (physician) "Good morning, Dave. How are you today?" (Moves off without waiting for a response.)

It is instructive to compare these data with data recently obtained at Stanford University. It has been alleged that large and eminent universities are characterized by faculty who are so busy that they have no time for students. For this comparison, a young lady approached individual faculty members who seemed to be walking purposefully to some meeting or teaching engagement and asked them the following six questions:

1. "Pardon me, could you direct me to Encina Hall?" (at the medical school: "...to the Clinical Research Center?").

2. "Do you know where Fish Annex is?" (there is no Fish Annex at Stanford).

3. "Do you teach here?"

4. "How does one apply for admission to the college?" (at the medical school: "...to the medical school?").

5. "Is it difficult to get in?"

6. "Is there financial aid?"

TABLE 1

Self-Initiated Contact by Pseudopatients with Psychiatrists and Nurses and Attendants, Compared to Contact with Other Groups

Contact	Psychiatric Hospitals		University Campus (Nonmedical)	University Medical Center Physicians		
	(1) Psychiatrists	(2) Nurses and Attendants	(3) Faculty	(4) "Looking for a Psychiatrist"	(5) "Looking for an Internist"	(6) No Additional Comment
Responses						
Moves on, head averted (%)	71	88	0	0	0	0
Makes eye contact (%)	23	10	0	11	0	0
Pauses and chats (%)	2	2	0	11	0	10
Stops and talks (%)	4	0.5	100	78	100	90
Mean number of questions answered (out of 6)	*	*	6	3.8	4.8	4.5
Respondents (No.)	13	47	14	18	15	10
Attempts (No.)	185	1283	14	18	15	10

*Not applicable.

285

Without exception, as can be seen in Table 1 (column 3), all of the questions were answered. No matter how rushed they were, all respondents not only maintained eye contact, but stopped to talk. Indeed, many of the respondents went out of their way to direct or take the questioner to the office she was seeking, to try to locate "Fish Annex," or to discuss with her the possibilities of being admitted to the university.

Similar data, also shown in Table 1 (columns 4, 5, and 6), were obtained in the hospital. Here too, the young lady came prepared with six questions. After the first question, however, she remarked to 18 of her respondents (column 4), "I'm looking for a psychiatrist," and to 15 others (column 5), "I'm looking for an internist." Ten other respondents received no inserted comment (column 6). The general degree of cooperative responses is considerably higher for these university groups than it was for pseudopatients in psychiatric hospitals. Even so, differences are apparent within the medical school setting. Once having indicated that she was looking for a psychiatrist, the degree of cooperation elicited was less than when she sought an internist.

POWERLESSNESS AND DEPERSONALIZATION

Eye contact and verbal contact reflect concern and individuation; their absence, avoidance and depersonalization. The data I have presented do not do justice to the rich daily encounters that grew up around matters of depersonalization and avoidance. I have records of patients who were beaten by staff for the sin of having initiated verbal contact. During my own experience, for example, one patient was beaten in the presence of other patients for having approached an attendant and told him, "I like you." Occasionally, punishment meted out to patients for misdemeanors seemed so excessive that it could not be justified by the most radical interpretations of psychiatric canon. Nevertheless, they appeared to go unquestioned. Tempers were often short. A patient who had not heard a call for medication would be roundly excoriated, and the morning attendants would often wake patients with, "Come on, you m......f......s, out of bed!"

Neither anecdotal nor "hard" data can convey the overwhelming sense of powerlessness which invades the individual as he is continually exposed to the depersonalization of the psychiatric hospital. It hardly matters *which* psychiatric hospital—the excellent public ones and the very plush private hospital were better than the rural and shabby ones in this regard, but, again, the features that psychiatric hospitals had in common overwhelmed by far their apparent differences.

Powerlessness was evident everywhere. The patient is deprived of many of his legal rights by dint of his psychiatric commitment (21). He is shorn of credibility by virtue of his psychiatric label. His freedom of movement is restricted. He cannot initiate contact with the staff, but may only respond to such overtures as they make. Personal privacy is minimal. Patient quarters and possessions can be entered and examined by any staff member, for whatever reason. His personal history and anguish is available to any staff member (often including the "grey lady" and "candy striper" volunteer) who chooses to read his folder, regardless of their therapeutic relationship to him. His personal hygiene and waste evacuation are often monitored. The water closets may have no doors.

At times, depersonalization reached such proportions that pseudopatients had the sense that they were invisible, or at least unworthy of account. Upon being admitted, I and other pseudopatients took the initial physical examinations in a semipublic room, where staff members went about their own business as if we were not there.

On the ward, attendants delivered verbal and occasionally serious physical abuse to patients in the presence of other observing patients, some of whom (the pseudopatients) were writing it all down. Abusive behavior, on the other hand, terminated quite abruptly when other staff members were known to be coming. Staff are credible witnesses. Patients are not.

A nurse unbuttoned her uniform to adjust her brassiere in the presence of an entire ward of viewing men. One did not have the sense that she was being seductive. Rather, she didn't notice us. A group of staff persons might point to a patient in the dayroom and discuss him animatedly, as if he were not there.

One illuminating instance of depersonalization and invisibility occurred with regard to medications. All told, the pseudopatients were administered nearly 2100 pills, including Elavil, Stelazine, Compazine, and Thorazine, to name but a few. (That such a variety of medications should have been administered to patients presenting identical symptoms is itself worthy of note.) Only two were swallowed. The rest were either pocketed or deposited in the toilet. The pseudopatients were not alone in this. Although I have no precise records on how many patients rejected their medications, the pseudopatients frequently found the medications of other patients in the toilet before they deposited their own. As long as they were cooperative, their behavior and the pseudopatients' own in this matter, as in other important matters, went unnoticed throughout.

Reactions to such depersonalization among pseudopatients were intense. Although they had come to the hospital as participant observers and were fully aware that they did not "belong," they nevertheless found themselves caught up in and fighting the process of depersonalization. Some examples: a graduate student in psychology asked his wife to bring his textbooks to the hospital so he could "catch up on his homework"— this despite the elaborate precautions taken to conceal his professional association. The same student, who had trained for quite some time to get into the hospital, and who had looked forward to the experience, "remembered" some drag races that he had wanted to see on the weekend and insisted that he be discharged by that time. Another pseudopatient attempted a romance with a nurse. Subsequently, he informed the staff that he was applying for admission to graduate school in psychology and was very likely to be admitted, since a graduate professor was one of his regular hospital visitors. The same person began to engage in psychotherapy with other patients—all of this as a way of becoming a person in an impersonal environment.

THE SOURCES OF DEPERSONALIZATION

What are the origins of depersonalization? I have already mentioned two. First are attitudes held by all of us toward the mentally ill—including those who treat them—attitudes characterized by fear, distrust, and horrible expectations on the one hand, and benevolent intentions on the other. Our ambivalence leads, in this instance as in others, to avoidance.

Second, and not entirely separate, the hierarchical structure of the psychiatric hospital facilitates depersonalization. Those who are at the top have least to do with patients, and their behavior inspires the rest of the staff. Average daily contact with psychiatrists, psychologists, residents, and physicians combined ranged from 3.9 to 25.1 minutes, with an overall mean of 6.8 (six pseudopatients over a total of 129 days of hospitalization). Included in this average are time spent in the admissions interview, ward meetings in the presence of a senior staff member, group and individual psychotherapy contacts, case presentation conferences, and discharge meetings. Clearly, patients do not spend much time in interpersonal contact with doctoral staff. And doctoral staff serve as models for nurses and attendants.

There are probably other sources. Psychiatric installations are presently in serious financial straits. Staff shortages are pervasive, staff time at a premium. Something has to give, and that something is patient contact. Yet, while financial stresses are realities, too much can be made of them. I have the impression that the psychological forces that result in depersonalization are much stronger than the fiscal ones and that the addition of more staff would not correspondingly improve patient care in this regard. The incidence of staff meetings and the enormous amount of record-keeping on patients, for example, have not been as substantially reduced as has patient contact. Priorities exist, even during hard times. Patient contact is not a significant priority in the traditional psychiatric hospital, and fiscal pressures do not account for this. Avoidance and depersonalization may.

Heavy reliance upon psychotropic medication tacitly contributes to depersonalization by convincing staff that treatment is, indeed, being conducted and that further patient contact may not be necessary. Even here, however, caution needs to be exercised in understanding the role of psychotropic drugs. If patients were powerful rather than powerless, if they were viewed as interesting individuals rather than diagnostic entities, if they were socially significant rather than social lepers, if their anguish truly and wholly compelled our sympathies and concerns, would we not *seek* contact with them, despite the availability of medications? Perhaps for the pleasure of it all?

THE CONSEQUENCES OF
LABELING AND
DEPERSONALIZATION

Whenever the ratio of what is known to what needs to be known approaches zero, we tend to invent "knowledge" and assume that we understand more than we actually do. We seem unable to acknowledge that we simply don't know. The needs for diagnosis and remediation of behavioral and emotional problems are enormous. But rather than acknowledge that we are just embarking on understanding, we continue to label patients "schizophrenic," "manic-depressive," and "insane," as if in those words we had captured the essence of understanding. The facts of the matter are that we have known for a long time that diagnoses are often not useful or reliable, but we have nevertheless continued to use them. We now know that we cannot distinguish insanity from sanity. It is depressing to consider how that information will be used.

Not merely depressing, but frightening. How many people, one wonders, are sane but not recognized as such in our psychiatric institutions? How many have been needlessly stripped of their privileges of citizenship, from the right to vote and drive to that of handling their own accounts? How many have feigned insanity in order to avoid the criminal consequences of their behavior, and, conversely, how many would rather stand trial than live interminably in a psychiatric hospital—but are wrongly thought to be mentally ill? How many have been stigmatized by well-intentioned, but nevertheless erroneous, diagnoses? On the last point, recall again that a "type 2 error" in psychiatric diagnosis does not have the same consequences it does in medical diagnosis. A diagnosis of cancer that has been found to be in error is cause for celebration. But psychiatric diagnoses are rarely found to be in error. The label sticks, a mark of inadequacy forever.

Finally, how many patients might be "sane" outside the psychiatric hospital but seem insane in it—not because craziness resides in them, as it were, but because they are responding to a bizarre setting, one that may be unique to institutions which harbor nether people? Goffman (4) calls the process of socialization to such institutions "mortification"—an apt metaphor that includes the processes of depersonalization that have been described here. And while it is impossible to know whether the pseudopatients' responses to these processes are characteristic of all inmates—they were, after all, not real patients—it is difficult to believe that these processes of socialization to a psychiatric hospital provide useful attitudes or habits of response for living in the "real world."

SUMMARY AND CONCLUSIONS

It is clear that we cannot distinguish the sane from the insane in psychiatric hospitals. The hospital itself imposes a special environment in which the meanings of behavior can easily be misunderstood. The consequences to patients hospitalized in such an environment—the powerlessness, depersonalization, segregation, mortification, and self-labeling—seem undoubtedly countertherapeutic.

I do not, even now, understand this problem well enough to perceive solutions. But two matters seem to have some promise. The first concerns the proliferation of community mental health facilities, of crisis intervention centers, of the human potential movement, and of behavior therapies that, for all of their own problems, tend to avoid psychiatric labels, to focus on specific problems and behaviors, and to retain the individual in a relatively nonpejorative environment. Clearly, to the extent that we refrain from sending the distressed to insane places, our impressions of them are less likely to be distorted. (The risk of distorted perceptions, it seems to me, is always present, since we are much more sensitive to an individual's behaviors and verbalizations than we are to the subtle contextual stimuli that often promote them. At issue here is a matter of magnitude. And, as I have shown, the magnitude of distortion is exceedingly high in the extreme context that is a psychiatric hospital.)

The second matter that might prove promising speaks to the need to increase the sensitivity of mental health workers and researchers to the Catch 22 position of psychiatric patients. Simply reading materials in this area will be of help to some such workers and researchers. For others, directly experiencing the impact of psychiatric hospitalization will be of enormous use. Clearly, further research into the social psychology of such

total institutions will both facilitate treatment and deepen understanding.
I and the other pseudopatients in the psychiatric setting had
distinctly negative reactions. We do not pretend to describe the subjective
experiences of true patients. Theirs may be different from ours,
particularly with the passage of time and the necessary process of
adaptation to one's environment. But we can and do speak to the
relatively more objective indices of treatment within the hospital. It could
be a mistake, and a very unfortunate one, to consider that what happened
to us derived from malice or stupidity on the part of the staff. Quite the
contrary, our overwhelming impression of them was of people who really
cared, who were committed and who were uncommonly intelligent.
Where they failed, as they sometimes did painfully, it would be more
accurate to attribute those failures to the environment in which they, too,
found themselves than to personal callousness. Their perceptions and
behavior were controlled by the situation, rather than being motivated by
a malicious disposition. In a more benign environment, one that was less
attached to global diagnosis, their behaviors and judgments might have
been more benign and effective.

References and Notes

1. P. Ash, *J. Abnorm. Soc. Psychol.* 44, 272 (1949); A. T. Becker, *Amer. J. Psychiat.* 119, 210 (1962); A. T. Boisen, *Psychiatry* 2, 233 (1938); N. Kreitman, *J. Ment. Sci.* 107, 876 (1961); N. Kreitman, P. Sainsbury, J. Morrisey, J. Towers, J. Scrivener, *ibid.*, p. 887; H. O. Schmitt and C. P. Fonda, *J. Abnorm. Soc. Psychol.* 52, 262 (1956); W. Seeman, *J. Nerv. Ment. Dis.* 118, 541 (1953). For an analysis of these artifacts and summaries of the disputes, see J. Zubin, *Annu. Rev. Psychol.* 18, 373 (1967); L. Phillips and J. G. Draguns, *ibid.* 22, 447 (1971).

2. R. Benedict, *J. Gen. Psychol.* 10, 59 (1934).

3. See in this regard H. Becker, *Outsiders: Studies in the Sociology of Deviance* (Free Press, New York, 1963); B. M. Braginsky, D. D. Braginsky, K. Ring, *Methods of Madness: The Mental Hospital as a Last Resort* (Holt, Rinehart & Winston, New York, 1969); G. M. Crocetti and P. V. Lemkau, *Amer. Sociol. Rev.* 30, 557 (1965); E. Goffman, *Behavior in Public Places* (Free Press, New York, 1964); R. D. Laing, *The Divided Self: A Study of Sanity and Madness* (Quadrangle, Chicago, 1960); D. L. Phillips, *Amer. Sociol. Rev.* 28, 963 (1963); T. R. Sarbin, *Psychol. Today* 6, 18 (1972); E. Schur, *Amer. J. Sociol.* 75, 309 (1969); T. Szasz, *Law, Liberty and Psychiatry* (Macmillan, New York, 1963); T.

Szasz, *The Myth of Mental Illness: Foundations of a Theory of Mental Illness* (Hoeber-Harper, New York, 1963). For a critique of some of these views, see W. R. Gove, *Amer. Sociol. Rev.* 35, 837 (1970).

4. E. Goffman, *Asylums* (Doubleday, Garden City, N.Y., 1961).

5. T. J. Scheff, *Being Mentally Ill: A Sociological Theory* (Aldine, Chicago, 1966).

6. Data from a ninth pseudopatient are not incorporated in this report because, although his sanity went undetected, he falsified aspects of his personal history, including his marital status and parental relationships. His experimental behaviors therefore were not identical to those of the other pseudopatients.

7. A. Barry, *Bellevue Is a State of Mind* (Harcourt Brace Jovanovich, New York, 1971); I. Belknap, *Human Problems of a State Mental Hospital* (McGraw-Hill, New York, 1956); W. Caudill, F. C. Redlich, H. R. Gilmore, E. B. Brody, *Amer. J. Orthopsychiat.* 22, 314 (1952); A. R. Goldman, R. H. Bohr, T. A. Steinberg, *Prof. Psychol.* 1, 427 (1970); unauthored, *Roche Report* 1 (No. 13), 8 (1971).

8. Beyond the personal difficulties that the pseudopatient is likely to experience in the hospital, there are legal and social ones that, combined, require considerable attention before entry. For example, once admitted to a psychiatric institution, it is difficult, if not impossible, to be discharged on short notice, state law to the contrary notwithstanding. I was not sensitive to these difficulties at the outset of the project, nor to the personal and situational emergencies that can arise, but later a writ of habeas corpus was prepared for each of the entering pseudopatients and an attorney was kept "on call" during every hospitalization. I am grateful to John Kaplan and Robert Bartels for legal advice and assistance in these matters.

9. However distasteful such concealment is, it was a necessary first step to examining these questions. Without concealment, there would have been no way to know how valid these experiences were; nor was there any way of knowing whether whatever detections occurred were a tribute to the diagnostic acumen of the staff or to the hospital's rumor network. Obviously, since my concerns are general ones that cut across individual hospitals and staffs, I have respected their anonymity and have eliminated clues that might lead to their identification.

10. Interestingly, of the 12 admissions, 11 were diagnosed as schizophrenic and one, with the identical symptomatology, as manic-depressive psychosis. This diagnosis has a more favorable prognosis, and it was given by the only private hospital in our sample. On the relations between social class and

psychiatric diagnosis, see A. deB. Hollingshead and F. C. Redlich, *Social Class and Mental Illness: A Community Study* (Wiley, New York, 1958).

11. It is possible, of course, that patients have quite broad latitudes in diagnosis and therefore are inclined to call many people sane, even those whose behavior is patently aberrant. However, although we have no hard data on this matter, it was our distinct impression that this was not the case. In many instances, patients not only singled us out for attention, but came to imitate our behaviors and styles.

12. J. Cumming and E. Cumming, *Community Ment. Health* 1, 135 (1965); A. Farina and K. Ring, *J. Abnorm. Psychol.* 70, 47 (1965); H. E. Freeman and O. G. Simmons, *The Mental Patient Comes Home* (Wiley, New York, 1963); W. J. Johannsen, *Ment. Hygiene* 53, 218 (1969); A. S. Linsky, *Soc. Psychiat.* 5, 166 (1970).

13. S. E. Asch, *J. Abnorm. Soc. Psychol.* 41, 258 (1946); *Social Psychology* (Prentice-Hall, New York, 1952).

14. See also I. N. Mensh and J. Wishner, *J. Personality* 16, 188 (1947); J. Wishner, *Psychol. Rev.* 67, 96 (1960); J. S. Bruner and R. Tagiuri, in *Handbook of Social Psychology*, G. Lindzey, Ed. (Addison-Wesley, Cambridge, Mass., 1954), vol. 2, pp. 634–654; J. S. Bruner, D. Shapiro, R. Tagiuri, in *Person Perception and Interpersonal Behavior*, R. Tagiuri and L. Petrullo, Eds. (Stanford Univ. Press, Stanford, Calif., 1958), pp. 227–288.

15. For an example of a similar self-fulfilling prophecy, in this instance dealing with the "central" trait of intelligence, see R. Rosenthal and L. Jacobson, *Pygmalion in the Classroom* (Holt, Rinehart & Winston, New York, 1968).

16. E. Zigler and L. Phillips, *J. Abnorm. Soc. Psychol.* 63, 69 (1961). See also R. K. Freudenberg and J. P. Robertson, *A.M.A. Arch. Neurol. Psychiatr.* 76, 14 (1956).

17. W. Mischel, *Personality and Assessment* (Wiley, New York, 1968).

18. The most recent and unfortunate instance of this tenet is that of Senator Thomas Eagleton.

19. T. R. Sarbin and J. C. Mancuso, *J. Clin. Consult. Psychol.* 35, 159 (1970); T. R. Sarbin, *ibid.* 31, 447 (1967); J. C. Nunnally, Jr., *Popular Conceptions of Mental Health* (Holt, Rinehart & Winston, New York, 1961).

20. A. H. Stanton and M. S. Schwartz, *The Mental Hospital: A Study of Institutional Participation in Psychiatric Illness and Treatment* (Basic, New York, 1954).

21. D. B. Wexler and S. E. Scoville, *Ariz. Law Rev.* 13, 1 (1971).

22. I thank W. Mischel, E. Orne, and M. S. Rosenhan for comments on an earlier draft of this manuscript.

Chapter Twenty-Nine

NURSES CAN CHANGE THE SOCIAL SYSTEMS OF HOSPITALS

Maxwell Jones

AT PRESENT, THE STATE mental hospital is seen as having a largely custodial function, lacking in interest, excitement, and effectiveness for most professional personnel. The enterprising registered nurse is usually far more attracted by the relatively new community mental health centers where her role relationship with the medical and other psychiatric disciplines is usually on a more egalitarian footing than often is the case in most of the state hospitals.

This need not be. Indeed, nurses might well be the pivotal force in turning the closed systems of these state hospitals into the open systems of truly therapeutic communities.

It is popular to prophesy the ultimate demise of state mental institutions, the argument being that even severely disabled mental patients can find a more varied and rewarding life in the outside community or in some form of hospital alternative—halfway houses, nursing or boarding homes, and so on. But the facts belie this, and many studies have stressed that patients in the community are often little, if any, better off than they were in the so-called back wards of the state hospitals.[1]

We seem to have forgotten that approximately 150 years ago we reacted against the punitive, prisonlike lunatic asylums of that day, and for a short time the so-called moral treatment approach was favored. Relatively small institutions were run by staffs who treated patients as people. Humane values prospered.

But the tide soon turned against the so-called insane who, without any compliance on their part, were labeled "sick" and compelled to be "treated" by doctors. What a pity the humanitarian moral treatment phase was not left to evolve in its own way. "The very matrix of moral treatment was the communal life of patients and hospital personnel."[2] Instead the huge state hospitals, usually hidden in the country away from public gaze, housing thousands of patients in prisonlike conditions with no real treatment, epitomized public distaste for the insane.

We had to wait until after World War II to see a new interest in the patient as a person. The concept of the therapeutic community started in a London hospital in 1947 and for 30 years my colleagues and I have been recommending this approach in any type of psychiatric facility.[3] Many other liberalizing concepts have emerged since that time in both the U.S. and Europe. The most dramatic example of a therapeutic community in this country was started at Fort Logan Mental Health Center 17 years ago.[4,5]). This center was organized as a therapeutic community with multidisciplinary teams that were largely autonomous. The team leader could be from any discipline provided he or she was seen as the most competent leader. Thus several registered nurses were team leaders with physicians accepting their leadership. The treatment was based on a systems approach rather than individual psychotherapy. Unfortunately, Fort Logan, a state hospital representing an immensely important new model of a democratic, egalitarian system, had few if any imitators, and the typical state hospital in the U.S. remains essentially hierarchical, dominated by physicians with registered nurses in relatively unimportant roles.

To me the problem is rooted in the hierarchy of status, responsibility, and authority, and the resistance to change in hospital systems generally. As already noted, there are hopeful signs, for example, the emergence of nonmedical directors trained in hospital management. But with few exceptions they, too, have tended to abuse their authority and have not involved all relevant personnel in shared decisions, and so forth.

Therefore, we need to take a new look at the mental hospital, particularly its function and social organization.

It could be said that anyone entering a mental hospital has failed to live up to his own and other peoples' norms and expectations of him as a competent individual, fit to survive by his own efforts in open society. Anyone who fails in this sense may find himself stigmatized as mentally "ill" and segregated, often against his will, in a mental hospital. The psychiatric examination, with its stereotyped questions, leading to the subject being given a label denoting some diagnostic category, may reinforce his own negative self-image.

A therapeutic community or social system approach would allow staff and patients to discuss the whole admission procedure and heighten staff's capacity to empathize with the patient. Already intensely upset by being handcuffed and driven in a sheriff's car or whatever else happened, the patient may have been kept in a waiting room until his admission interview. What a chance for a welcoming committee of patients or caring nurses to reassure him and correct many of his distorted fantasies about hospitals. Perhaps one or two of this group might accompany him to the admission interview, or better still, a relative or friend.

"Fact finding" for case records is far less important at this stage than giving the new patient a feeling of belonging and establishing a base for social relationships. The ultimate outrage, in my opinion, is the tendency to demonstrate new patients to a room full of students or staff, without any support system, for instance, without the nurses who are familiar to him and can help to clarify misunderstandings that such an asocial situation invites.

By using open-system lines, the community of staff and patients can look at the strategy, or plan, to help the patient to overcome his negative self-image. If the whole community meets daily for an hour to discuss intraward problems, the new patient can be introduced at that time, and if he feels inhibited, he can be helped by nurses who know him or by the patient welcoming committee. Ideally, everyone in the ward will get some idea of his problem. This gives clues to appropriate role relationships that will help provide him with support and guidance.

If the new patient refuses to use the opportunity presented by the ward meeting, then his wish must be honored, although often a staff member may obtain his permission to give at least some information. For example, if the problem has to do with an overdependent young girl whose widowed mother has tended to live her life for her, and the mother died leaving her daughter relatively helpless, then the community has an idea how to help the girl to evolve her own coping mechanisms.

This social system approach to treatment differs greatly from individual psychotherapy. Instead of the patient's conflicts being worked through in the traditional doctor-patient relationship (individual psychotherapy), the patient's social environment is used to make the subject aware of his behavior as seen by others, and more appropriate and effective behavior patterns are learned.

We are all significantly influenced by our environment and we are talking about using a social system for change. Up to now, the training of both nurses and physicians has largely ignored communication theory, learning theory, and systems theory. While this is changing rapidly in nurse training programs, I am unaware of a similar reorientation in the training of doctors and psychiatrists.

This training dimension can readily be added by holding a staff review for at least 45 minutes immediately following the community meeting. For a good process review, it is best to have a facilitator who may be an outsider. His or her function is to keep the staff to the "here and now" and avoid reminiscing or other irrelevancies.

To relive the community meeting in a sequential manner is more difficult than it sounds. The staff tries to remember how the meeting started, who said what, and what happened. Did the staff tend to dominate the meeting and miss opportunities to involve patients? To confront a psychiatrist who tended to dominate the meeting takes courage. By the same token a well-timed comment that led to a discussion of important problems affecting the ward should be praised. In both instances criticism helps to develop a learning situation. Society has come to see criticism in a negative context, but through time, when the team develops a high trust level, any kind of confrontation or criticism is seen as an essential part of social learning or growth.

Social learning is a two-way communication in a group situation, motivated by some inner need or stress, leading to the overt or covert expression of feeling, and involving cognitive awareness and change. Such learning may relate to the individual, group, or system. Confrontation as already described has the potential for social learning, but this can be realized only when the attributes of an open system are available and a skilled facilitator or interventionist is available.[6]

To "process a meeting" means that the participants' performance is examined by the whole staff, an experience that can be painful, but nonetheless rewarding. The quality of an input, the timing, the sensitivity to group climate, the skill at picking up nonverbal communication, and many other aspects of effective or ineffective intervention are discussed.

The day in, day out analysis of staff performance at a community meeting inevitably leads to learning. The silent staff member is not overlooked. For example, a newly employed nurse may be asked what she felt about some interchange and, in a supportive staff climate, may find that what she felt was appropriate. She may also learn that to express what one feels cannot be wrong. But it takes time and practice to know how to express such feelings so that they contribute to social learning.

A further stage of this learning process is to institute weekly staff meetings that focus on interpersonal feelings within the staff. Here the role of the nurse and her role relationships with the physician and other disciplines can be discussed openly. If the physician is making treatment decisions without involving the relevant staff members, then someone has to confront him. If criticism never reaches the person or persons mainly responsible for discord or strife nothing is learned. "Risk takers" are invaluable members of a team and should be cherished and encouraged. Often we "speak our minds" only when in the company of our trusted friends.

The basic principles of an open-system approach to a psychiatric ward are two-way communication of content and feeling (information sharing), and listening, interacting, and discussing with a view to social learning and growth.

Similar principles apply to top administrative meetings and at all levels of the hierarchy. The social organization of the whole hospital can be reviewed. Ideally any decision to change structure should involve all persons involved in carrying out a new plan. In this way everyone has a vested interest in the plan and will not feel "put upon" by some administrative fiat from above. Such fiats usually are regarded as lacking many of the factors, which if asked, staff would have contributed. Decision making by consensus is time consuming, but on important issues it is well worth the time spent.

To evolve an open system in a hospital or even a ward may take years because many of the attitudes and beliefs that permeate society have to be changed. By and large we all grow up in closed systems where conformity, rigid role prescriptions, hiding one's true feelings, and a passive acceptance of authority, status, and power are ingrained. One furthers one's career usually by conforming to the expectations of the system. This is beginning to change, particularly in the nursing world, where the role of the nurse is becoming more fluid and nurses are participating in treatment and assuming leadership roles.

An open system will, by its very nature, change our concept of a mental hospital. Why have the usual hospital hierarchy with most of the power in the hands of the physicians? Why not evolve a social system where all, including patients, feel free to comment and plan? I'd like to see a group of social-system-trained nurses run a new experimental unit, using psychiatrists as consultants and other professional groups as needed. Their proximity to the patient world inevitably makes them patient centered. Home visits, family involvement, and productive functional roles for patients might well follow. We must get away from the stereotype of deviancy and badness tied to the idea of madness. In my opinion, we have only begun to recognize the potential of nurses as facilitators of change in the social systems of mental hospitals.

References

1. U.S. National Institute of Mental Health. *Deinstitutionalization—an Analytical Review and Sociological Perspective,* by L. L. Bachrach. (DHEW Publ. No. (ADM) 76–351 (Series D. No. 4) Washington, D.C., U.S. Government Printing Office, 1976.

2. Almond, Richard. *The Healing Community: Dynamics of the Therapeutic Milieu*, New York, Jason Aronson, 1974.

3. Jones, M. S. *The Therapeutic Community: A New Treatment Method in Psychiatry*. New York, Basic Books, 1953.

4. Schiff, S. B. A therapeutic community in an open state hospital: Administrative framework for social psychiatry. *Hosp. Community Psychiatry* 20:259–268, Sept. 1969.

5. Jones, M. S., and Bonn, E. M. From therapeutic community to self sufficient community. *Hosp. Community Psychiatry* 24:675–680, Oct. 1973.

6. Jones, M. S. *Maturation of the Therapeutic Community*. New York, Human Sciences Press, a Division of Behavioral Publications, 1976.

Chapter Thirty

INFLUENCE OF GROUP PROCESS ON THE UNIT MILIEU

Cecilia M. Tuohey

IN THIS PAPER, *MILIEU* is used to refer to the primary *affective* state of a group of people, taking into consideration that the affect may be deduced from *both* the physical environment and the behavior of the group members. While in a strict sense the term "milieu" means environment, for the purposes of this paper it primarily means the emotional environment.

In discussing the influence of group process on the milieu, my primary frame of reference will be the inpatient psychiatric unit, which is composed of patients who have serious emotional problems that prevent their living outside the hospital. The units to which I will refer have some mixture of patients in terms of variety of problems; that is, there are people with addictive disorders, severe affective problems, psychotic illness, and problems that are shown in acting-out behavior of an antisocial nature. The therapeutic community philosophy is the belief system that influences the interaction pattern between patients and staff as well as determining the structural aspects of the unit. I will refer here primarily to the role of nursing staff in dealing with patients, although the interrelationships with other disciplines are considered.

The group process of a unit might be described as including both the communication or message, usually unconscious, of the patient group to the staff, and the staff group's response to the communication from the

From "Influence of Group Process on the Unit Milieu," by Cecilia M. Tuohey, *Nursing Clinics of North America*, December, 1978, Vol. 13, No. 4, pp. 665–671. Reprinted by permission.

patient group. The main thesis of this paper is that a group process exists on a psychiatric unit, no matter what the structure or philosophy of the unit, and that this group process is a strong force in determining the milieu or emotional environment of an inpatient unit. A further position is that one of the most important tasks of nursing staff and, primarily, those responsible for nursing leadership on a unit is to constantly assess the group process of a unit—both the message that the patient group transmits to staff and the response of the staff to that message. The task after making the assessment is to intervene in the group process, if necessary, to facilitate the maintenance of an emotional environment conducive to patients' understanding and coping with their problems and staff's finding satisfaction and growth in their work.

DOCUMENTATION OF PATIENT-STAFF INTERACTION

A review of the literature indicates that the interdependency between the staff and patient group is well documented. The stresses present on a psychiatric ICU engender intense emotions, which may lead to a state of emotional exhaustion on the part of staff.[3] A lack of self-scrutiny, and dissension, can cause the staff to become distant and emotionally unavailable to patients. Not identifying the problem situation can result in deterioration of the therapeutic effectiveness of the unit until the well-being of the patient is seriously threatened or staff members are lost. Rosen suggests that the most important task is to increase awareness of the staff that such adverse effects do occur, so that open discussion of the patients' responses is encouraged and the sources of stress are identified and diminished. Further, it was suggested that staff be selected partially on their willingness and ability to tolerate high levels of stress, and that consultation be provided to stimulate self-scrutiny on the part of the staff and to prevent the destructive effects of staff exhaustion.

An Article by Ravenscroft on milieu process during the residency turnover period describes the following:

> In essence because of the overdetermined and conflictual staff pressures and problems during the turnover, there is a recurrent and observable tendency on the part of staff to lose their objectivity, overlook their own emotional and behavioral contributions to patient behavior, and displace their problems onto the patients. By externalizing these issues, staff disown their contributions to and compound the burden of the patients: the staff also work on their

own problems by means of this process of temporary displacement onto the patients.[1]

One of the recommendations made by the author to prevent deterioration of the therapeutic process is that workshops be structured to provide tools for acknowledging the issues and effects of the turnover, for following the process throughout its course, and for working through the fantasies, feelings, and facts involved. Again, emphasis is placed on the staff's becoming aware of the group process during a stressful period and on setting up a structure to be used to cope with the tensions.

In *The Mental Hospital,* Stanton and Schwartz describe the structure of a collective disturbance on a ward.[5] They see the collective disturbance as being an institutional phenomenon, characterized by the fact that the failure in function of each person is integrated with the failure in function of the next one. All failures are integrated in such a way that the disorganization or reorganization gains impetus like a snowball going downhill, with increasing size, spread, and seriousness of effects. The authors describe an acute crisis as always being preceded by a period of less acute partial disorganization among the staff. This disorganization might be manifested by errors in technique, absenteeism, or staff preoccupation with the problems of other staff members, so that less effective staff time is available for patient care. Withdrawal from the ward is prominent.

This brief review of the literature confirms what those of us who work with groups of patients know at both an emotional and intellectual level—that there is a system of reciprocity of feelings operating between the patient group and staff group and, if we are in clinical leadership positions, between ourselves and both groups.

DETERMINATION OF GROUP PROCESS

Before talking about ways to determine the group process of a unit, we should realize that there *are* periods of time when patients are working quite well on their problems and staff are facilitating this process. At these times, I don't think it is necessary to spend energy on trying to analyze a process that is obviously facilitative. Instead, the periods when close attention needs to be paid to the process are those when work is floundering and patients and staff are having difficulty exercising their roles. While I am not limiting the form a large group process can take to the three basic assumption groups described by Bion, some of his descriptions can be helpful in determining the group process that is hindering work.[2]

Orientation: Reality vs. Fantasy

Bion sees life as being oriented not toward reality, but fantasy, which is then acted out. Staff and patients both act "as if" something is the case. An example of such a fantasy is that staff have the responsibility for controlling the impulses of patients. In attending a community meeting on an adolescent service, I heard a discussion of how irresponsible the staff was in not fixing a broken lock on a window. The staff made valiant efforts to defend themselves by explaining the difficulties they had with the maintenance department, and they counterattacked by pointing out that the adolescents had broken the lock. I was impressed by the energy that was being devoted to this issue and by the defensiveness of the staff. Finally, one staff member pointed out that the staff had not forced the child who was leading the attack to climb out the window. The message to staff that I heard was that they were responsible for controlling all the impulses of these kids, and the nursing staff had agreed with this fantasy. Thus, one can see how misdirected staff energy can become when it is based on an illogical proposition.

Attitudes and Emotions

Bion also characterizes a basic assumption group as having little patience for an inquiring attitude or for testing consequences. Meetings that reflect this are often characterized by staff blaming each other for patients' actions. This was seen in one meeting in which the psychiatrists and social workers were on one side and nursing staff was on the other, both trying to determine which side was responsible for kids running away from the hospital. Nursing staff saw what they characterized as the permissiveness of the psychiatrists and social workers as being the cause of the acting out, while the others saw the harshness of the nursing staff as the impetus. One staff member suggested that before coming to the hospital, these kids had acted out by running away, and the fact that they were running away now was neither surprising nor the result of the incompetence of staff. Because the group had bought the kids' message, their thinking now involved loose generalizations and illogical thinking. In describing the basic assumption group, Bion stresses that it is mainly recognizable from the emotional state of the group.

Communication and Response

There are some other cues one can use in determining the nature of the group process. One is the language of the group. How do staff describe patients—hopeless, destructive, helpless, dependent, and so forth, and what are the data that are supporting these characterizations? In other words, are we picking up a cue from supporting data, or are we making some assumptions based on the patients' fantasy? This is not suggesting that the fantasy of a group of patients is not important, but rather that our intervention in the group process should reflect what is truly happening.

Of crucial importance is the manner in which staff respond to the communication of the patient group. We often hear comments about whether patients are really acting out some covert staff problems, as described by Stanton and Schwartz.[5] While the question is an irritating one if it is being asked of us—especially if we are trying to make some order out of chaos—I also think it has limited value on an operational level. It seems to me to be a more useful proposition that it is the patient group that most often initiates the particular message, with staff responding to that message. Since the patient group is dealing with a patient role, with its accompanying dependency, in addition to the disorganized psychologic process of its members, its capacity to communicate an anxiety-producing message is quite strong.

Therefore, an important cue to defining the group process, and one that nursing staff often neglect, is our own emotional state, which is a cue to the patients' emotional state. The work of Harold Searles with schizophrenic patients can be very useful in this regard. Searles describes a phenomenon that he labels the "reflection process."[4] He postulates that in the supervision of a therapist, if a supervisor finds himself experiencing some particular emotion, he should consider the possibility that the source of this emotion may lie chiefly in the therapist-patient relationship and, basically, in the patient himself. Several other contributors to psychoanalytic literature emphasize how much the analyst can learn about the patient by noticing his own feelings.

While some nursing staff may lack the sophistication in terms of theory and skills as well as the personal maturity and security to attain this level of objectivity, it is a posture that nurse clinicians can assume. Essentially, we can theorize that the primary emotional attitude of ourselves and our staff toward the patient group says something about the process of the patient group and should be received as data. For instance, the anger we experience as a group of patients express, in a reasonable, logical and helpful manner, the deficits in our system of unit management should serve as a piece of data in terms of the unit's group process. Our feeling that the constant somatization of a group of patients that has resulted in the ordering of numerous tests, medications, and treatments is malevolently designed to drive us to an early grave should be viewed as data. Our staff telling us that the patient group is malingering and is not troubled by serious emotional problems is again data about what the patient group is communicating. For example, are patients feeling as if their problems are the result of their evil natures and that they deserve to be punished?

Nonverbal communications also serve as data in determining the group process: body language in meetings, assaultive or isolative behavior, tone of voice, the regression of patients, absences of staff, and timing of resignations.

GROUP PROCESS AND STRESS

It was mentioned earlier that if the unit group, both patients and staff, are going about their work in a reasonable fashion, it is not necessary to be concerned about the group process. It is only if work is floundering that one needs to take action. It would be useful to review some of the stresses that a unit may experience that may require close attention to the group process. One familiar example is the loss of significant members of the group, whether patients or staff, with senior clinical staff probably being as important a loss as a patient suicide. Another is the admission of a different type of patient from those a unit is familiar with, or the numbers of a particular kind of patient becoming particularly high. For instance, I heard a tape recording of a therapy group in which five of the eight patients were diagnosed as paranoid schizophrenics. This particular personality organization was very strongly affecting that group and those of us listening to the tape became more isolated and silent as the group went on. We are all familiar with this phenomenon—our own emotional cues as to where a group is—but use it less often than we might.

Entry of new staff into a unit, especially as roles become defined, is another stressful time. A particularly strong influence on the group process of a unit is the interference with its system from the larger institution in which it is located, or from the community at large. For instance, any threat to a group's existence will be met with a strong response. These stressful times should be watched more carefully.

"LACK" OF GROUP PROCESS

I had mentioned earlier in the paper that a group process exists on any unit regardless of its particular structure. A unit that reflects an individual treatment approach in which neither staff nor patients ever meet in a formal group will share a covert communication process. Characterizing such units as angry, depressed, pleasant, and so forth is a reflection of a large group process, unless we are being terribly imprecise and talking about one or two patients. We have also characterized staff groups in much the same way—as reflecting a change in affective state from day to day or being fixed in certain positions (they're a very angry staff, they're not a cohesive group, and so forth).

While the group process operates in any large group, it is much easier to determine on units where group meetings are a part of the structure, especially in the setting where all patients and staff meet together. The community meeting can be conceptualized as a microcosm of the group process and, therefore, an additional source of data.

SUMMARY

The purpose of this paper has been to discuss one clinical phenomenon, that of the group process, the determination of which facilitates the provision of nursing care on an inpatient psychiatric unit. Both the phenomena that engender a stressful group process and the cues to determining a group process were discussed.

References

1. Ravenscroft, K.: Milieu process during the residency turnover: The human cost of psychiatric education. *Amer. J. Psychiatry*, May, 1975.

2. Rioch, Margaret: The work of Wilfred Bion in groups. *Psychiatry*, 33:56–66, 1970.

3. Rosen, H.: Impact of psychiatric intensive care unit on patients and staff. *Amer. J. Psychiatry*, May, 1975.

4. Searles, H.: *Collected Papers on Schizophrenia*. New York. International Universities Press, 1966.

5. Stanton, A. H., and Schwartz, M. S.: *The Mental Hospital*. New York, Basic Books, 1954.

Chapter Thirty-One

THE EFFECT OF INSTITUTIONAL RACISM ON THE THERAPEUTIC RELATIONSHIP

Lula D. Hankins-McNary

BLACK PEOPLE CONSTITUTE THE largest racial minority group in the United States, which means that the racial minority client with whom the psychiatrist/therapist is most likely to come in contact will be black. Because most therapists in this country are Caucasian, and because of the increased demand of black people for therapy, there exists an increased need to develop effective skills in providing this therapy. However, most therapists, white and black, have not been intellectually or culturally prepared to conduct effective therapy with the average black client.

Psychiatry has been described as having a pattern of institutional racism that creates barriers to the full participation of blacks as equals in all areas of psychiatry. Sabshin, et al. maintain that "Such structuralization leads to a relative diminution of the status of black members as well as to a depreciation of the black community as a whole, circularly providing renewed force and justification for the original barriers." (1970:787)

Although overt, individual racist behavior may occur between white therapists and black clients, institutional racism in psychiatry is the

From "The Effect of Institutional Racism on the Therapeutic Relationship," by Lula D. Hankins-McNary, *Perspectives in Psychiatric Care*, January/February, 1979, Vol. 17, No. 1, pp. 25–31. Reprinted by permission.

primary basis for individual acts of racism. Hence, institutional racism is one of the most significant influences on the relationship between a therapist—both black and white—and a black client. This paper demonstrates how institutional racism influences the client-therapist relationship.

Institutional racism involves the notion that those who are not white are inferior. Consequently, non-white subcultural groups in this country have historically been rejected by the dominant (European) cultural group. Instead of perceiving them as being culturally different, they have been viewed as culturally disadvantaged, deprived, or underprivileged. As a result, therapists are confronted today with cultural barriers which impair their ability to establish a positive relationship with their clients.

Vontress (1969) maintains that the polarization of racial attitudes in this country has increased in direct proportion to physical racial separation. As the separation becomes greater, both therapist and client have fewer opportunities to share experiences and know each other's values, lifestyles and attitudes. The reinforcement of negative attitudes toward blackness causes them to become ingrained in American culture.

Vontress identifies these cultural barriers in the counseling relationship as being "the counselor's and client's reciprocal racial attitudes, the counselor's ignorance of the client's background, the language barrier of poor people in general, the client's lack of familiarity with counseling, the Negro's reservation about self-disclosure, and the sex and race taboo." (1969:11)

Lowinger and Dobie (1966), in their study of the patient-therapist relationship, found a significant difference in the attitudes of the white therapist toward white and black clients at the time of the initial interview. Responses to their questionnaire indicated bias when white therapists confronted psychiatric patients of different races and religions. Also affecting the therapists' attitudes were such variables as the patient's social class and source of referral.

"Lack of understanding of the socio-psychological background of the client can be the greatest blockage in the [therapeutic] relationship," states Vontress. (1969:14) For example, many therapists expect their clients to be able to verbalize feelings fluently, especially during the working phase of the relationship. They do not take into consideration that the speech of the lower socio-economic-class is characterized by the use of fewer modifiers than is the speech of the middle-class, particularly when feelings are being discussed. As a result, middle-class therapists interacting with poor people may be rendered professionally helpless because of their inability to penetrate the language barrier. Moreover, the average poor black client has had little experience with professionals or counseling. Hence, when the black client approaches a therapist this may be a first attempt to establish a relationship with a professional for the purpose of receiving counseling.

The identification of the client's core problem, the establishment of trust, and the process selected to alleviate the client's problem are important in a therapeutic counseling relationship. The client is encouraged to make his or her feelings and experiences known to another through the process of self-disclosure. However, the ability to reveal oneself to another seems directly related to the way the person has been treated by society. Vontress observes that, "Individuals who have been treated harshly and have experienced hardships are very reluctant to self-disclose their pain." (1969:14) He noted a difference in self-disclosure between northern and southern reared blacks. Both were reserved in disclosing themselves within the counseling relationship, but blacks reared in the North were often overtly hostile in the counseling relationship; whereas blacks reared in the South tended to conceal their hostility, and disguise their antagonism and feelings of contempt with a demonstration of extreme passivity.

Institutional racism also influences the quality of the relationship that develops between a white therapist and a black client because it affects the development of trust. Trust is crucial to the constructive progress of a therapeutic relationship. According to Vontress, rapport is difficult to establish whether the therapist is white or black. Even though a white therapist may initially approach a black client with genuine empathetic understanding and unconditional positive regard, if trust has not been established, the client will reject the therapist's attempt to apply his or her skills. As a consequence, the therapist is rendered therapeutically ineffective. And, because of the effects of institutional racism, the antipathy to all whites demonstrated by some black clients will not allow them to evaluate and react to white persons as unique individuals.

Some black clients openly state they would prefer or would accept a black therapist simply because the therapist is black. (Vontress, 1969) On the other hand, if the client perceives the white therapist as the enemy, he or she may perceive the black therapist as a traitor and collaborator with the enemy. The black therapist who is accepted by the client simply because he or she is black must be able to "assist the client with the problems he experiences or his blackness will be of fleeting value." (Vontress, 1969:13)

Institutional racism may also have a negative effect on the attitude of the black therapist toward his or her black client. Because of the universal images and stereotypes associated with blacks, administering therapy to a black client may be considered a low status task to both black and white therapists. As a result of working with what they consider low status clients, black therapists may become frustrated and angry because their own self-image is threatened. Their anger "may then be displaced onto the client in an unconscious effort to drive him away." (Calnek, 1970:44) Also, when comparing themselves with white therapists, black therapists may consider themselves as possessing low status because they are black. Having adopted a negative self-image and possessing a diffused identity, they may also possess unconscious negative white prejudices. They may view a black client as being a "dumb nigger"; the stereotype of the inarticulate and usually passive black who is seemingly of low intelligence. Therefore, they may proceed to reject black clients, using labels such as untreatable, poor prognosis, or unreachable. This attitude paralyzes the black therapist's skill, and impairs the accuracy of his or her assessment of the black client's level of mental health and corresponding need for therapy. (Calnek, 1970:44)

Therapists, both black and white, should be able to determine when the source of their clients' problems is racial and socio-economic, or personal and independent of race and socio-economics. However, Calnek (1970) identifies and analyzes three problems of the black therapist which originate in the white societal value system. Two of the problems relate to the therapist's denial of identification and over-identification. Denial of identification can impair the therapeutic relationship either by the therapist identifying with the client only on a therapeutic level or by not attributing any of the client's problems to racial discrimination. In over-identification, there is a bond with the black client whom the black therapist sees as an extension of himself or herself because of a common racial experience. The therapist uses the relationship to achieve personal satisfaction.

When therapists tend to identify with clients only on a racial level, they have a corresponding tendency to under-estimate the significance of those client difficulties unrelated to race. Consequently, they may attribute the cause of most, if not all, of the client's problems to external societal factors. Or, the therapist may go to the opposite extreme and deny identification with the black client by attributing all the problems to the client, rather than to the possible external effects of racial discrimination.

Calnek (1970) identifies the third problem among black therapists as the tendency of traditional, conservative therapists to prefer black clients who are passive and non-assertive, and the tendency of black consciousness therapists to be intolerant of this type of client. The implication is that the assertive client may threaten the values of the traditional therapist, whereas a therapist who readily accepts assertive behavior in a black client may negatively react to a passive client. Black therapists may also be judgmental with the black clients who "act white," because these clients may remind therapists of their own concealed tendencies.

Just as institutional racism exerts a negative effect on the attitude of white and black therapists toward black clients, it also has a negative effect on the attitude of black clients toward their therapists—white or black. Being a member of an oppressed minority group, and having experienced acts of discrimination, black clients enter into therapy with at least three negative attitudes which influence their treatment: resentment, distrust, and self-hatred. Owing to past experiences of discrimination, a black client may be resentful and anxious when approached by a white therapist. (Rosen and Frank, 1962) Because of their experiences with discrimination, most

310

blacks distrust all whites, which carries over to the black client/white therapist relationship. The clients' attitudes inhibit their willingness to reveal their core problems. The most malignant attitude found in black clients is self-hatred. Often a direct result of institutional racism, it immobilizes the client. Self-hatred may be difficult to disclose to a white therapist or white group members, thus retarding and impairing the progress of therapy.

Racist attitudes of white people have repeatedly advanced the notion that everything affiliated with black is bad, whereas everything associated with white is good. Therefore, the black person, in an attempt to be accepted as equal to the white person, may inappropriately strive to attain and imitate all those things that represent whiteness. In doing so, he or she rejects all those things that represent blackness. Rosen and Frank attempt to explain this occurrence in their comment: "Whiteness represents full personal dignity and complete participation in American Society." (1962:457)

Some blacks—those most nearly white in appearance, class, educational status, and attitude—tend to look down on blacks who closely resemble the white stereotype of the black man or woman. Whereas blacks who are closely associated with the white stereotypes of their group may outwardly demonstrate feelings of resentment toward "assimilated" blacks, of whom they may also be secretly envious.

The therapist's attitude, evaluation, diagnosis, and the type of therapy administered to the black client are all interrelated. The effect of institutional racism on the therapist's attitude may adversely affect the accuracy of the therapist's evaluation and diagnosis of the black client. Clements, et al. (1969) state that the leading cause of inaccurate evaluation is the influence that cultural differences exert on a white therapist's evaluation of a black client. Rejection of clients, negative responses to tests, mistrust between client and tester, lack of understanding as to the purpose for testing, inadequate norms, and insufficient or erroneous interpretation of test performances—all reduce the accuracy and meaningfulness of standardized evaluations.

Jones, et al. give additional support to the observation that cultural differences have a negative influence on evaluation. They state: "We feel that too many intake workers are not empathetic enough to make accurate assessments of black patients because they are unable or unwilling to deal with the subtleties and nuances present in the material presented by these patients." (1970:801)

The diagnosis and labels attached to the black client seem also to be influenced by the effects of institutional racism and cultural stereotypes. The most commonly held white stereotypes are that black people are lazy, happy-go-lucky, always smiling; are ignorant and have difficulty in learning because their brains are smaller; have the intelligence of monkeys; stink; are sexually endowed with superior genitals; and are always singing and dancing. According to Sabshin, et al. (1970:788), white American psychiatry has its equivalent racist stereotypes about black psychiatric patients; that is, they are hostile and not motivated for treatment, having primitive character structure; are not psychologically-minded, and are impulse-ridden.

Assumptions evolved from the psychoanalytic theoretical framework indicate that individuals who will most benefit from intensive psychotherapy are those who are highly motivated, intelligent, can tolerate a delay of gratification, are introspective, and repudiate action in favor of thought. Most black clients are rated as possessing few of these ego strengths; consequently, are not considered good candidates for anything more than supportive therapy.

Jones, et al. have insisted that because of covert institutional racism, "Predominantly white psychoanalytically-oriented residency programs are failing to produce psychiatrists, black or white, who are motivated or prepared to address themselves to the mental health needs of the black community." (1970:798) Fewer doctors practice in predominantly black communities, and of all the health specialties, psychiatry is the least available to clients. Churches, not psychiatrists or clinics, provide most of the mental health services to the black community.

In addition, since admission policies of many psychiatric clinics are dictated by training needs of the staff and research projects, patients selected for admission are often those considered "good" treatment cases. They usually include young, motivated, introspective students, suburban housewives, or career-motivated junior executives, with few reality difficulties. The design of this selection process further limits the number of blacks seen and treated in clinics. The observation supports Sabshin, et al. (1970), who contend that patients from backgrounds culturally different from their therapists receive the least amount of intensive therapy. And, it would appear, that "once a psychiatric facility is reached, blacks are more likely than whites to be diagnosed as psychotic, schizophrenic and paranoid." (Miller, et al., 1973:462)

The number of blacks engaged in individual, group, and family therapy is small, yet the need for treatment is obvious. Because early intervention or sustained clinic treatment is less likely for the black psychiatric patient than the white, the result is a greater need for hospitalization, longer hospitalization, and chronicity.

Although Calnek and Sabshin, et al. have suggested that black therapists may have greater success with black clients because they share the communality of culture, race, and similar experiences, Grier and Cobbs disagree. They state, "Even though the experiences of black people in this country are unique, the principles of psychological functioning are universal to all men" (1968:129); that is, a white therapist, given knowledge of the cultural differences of a black client can develop true empathy toward this client and administer therapy as effectively as a similarly skilled black therapist.

However, the issue of race cannot and should not be ignored when the client is black, regardless of the therapist's color. For a therapeutic relationship to develop and progress, all feelings about race which might negatively influence the therapy process should be acknowledged, discussed, resolved, or controlled for the benefit of the client. Black clients who bring feelings of resentment into the relationship must be assisted to identify and discuss these feelings before therapy can promote a higher degree of mental health. If not identified by the therapist, the black client's defense mechanism can retard the progress of therapy and lead to erroneous assessment, evaluation, diagnosis, and treatment.

Recommendations

As a result of cultural barriers in the counseling relationship, counselor education programs should be revised. White educational institutions are not preparing students to provide therapy to black clients. Therapist trainees must be given the opportunity to experience therapeutic encounters with clients who are culturally different from themselves, and to explore their negative or inaccurate feelings and perceptions. As Vontress (1969) suggested, one way to accomplish this goal is to require that students live or work in the black community as part of their training so they may learn to communicate with black people in their own setting. Also, if the employment of black professional and non-professional workers in neighborhood community health centers were increased, therapists and trainees could share experiences and know each other's values, lifestyles, and attitudes, as recommended by Vontress (1969). "Perhaps," as Kincaid suggests, "the final challenge for the white counselor is his willingness and ability to fulfill a role as interpreter and change agent in the white community, where he faces the sanctions of his peers and more often looks upward rather than downward at his clients." (1969:890)

THE GENESIS OF RACISM

Lula D. Hankins-McNary

In 1619, twenty immigrants arrived in Jamestown on the Mayflower. For approximately forty years, black settlers experienced all the freedoms of white settlers. They had equal opportunity and freedom to purchase land, vote, testify in court, and socialization with settlers was commonplace.

During this period whites, Indians, and blacks were used in a system of "indentured servitude"; the original purpose of which was to encourage poor whites to settle in America in exchange for labor for a defined number of years. As the economical significance of tobacco and cotton crops increased, so did the need for cheap and abundant physical labor.

The system of indentured servitude failed because many large crop owners tried to permanently enslave their servants. The attempt to force white men and women to continue serving, after their contracts had expired, failed because the protective laws of their mother country legislated their release when they had worked the designated period of time, or had acquired the money necessary to compensate the crop owners for their services. If the agreement was not respected, the white indentured servant could appeal to the courts of England and be protected.

When white indentured servants escaped they could easily be mistaken for free white settlers. The enslavement of the Indian also failed because he was more familiar with the land and could easily escape to his tribe. Black indentured slaves, unfortunately, were a visible color, therefore, could not blend in with the settlers and be mistaken for free men. They were not protected by the government of a mother country, hence, had no means of appeal. Finally, large quantities of black captives could be supplied from the continent of Africa.

In the 1660s, Virginia and Maryland formulated laws which declared black people slaves for life: "Children born of Negro women were ruled bond or free, according to the status of the mother, and intermarriage forbidden because black people were not Christians." In 1667, Virginia passed a law which indicated that baptism, "Does not alter the condition of the person as to his bondage or freedom." As a direct result, black people experienced a loss of self-esteem and the destruction of their families, which further resulted in psychological castration of the male and escalation of the female.

Even though chattel slavery was technically "abolished" by 1863, perpetuation of racism continues to influence all aspects of the lives and identity of most black people.

References

Calnek, Maynard, "Racial Factors in the Countertransference: The Black Therapist and the Black Client," *American Journal of Orthopsychiatry*, Vol. 40, No. 1 (January) 1970, pp. 39–46.

Clements, Hubert M., Jack A. Duncan, and Wallace M. Taylor, "Towards Effective Evaluation of the Culturally Deprived," *American*

Personnel and Guidance Association, Vol. 47, No. 9 (May) 1969, pp. 891–896.

Grier, William H. and Price M. Cobbs, *Black Rage*, New York: Bantam Books, Inc., 1968, p. 129.

Jones, Billy E., Orlando B. Lightfoot, Don Palmer, Raymond G. Wilderson, and Donald Williams, "Problems of Black Psychiatric Residents in White Training Institutes," *American Journal of Psychiatry*, Vol. 127, No. 6 (December) 1970, pp. 798–803.

Kincaid, Marylou, "Identity and Therapy in the Black Community," *Personnel and Guidance Journal*, Vol. 47, No. 9 (May) 1969, pp. 884–890.

Lowinger, Paul L. and Shirley Dobie, "Attitudes and Emotions of the Psychiatrist in the Initial Interview," *American Journal of Psychotherapy*, Vol. 20, (January) 1966, pp. 17–34.

Miller, Kent S. and Ralph M. Dreger, *Comparative Studies of Blacks and Whites in the United States*, New York: Seminar Press, 1973, p. 462.

Rosen, Harold and Jerome D. Frank, "Negroes in Psychotherapy," *American Journal of Psychiatry*, Vol. 119 (July-December) 1962, pp. 456–460.

Sabshin, Melvin, Herman Diesenhaus, and Raymond Wilkerson, "Dimensions of Institutional Racism in Psychiatry," *The American Journal of Psychiatry*, No. 127, No. 6 (December) 1970, pp. 787–793.

Vontress, Clemont E., "Cultural Barriers in the Counseling Relationship," *The Personnel and Guidance Journal*, Vol. 48, No. 1 (September) 1969, pp. 11–17.

Bibliography

Adams, Paul L., "The Social Psychiatry of Frantz Fanon," *American Journal of Psychiatry*, Vol. 127, No. 6 (December) 1970, pp. 809–814.

Carmichael, Stokely and Charles Hamilton, *Black Power: The Politics of Liberation in America*, New York: Vintage Books, Random House, Inc., 1967.

Chethik, Morton, Elizabeth Feming, Morris F. Mayer, and John N. McCoy, "A Quest for Identity: Treatment of Disturbed Negro Children in a Predominantly White Treatment Center," *American Journal of Orthopsychiatry*, Vol. 37, 1967, pp. 71–77.

Coleman, James C., *Abnormal Psychology and Modern Life*, (5th ed.) Chicago, Illinois: Scott, Foresman and Company, 1976.

Crisp, A. H., "Therapeutic Aspects of the Doctor/Patient Relationship," *Psychotherapy and Psychosometrics*, Vol. 18 (1–6), 1970, pp. 12–33.

Fischer, Newell, "An Interracial Analysis: Transference and Countertransference Significance," *Journal of the American Psychoanalytic Association*, Vol. 19, No. 4 (October) 1971, pp. 736-745.

Friedman, Neil, "James Baldwin and Psychotherapy," *Psychotherapy: Theory, Research and Practice*, Vol. 3, No. 4 (November) 1966, pp. 177–183.

Hirsch, Selma G., *Fear and Prejudice*, (1st ed.) Public Affairs Committee, Inc. (January) 1967, p. 10.

Hirsch, Selma G., *The Fears Men Live By*, New York: Harper and Brothers, 1955.

Jones, Reginald L., *Black Psychology*, New York: Harper and Row Publishers, 1972.

Kaplan, Seymour R. and Melvin Roman, *The Organization and Delivery of Mental Health Services in the Ghetto*, New York: Praeger Publishers, Inc., 1973.

Kini, Joan F., "The Effects of Patient Social Class on the Judgments of Public Health Nurses," *Nursing Research* (May-June) 1968, pp. 261–263.

Lerner, Barbara, *Therapy in the Ghetto: Political Importance and Personal Disintegration*, Baltimore: The Johns Hopkins University Press, 1972.

Lind, J. E., "The Dream as a Simple Wish Fulfillment in the Negro," *Psychoanalytic Review*, Vol. 1, No. 4, 1913, p. 300.

Payne, R. L., "The Psychology of Racial Prejudices," *Nursing Mirror*, (June 17) 1966, pp. 1–111.

Prudhomme, Charles and Chester Pierce, "Reflections on Racism," *American Journal of Psychiatry*, Vol. 127, No. 6 (December) 1970, pp. 815–818.

Reissman, Frank, Jerome Cohen, and Arthur Pearl, *Mental Health of the Poor*, New York: The Free Press, 1964.

Sager, Clifford J., Thomas L. Brayboy, and Barbara R. Waxenberg, *Black Ghetto Family in Therapy: A Laboratory Experience*, New York: Grove Press, Inc., 1970.

Thomas, Alexander and Samuel Sillen, *Racism and Psychiatry*, New York: Brunner/Mazel, 1972.

Wesson, Alan K., "The Black Man's burden: The White Clinician," *The Black Scholar*, Vol. 6, No. 10 (July-August) 1975, pp. 13–18.

William, Charles, Bernard Kramer, and Bertram Brown, *Racism and Mental Health*, Pennsylvania: University of Pittsburgh Press, 1973.

Wilcox, Roger, *The Psychological Consequences of Being a Black American: A Sourcebook of Research by Black Psychologists*, New York: John Wiley and Sons, Inc., 1971.

Yalom, Irvin D., *The Theory and Practice of Group Psychotherapy*, (2nd ed.) New York: Basic Books, Inc., Publishers, 1975.

Yamamoto, Joe, Quinton C. James, and Norman Palley, "Cultural Problems in Psychiatric Therapy," *Archives of General Psychiatry*, Vol. 19 (July) 1968, pp. 45–49.

Chapter Thirty-Two

LEGAL AND ETHICAL ASPECTS OF PSYCHIATRIC NURSING

Ann Marie Leichman, R.N., M.S.N.

RECENTLY, HEALTH PROFESSIONALS HAVE expressed a growing interest in clients' rights. This seems to reflect an overall trend in society to define the rights of its members more clearly. Legislation, such as the Civil Rights Act of 1964 and the recently defeated Equal Rights Amendment, are examples of attempts to clarify society's position on the matter of guaranteeing rights to certain groups of people. The mentally ill, a group of citizens who have long borne the brunt of societal neglect, are in the midst of a heated debate about their rights. Within the past decade, the American judicial system has handed down several landmark decisions regarding the rights of the mentally ill. It is important for psychiatric nurses to be aware of these decisions and ways they affect clinical practice. It is of equal importance for psychiatric nurses to increase their awareness of ethical principles underlying a competent practice. This article will outline some basic ethical principles used in decision making and highlight the legal rights of psychiatric clients.

LEGAL RIGHTS OF THE MENTALLY ILL

The status of the rights of the mentally ill has changed drastically within recent years. Not long ago, the mentally ill were shut away in institutions that offered little more than custodial care and that deprived them of basic human rights. Perhaps the trend toward increased consumer advocacy in our society has made the plight of these individuals of concern.

An Alabama federal judge handed down a historic decision in the Wyatt v. Stickney (1971) case. The judge ruled that state hospitals must provide adequate treatment for the involuntarily hospitalized mentally ill. The court mandated strict guidelines to meet the requirement of "adequate treatment," thereby recognizing a citizen's constitutional right to treatment (Byrne, 1981).

Lately, the focus has been on the right to refuse treatment. In two landmark cases—Rennie v. Klein (1978) and Rogers v. Okin (1979)—the court acknowledged that under certain circumstances individuals have a constitutional right to refuse treatment. Both cases support the right to refuse medication in nonemergency situations. The Rogers v. Okin case declared that this right can be overturned only after a client has been declared incompetent by a judicial hearing. The Rennie v. Klein proceeding determined that the client can be pronounced incompetent by the treating physician after the case is reviewed by a client advocate. A legal guardian or a family member must then give permission for the client to be medicated against his or her will. The court is still hearing appeals in the Rennie v. Klein case.

These cases highlight constitutional right of the mentally ill to due process and equal protection of the laws as set forth in the Fourteenth Amendment, and they demonstrate that the mentally ill should not be judged incompetent by virtue of their need for hospitalization. Competency is purely a legal term, and determination of competency is in the hands of a judge.

What rights do psychiatric clients have if they are guaranteed equal protection of the law? Specifically, they are entitled to all civil rights, including the right to vote, to hold office, and to have civil service rank and appointment. They are eligible for a license, permit, privilege, or any other benefit provided by law. It also means that they are entitled to manage their property and to wear their own clothes.

The right to due process of the law enables a mentally ill person who is threatened with an involuntary commitment to petition the court for a hearing. The individual is entitled to all privileges associated with a court hearing, such as the right to counsel, the right to be present, and the right to cross examine witnesses. If committed, the person continues to have the right to petition the court and is entitled to a periodic judicial review, testing the need for continued hospitalization. This process prevents unnecessary, long-term hospitalization.

Due process binds the court and hospital to use "the least restrictive alternative" for clients requiring psychiatric care, a mandate that has many implications for treatment. First, a mentally ill person cannot be committed if alternatives, such as outpatient treatment or supervised residential living, are available and will meet the needs of that client.

Second, a hospitalized client cannot be restricted in freedom any more than is necessary to provide adequate treatment. Therefore, locked units, seclusion rooms, quiet rooms, and restraints should only be used as a last resort in treatment. They cannot be utilized as part of a behavior modification plan, as a punishment, or as a threat when a client is noncompliant with treatment.

Due process not only grants the right to treatment but also entitles the client to be an active participant in the care plan. Unless a client is declared incompetent or the hospital has a court order mandating treatment, the client must give informed consent to all proposed medical procedures, such as electroconvulsive therapy and research drugs.

The First Amendment protects the individual's rights associated with freedom of speech and association. These rights allow the client to have visitors, write and receive letters, use the telephone, and visit outside the facility. Any limitations placed on these rights must be justified by exceptional circumstances and must be based on therapeutic reasons. Careful documentation of the limitations must be recorded on the chart. Furthermore, the client must be notified of the decision—orally if the limitation concerns visiting rights and in writing if the limitation is imposed on correspondence or on the use of the telephone. These limitations can be appealed by the client to the director of the facility. The only exception to these limitations is the client's right to correspond with the Mental Health Information Service, a lawyer, a clergyman, or a public official; no restriction whatsoever can be placed on these rights.

These laws have a tremendous impact on clinical practice for the psychiatric nurse. Some nurses continue to blindly follow doctors' orders to medicate a client against his or her will or use quiet rooms as part of a behavior modification plan. Nursing care plans, more often than not, are developed without input from the client, thereby denying the right to be an active participant in the treatment. They also contain approaches that sometimes impinge upon the rights of a client. Consider the approach, "set limits on inappropriate behavior." In practice, this could mean restricting phone calls made at 3 A.M. by a manic client. If this is the case, then the nurse is responsible for having the proper written notification of this decision delivered to the client. As nurses themselves strive to be recognized as autonomous professionals, they must realize that the term *autonomous nurse* is a misnomer, unless they are willing to become accountable for their behavior and actions.

A working knowledge of the mental health laws is a good first step to becoming accountable in practice, but it does not stop there. One must remember that the law is often vague in this area and varies from state to state. An individual's right to refuse medication except in an emergency situation leaves open to question what the term *emergency* means. For these cloudy areas of the law, practitioners are obliged to have a working knowledge of ethical decision making so they will always act in the best interest of the patient. A fit beginning point for becoming acquainted with this subject is to explore the complex concept of rights. When nurses understand the meaning of rights, they are on the road to using sound ethical reasoning as part of the decision-making process.

THE MEANING OF RIGHTS

Let us first examine those rights considered absolute. All citizens of the United States are guaranteed certain unconditional rights by the Constitution, such as the right to life, liberty, and the pursuit of happiness. Citizens are also entitled to freedom of speech, religion, and press and to the right of assembly. These rights can never be set aside unless the state can prove a compelling interest.

Not all rights are guaranteed or so clear-cut. Philosophers have argued for centuries about the definition and meaning of rights. As Bandman and Bandman (1978) point out, "rights have variously been defined as needs, interests, powers, claims, and entitlements" (p. 7). To simplify matters, the view that rights are claims will apply here. In this context, the right holder presses a claim for something to which he or she feels entitled. A depressed client who refuses to consent to electroconvulsive therapy is pressing a claim for the right to refuse treatment. Moreover, there is a corresponding duty for others to see that this claim is upheld (Feinberg, 1978). Therefore, the health professionals caring for this person have a corresponding duty to withhold the electroconvulsive therapy and offer other treatment options.

There are limits to rights, however. Brandt (1959) highlights how "prima facie" rights can be overridden in interest-balancing situations. A suicidal client who claims to be entitled to kill himself or herself could have this right legitimately overturned by a member of the hospital staff. Any person denying this patient's right to kill himself or herself takes justified action, according to the prima facie viewpoint, since a person's "right to life" outweighs the "right to decide." How does one decide, then, how to balance rights? The answer lies in supporting decisions regarding rights with sets of ethical principles.

DECISION MAKING AND ETHICS

According to Davis (1982), rights are derived from the ethical principle of autonomy. An autonomous person is capable of making decisions that affect personal welfare without interference from others. If we respect a client as an autonomous agent, we honor personal decisions regarding treatment, even if we do not agree with them. This is true for all clients, regardless of diagnosis. The presence of a mental illness does not preclude autonomy; only those individuals who have diminished mental capacity and are unable to make a rational choice are nonautonomous. A psychotic client who is smashing objects and threatening to kill other people is clearly not an autonomous agent, since the person is acting in an irrational manner that prevents making sound decisions. When a nurse must intervene on behalf of a nonautonomous individual and block irrational decisions made by that person, the greatest degree of care needs to be exercised so the individual is not exploited or abused. In terms of providing appropriate health care to nonautonomous individuals, the nurse must act according to the ethical principles of nonmaleficence and beneficence.

The principle of nonmaleficence requires the nurse to act in a manner that avoids inflicting intentional harm and the risk of inflicting harm. A nurse who adheres to established guidelines for practice, such as performing range of motion exercises every two hours on a patient in restraints, is complying with the duty of nonmaleficence. Unfortunate atrocities that we read about in newspapers, such as staff leaving patients in seclusion rooms for days on end, are certainly in violation of the ethical principle of nonmaleficence.

Beneficence mandates the duty holder to act in the best interest of another person. Furthermore, the actions of the duty holder must contribute to the welfare of that person. This ethical principle should always govern the actions of a nurse in a situation where he or she is unsure whether the action violates a client's rights. For example, psychiatric nurses are often faced with an ethical dilemma when a voluntary psychiatric client becomes agitated and refuses medication that might help to regain control. Legally, this person has the right to refuse treatment except in an emergency situation where an individual is considered a danger to himself or others. The nurse is in the position of deciding if the patient's level of agitation poses enough of a threat to himself or others to override the guaranteed right to refuse medication. Surely, one can see there is room for individual interpretation. Some people would accept a verbal threat as a danger, whereas others would argue that only an aggressive act in itself is evidence of danger. In this situation, the nurse must balance this client's right to appropriate health care against the right to refuse treatment and against the staff and other clients' right to a safe environment. If this nurse, in his or her best judgment, feels this person will lose control and inflict harm on himself or others, the nurse must take positive action to prevent this. Medicating such clients against their will so they can benefit from a calmer, more rational state of mind is frequently thought to be in the clients' best interest and therefore meets the criteria of the duty of beneficence.

Unfortunately, the problem of balancing rights raises many ethical dilemmas for the long-term treatment of clients. Most health professionals would feel comfortable overriding a dangerous client's right to autonomy. Yet, what happens to the psychotic or severely depressed individual who is not dangerous but refuses all forms of treatment? Is this client truly autonomous or is the decision to refuse treatment a reflection of the illness? Are voices telling the client not to accept medication? These questions are the hardest to answer in a discussion on the rights of the mentally ill and lead us to seriously question how rights will be balanced. The community, for instance, might not want to recognize a corresponding duty to uphold a psychotic client's right to refuse treatment, if it means an excessive financial burden on their resources through such things as disability payments, frequent hospital admissions, and so forth.

The right to refuse treatment is probably the most controversial present-day issue in the field of forensic psychiatry, and there are no pat solutions or answers to this problem. Ultimately, as Michels (1981) points out, imposing treatment on people afflicted with a mental illness would be an unfair discrimination against one class of citizens. He goes on to say that forced treatment of a mentally ill person deemed competent by accepted legal standards borders on associating competency with agreement with the doctor.

APPLICATION OF ETHICAL PRINCIPLES AND THE LAW

The following case example will help illustrate the resolution of an ethical dilemma. Mark is a 28-year-old, 6'2", 220 lb., chronic schizophrenic who is put into restraints at 9 A.M. after hitting a staff member. At 6 P.M., Mark is calm and asking to be released. He says that he realizes his actions were wrong and feels he can now control himself. The charge nurse feels comfortable in recommending to the doctor that Mark be released, but the other staff are strongly opposed. They are afraid of Mark and feel he should be kept in restraints until the morning when more staff will be present. They think that if Mark becomes agitated again they will be unable to prevent him from hurting someone. The charge nurse stands firm on the belief that Mark should be released and explains the rationale to the staff. The nurse views Mark as an autonomous person because he is now rational. Continuing the restraints would be violating the duty of beneficence, since it would not contribute to his welfare. Furthermore, restraints pose a risk of inflicting harm, which is a violation of the duty of nonmaleficence. Finally, the nurse points out to the staff that legally this person cannot be restricted in his liberty any more than necessary. The fact that a client might exhibit violent behavior at a future time is an unpredictable variable; therefore, it is not a justifiable reason to override his rights.

In conclusion, nurses must be aware of the complexity of the legal and ethical problems involved in treating the mentally ill. They should be able to support their decisions and opinions with sound ethical reasoning. In the final analysis, it will be their clients who benefit from this knowledge; when one person respects another's rights, he or she is treating that person with dignity and self-respect. A psychiatric client who senses that personal rights have been respected is likely to view himself or herself as others do—an autonomous individual capable of self-determination. Only under these circumstances can the client enter into a trusting and therapeutic nurse-client relationship.

References

Annas, G., and Healy, J. (March 1974). The patient's rights advocate: Redefining the doctor-patient relationship in the hospital context. *Vanderbilt Law Review, 27,* 243–269.

Bandman, E., and Bandman, B. (eds.) (1978). *Bioethics and human rights: A reader for health professionals.* Boston: Little, Brown and Company.

Brandt, R. (1959). *Ethical theory.* Englewood Cliffs, NJ: Prentice-Hall.

Byrne, G. (February 1981). Conference report: Wyatt v. Stickney: Retrospect and prospect. *Hospital and Community Psychiatry, 32,* 123–126.

Davis, Anne. (February 1982). Helping your staff address ethical dilemmas. *The Journal of Nursing Administration, 11,* 9–13.

Feinberg, Joel. (1978). The nature and value of rights. In E. Bandman and B. Bandman (eds.), *Bioethics and human rights,* (pp. 19–31). Boston: Little, Brown and Company.

Michels, R. (1981). The right to refuse treatment: Ethical issues. *Hospital and Community Psychiatry, 32,* 251–254.

Rennie v. Klein, 462 F. Supp. 1131 (D. NJ 1978), No. 79-1648 (1st Cir., 1980).

Rogers v. Okin, 478 F. Supp. 1342 (D. MA 1979), No. 79-1648 (1st Cir. Nov. 25, 1980).

Chapter Thirty-Three

THE CHRONIC PSYCHIATRIC PATIENT IN THE COMMUNITY— A MODEL OF CARE

Judith B. Krauss

THE IMPACT OF DEINSTITUTIONALIZATION on chronic psychiatric patients, their families, and the communities into which they are discharged has been profound. Communities are increasingly faced with men and women released from state hospitals on large doses of therapeutic medication—persons who suffer constant low level symptomatology and periodic exacerbation. Many of them live in social isolation, unemployed, and in despair or apathy.[1] Recent studies have shown also that discharged patients are often a health and financial burden to their families. And there is evidence that certain types of families can precipitate relapse in former patients.

Nurses already play key roles in caring for the needs of this population. But what do we actually know about managing this population of chronic patients in the community? How can we help make community care for the deinstitutionalized patient and his family more effective and humane? A brief review of the recent history of caring for the mentally ill may help make the picture clearer and provide direction for care services in the community.

The treatment of people with chronic psychiatric illness has improved greatly over the past 25 years, since the discovery of psychopharmacologic methods of suppressing psychotic symptoms. During that time, the resident population of large state mental hospitals has been reduced by two thirds, and new forms of outpatient and aftercare therapy have been developed. In addition, the need for community-based transitional living facilities and social/vocational programs to assist the scores of lonely patients being discharged into localities ill equipped to deal with them has been recognized—although it is a long way from being implemented adequately.

But institutional care has not been ruled out for some patients such as those with chronic schizophrenia. Wing believes, for instance: "A good hospital is better than a poor hostel, nursing home, or hotel and is just as much a part of community care. Even the concept of community itself can be challenged if the patient has no social roots, is markedly withdrawn, and is unable to make spontaneous social contacts."[2]

DEINSTITUTIONALIZATION

Deinstitutionalization is the term used to describe the relocation of a "long-stay" patient from a large public mental hospital into a community, to be supported there by a formal network of clinical, social, and vocational agencies, as well as an informal network of family, neighbors, and local community resources.

Deinstitutionalization stems from the unintended negative effects of confinement in large public institutions devoted to the care and treatment of the mentally ill. Criticisms of these hospitals first led to attempts at internal reform and then to policies of deinstitutionalization advocated by community mental health movements and legislated by the Federal government in the early sixties.

The change that took place can be seen in the fact that in 1955, 77 percent of services were provided in inpatient settings and 23 percent in outpatient settings, while in 1975 the situation was reversed, with 76 percent of services being provided on an outpatient basis and only 24 percent in inpatient settings. The greatest reduction occurred in inpatient services of state mental hospitals, which provided 49 percent of all services in 1955 and only 9 percent in 1975.[3]

However, as Bassuk and Gerson point out, these statistics are illusory. "Although the annual census was decreasing, admissions to state hospitals increased from 178,000 in 1955 to a peak of 390,000 in 1972 and declined only to 375,000 by 1974.... Moreover, a growing proportion of the admissions were readmissions...about half of the released inpatients are readmitted within a year of discharge."[4]

The reduction in hospital census and the concomitant increase in the

annual number of admissions are most likely the result of two factors: a
new philosophy of briefer hospitalization, and an increase in readmissions
due to the inability of both patients and communities to adjust to each
other. In a five-year follow-up study of all patients discharged from
California state institutions, Miller found that 100 percent were readmitted
at least once during that time.[5] And in a review of 28 different
populations, Rosenblatt and Mayer found that the one factor consistently
related to readmission was the previous number of hospitalizations.[6]

Solomon and Doll argue the case against the use of recidivism rates
as a measure of program effectiveness. They suggest that recidivism is
related to a complex of variables that cannot be reflected in statistics
alone. They postulate that readmission can reflect any one or a
combination of the following factors: 1) the patient's solution to
emotional problems; 2) a function of demographics (age, sex, race, marital
status, social class); 3) family tolerance; 4) community tolerance; 5)
caregivers' reactions to deviant (noncompliant) patient behavior; 6) patient
characteristics (attractiveness, previous history, likeability); 7) caregiver
characteristics (attitudes, experience, status in system); and 8) the nature
of the mental health delivery system (policies, census, available
alternatives).[7]

The outpouring of literature concerning the aftermath of
deinstitutionalization tends to confirm this thesis and to suggest that these
causes of recidivism are related to existing gaps in the networks of support
available to discharged patients.

WHAT HAPPENS TO THE
DISCHARGED PATIENT?

The "careers" of many chronic psychiatric patients have changed from
stable, long-term residence in state mental hospital facilities to a transient
existence in a community and multiple hospital readmissions. Several
follow-up studies of such discharged patients indicate that over 50 percent
of any chronic population will relapse within a year of discharge, and that
most patients do not return to their community of origin but cluster in
low-income, poor housing areas, suggesting a "ghetto-ization" of
ex-patients.[8]

My colleagues and I found in interviews with 200 discharged
patients that many were socially isolated and socially deficient. Few had a
treatment source; they were shuffled from hospital to hospital, from
doctor to doctor, unwanted and undesirable as candidates for
psychotherapeutic treatment.[9]

A demographic study of the Bowery in New York, formerly a last refuge of alcoholics, revealed that the population has altered drastically since deinstitutionalization. Over 50 percent of the Bowery population is now 19-39 years of age, nonwhite, nonalcoholic, and characterized by primary psychiatric disorders of the psychotic or personality disturbance type.[10]

Another author suggests that the reason loneliness and asocialization increase in chronic patients after they are discharged is that the stigma of the illness and associated myths of violence and impulsiveness, coupled with the real social inadequacies of patients, cause others to shun them or to take advantage of them.[11]

Still another writer documents that briefer inpatient stays parallel an increased tendency to discharge patients on large therapeutic doses of phenothiazines before proper maintenance dosages are established.[12]

A study of acute schizophrenics discharged to a community mental health center confirms what many health care professionals know from experience: that many deinstitutionalized patients do not find their way to outpatient treatment. More than 40 percent of the patients in this study never appeared at the outpatient clinic. Of those who did, 36 percent showed up from one to five times, and only 21 percent appeared six or more times. On the basis of their findings, the authors suggest that the usual process of casual outpatient referral does not work for almost 80 percent of all chronic patients.[13]

Klerman has noted that patients have developed new forms of chronicity as represented by dependencies on community institutions, ghetto-type living, poor quality of life, and increasing neurologic complications resulting from long-term maintenance on potent drugs.[14]

Reviewing a study of 162 adult patients of three Pennsylvania State hospitals who had been discharged for one year, Ozarin and Sharfstein report that:

- 94 percent preferred living in the community

- patients with long previous hospitalizations fared less well than those with shorter hospitalizations

- only 2.5 percent were gainfully employed

- the majority felt that the hospital provided more social outlets than the community did

- 70 percent were dependent on public funds

- 8 percent had had police involvement

- 69 percent reported no emotional disturbances

- 75 percent were taking psychoactive drugs [15]

In general, then, although the psychiatric patient of today may fare better than the patient of 25 years ago, the picture of the deinstitutionalized patient in the community reflected in these studies is a bleak one. We see individuals with low levels of social competence living isolated lives in impoverished, ghetto-ized areas. They suffer constant chronic symptomatology with periodic exacerbation, are on large therapeutic doses of psychotropic drugs, and often do not find their way to outpatient treatment.

IMPACT ON FAMILIES

Patients who return home present their families with a range of troublesome behaviors. It is also apparent that little is being offered these families in the way of supportive guidance. Grad and Sainsbury conducted a follow-up study of patients treated in two psychiatric service areas with different admissions policies: the more traditional one favored inpatient hospitalization, while the other favored community-based treatment. The effect of patient behavior on families was measured at the beginning, during, and at the end of a two-year period. All the findings showed that the community service, which favored extramural care, left families more burdened.

"Burden" was measured in terms of alterations in household routines, social and leisure life, income, family employment, mental health, physical health, and behavior of children. The community service families experienced significantly more financial problems and effects on mental health of family members. Patient behaviors most often mentioned as troublesome by all families were: patients' preoccupations with bodily ailments; family fears that patients might harm themselves accidentally or purposefully; and patients' excessively demanding behavior. Dangerous behavior or behavior that might provoke comments from neighbors was least often mentioned. While patients with serious socially deviant behavior problems were found to be equally burdensome, those with less conspicuous but annoying behavior caused more burden to the community service families.[16]

In a survey of the families of 56 unemployed psychiatric patients in England, 29 of them, most of them chronic schizophrenics, were living with parents or siblings. Results indicated that dependence on parents of pensionable age was an obstacle to patient rehabilitation. Relatives experienced considerable financial burden and symptoms of reactive anxiety and depression. The study revealed a need for special services to assist patients toward a more independent existence when elderly relatives die.[17]

A study of the relatives of 80 patients from two London districts demonstrated major gaps in available supportive services. These included a lack of guidance on how to deal with a patient's withdrawn or disturbed behavior, lack of assistance in finding help, and lack of local alternatives to long-term hospitalization.

The most disturbing set of patient behaviors to relatives was described as social withdrawal, underactivity, lack of conversation, and minimal leisure interests. The next disturbing set consisted of slowness, overactivity, odd ideas, depression, odd behavior, neglect of appearance, and odd postures and movements. Less frequently mentioned were threats or violence, poor mealtime behavior, socially embarrassing behavior, sexually unusual behavior, suicide attempts, and incontinence.

Relatives had to learn by trial and error which behaviors to try to alter and which to ignore. They appreciated even the most minimal guidance in this area. There was a general failure on the part of professionals to recognize relatives as important primary caregivers who were often more skilled in dealing with difficult management problems than the professionals were.[18]

Families can present problems to patients, also, jeopardizing their already tenuous ability to survive community life. Brown and others followed ill patients and their families over a two-year period to measure whether a high degree of expressed emotion in relatives is likely to cause a recurrence of florid symptoms in patients living at home. They found that there was a significant relationship between high expressed emotions and relapse. They also found that marked warmth on the part of relatives, free from overemotional involvement, was associated with a low rate of relapse. Through a series of complex analyses, they determined that patients who reject hospital readmission, take drugs regularly, and have little face-to-face contact with relatives after discharge remain in the community longer. In contrast, patients with "typical" schizophrenic symptoms who are male, accept hospital admission, are irregular medication-takers, and have high face-to-face contact in the home are more likely to relapse. Relatives' expressed emotion, however, was the greatest predictor of patient relapse when these variables were controlled.[19]

Another study of a group of schizophrenic and depressed patients yielded similar findings—that is, for schizophrenic patients high levels of expressed emotion on the part of relatives were associated with relapse, but that medication and decreased face-to-face contact with relatives provided added protection against relapse. Depressed patients, however, proved to be more sensitive to relatives' criticisms and were not helped by the additive effects of medication and decreased face-to-face contact.[20]

The negative aspects of the impact of deinstitutionalization on patients' community adjustment, on the health and well-being of family members, and on patient-family interactions have been clearly defined. Community-based treatment must be concerned with counteracting them.

BASIC NEEDS TO BE ADDRESSED

Most experts agree on the basic needs of chronic psychiatric patients that must be addressed by any community treatment network. These needs can be organized under five categories:

1. *Basic life necessities:* food, clothing, housing (including transitional living arrangements), income maintenance, health care (both physical and psychological), and legal protection.

2. *Meaningful use of time:* social and vocational rehabilitation, employment, sheltered workshops, leisure/recreational activities, education, spiritual activity, and resocialization.

3. *Access to medication:* availability, motivation to comply, proper dosage, and coordination with other treatment.

4. *Support for family members.*

5. *Integrated medical, nursing, and social services.*

Obviously, no one service can possibly meet all these needs. While treatment may appropriately be initiated at a community mental health facility, it must extend beyond that to involve a network of professional and neighborhood helpers.

Naparstek and Haskell suggest that there are two distinct helping networks available to patients—the "professional" and the "natural." The first includes public welfare agencies, general hospitals, mental health centers, courts, schools, religious institutions, child guidance centers, nursing homes, social service agencies, and emergency/crisis service. The second encompasses family, friends, neighbors, neighborhood organizations, voluntary associations, social clubs, self-help groups, clergy, teachers, police, pharmacies, and other informal helpers.[21]

The key to any successful community treatment model is proper placement of the patient in the community and adequate linkage between the professional and natural helping networks. This linkage can be achieved through shared goals for treatment and communication between primary caregivers in both networks.

ELEMENTS OF TREATMENT
COMPONENT

Based on what we know of the needs of the chronic psychiatric patient in the community, the following five elements must be included in the treatment components of any service delivery network designed with this population in mind:

1. Maintaining a stable level of functioning at the patient's current level of adjustment.

2. Meeting the patient's dependency needs (and recognizing that dependency is a comparatively healthy adjustment to life where the alternative is an acute exacerbation of illness).

3. Assisting the patient to cope with crisis.

4. Providing social/vocational rehabilitation opportunities.

5. Coordinating the helping networks.

Maintenance

The maintenance component of the service network must include medication management, family support intervention, and patient support intervention. While we have little empirical evidence that any of our treatment technologies work with chronic patients, we know that the neuroleptic drugs are capable of reducing florid psychotic symptoms, forestalling symptom exacerbation, and reducing relapse in a significant proportion of the chronic psychiatric population.[22]

However, studies have shown that a small group of patients do not seem to benefit from drugs: men whose families were disrupted early in life; patients who live alone or with families whose attitudes toward treatment are negative; and irregular medication takers.[23] We are also aware of the Parkinsonian side effects of the major phenothiazines and the additive negative effects they can have on already socially dysfunctional behavior.

A comprehensive medication maintenance program requires both psychiatrists skilled in psychopharmacologic management and psychiatric nurses skilled in the observation of symptoms and side effects, as well as in the day-to-day management of the medication ritual and its fit with other aspects of treatment. The nurse-physician team can provide inservice education programs for nonmedical caregivers that are geared toward early detection of patients who do not respond to the drug. Such patients may be managed more successfully with long-acting, parenteral medication or by being referred to a public health nursing agency for follow-up supervision of medication-taking at home.

Anyone who has cared for a chronic psychiatric patient is aware of the importance of the drug-taking ritual and its effects on compliance and attitudes toward treatment.[24] For patients for whom the drug-taking ritual is as therapeutic as the drug itself, steps can be taken to coordinate the prescription regimen with the ritual. When such coordination is impossible, clinicians can be alerted to initiate supportive intervention designed to provide another way of dealing with the need the drug ritual fulfilled while gradually adjusting management of the patient's medication.

Several studies confirm that family members can be the single greatest facilitator or deterrent to a patient's successful community adjustment and that certain patient behaviors can be identified as more troublesome than others to family members. This information can be used in conducting routine, periodic family assessments for patients and families who live together to determine the level of intervention required to maintain a stable environment for the patient. Intervention requires the availability of community and treatment-center based services. It can take place on one of four levels:

1. *Education level.* Families judged to be stabilized at higher levels of adjustment may benefit from programs located in the community (in churches, schools, local YMCAs, etc.) which use an educational model to present issues common to people coping with chronic psychiatric illness. A community series on chronic psychiatric illness—what it is, whom it affects, *and* what community members can do to help—may be organized collaboratively by caregivers and patients and their families. A series on how to manage behavioral problems common to people with chronic psychiatric conditions could be enormously helpful to families who have to deal with annoying behavior on a daily basis.

2. *Self-help level.* Some families will not require professional intervention but will need regular support in order to be able to continue to provide a stable environment for the patient. Caregivers can help organize groups of families in the community who share common problems and are capable of exchanging information and offering support to each other. Often local clergy can be enlisted to assist in sustaining such self-help programs. Periodic consultations with mental health professionals can be made available to these groups and their individual members.

3. *Extended support level.* Some families will require the continuing help of health care providers to assess their home performance and to provide support, encouragement, and suggestions for managing a patient's problem behavior. These services are best provided through the use of community agencies such as local public health nursing or visiting nurse associations, although home visits by mental health clinicians can also serve these needs.

4. *Supportive therapy level.* Brief supportive family therapy is best reserved for those families with identified high levels of expressed emotion or where the patient has severe behavior problems which require special management and constitute an added burden to the family. Such therapy is aimed at shoring up family members and modifying behavior which is likely to provoke relapse. For instance, face-to-face contact with relatives high in expressed emotion can be reduced by imposing a schedule which requires the patient to be out of the house more often. Finally, some patients will require group and/or individual supportive therapy in order to remain in the community. These therapies should be distinguished from rehabilitative therapies which also employ group and individual modalities.

The goals in supportive therapy are symptom management, relationship building, and ego support. Assessment should focus on the patient's ego strengths, ability to tolerate intimacy, and capacity to interact in groups of varying sizes in a relatively asymptomatic fashion. The decision to place a patient in supportive therapy should be based on the judgment that his deficits in these areas are sufficient to put him at risk for relapse if rehabilitation therapy were initiated. Services must provide a choice of group or individual therapy to take into account both the patient's ability to respond more easily to one modality or the other and the type of therapy needed to shore up deficit areas. For example, a patient who has major problems tolerating the intimacy of a one-to-one relationship may be placed in a group initially with the intention of gradually building such a relationship between him and the group therapist.

Dependency

The encouragement of dependency runs counter to most psychotherapeutic interventions. Actually, it was the recognition of the deterioration effects of institutional dependency that sparked the move toward deinstitutionalization. As a result of deinstitutionalization, however, many patients were transferred from a position of total dependence to a situation where independence was the norm. But expectations of independent performance can precipitate symptom exacerbation and/or relapse even in patients who have not experienced prolonged hospitalization. For that reason, in caring for chronic psychiatric patients, the clinician must accept, and in some cases encourage, varying levels of dependency.

Services designed to take dependency needs into account might well adopt a model of care similar to the primary nursing model developed by Manthey.[25] It is the responsibility of the primary nurse to assess patient needs, negotiate and coordinate treatment, and provide 24-hour "on call" coverage. Such a system provides for dependency needs while simultaneously assisting a patient toward more independent behavior.

Patients will necessarily encounter multiple caregivers in the support network, but it is comforting to them to know that one person is consistently available in an emergency or when a question about care arises. Using the primary nursing model in chronic care programs provides structure to otherwise large, disorganized caseloads and allows staff to communicate essential patient data through team meetings, charting, and other formal and informal channels.

Dependency needs are crucial when decisions are being made to move patients into the community. Where the patient lives and the kinds of resources that will surround him will affect how successfully he will adjust; they must fit with his capacity to make independent decisions. Assessment of a patient's daily living skills, problem-solving ability, available personal support systems, and social/vocational skills will help determine whether he should return to his family, move into a half-way residence, a board-and-room facility, a cooperative apartment, a foster family, a nursing home, or attempt to live alone. The greater the patient's dependency needs, the more structure he will require.

For this reason, a successful service network needs to have a full range of living arrangements available. Caregivers should actively lobby for this in situations where some types of placements are lacking.

Crisis Intervention

In a population with chronic psychiatric illness, symptomatic exacerbation is the most common response to stress or change. The chronic care clinician must be vigilant and aggressive in assessing for actual or potential life changes. Clinicians must be well versed in the commonly occurring life events and conduct monthly interviews designed to screen for their existence and to date their occurrence. Chronic patients will not voluntarily offer information concerning such events, frequently believing, as many clinicians do, that their symptom exacerbations are simply cyclical in nature and not linked with precipitating causes. Very often anticipatory guidance toward a pending life event will be enough to enable a patient to cope with it.

Community-based, ex-patient, self-help groups, similar to Alcoholics Anonymous, can be of enormous help in staving off untoward reactions to stress. As with the self-help groups of family members, local clergy or other identified community helpers will often be willing to help keep such groups going, and a system of periodic consultation and available referral can be established in conjunction with these groups.

In cases where patients must be removed temporarily from their community setting, it is essential that community-based services, including day treatment, night treatment, and brief hospitalization, are available and easily accessible. If possible, arrangements should be made to allow the primary clinician to be involved in the patient's admission and discharge.

Day and night treatment programs can be located on the aftercare service to allow maximum staff crossover.

A formal system of notification and back-up calls between the chronic care service and local emergency rooms will help prevent precipitous and unnecessary hospital admissions. Properly alerted emergency room staff can provide medication, holding beds, or intervene supportively with patients and significant others to avoid hospitalization. They can also, when warranted, make a more informed inpatient referral, initiating discharge planning from the beginning and communicating with the primary clinician as soon as possible.

Rehabilitation

The rehabilitation process, unlike the supportive therapy process, is aimed not at stabilization, but at movement toward higher levels of adjustment. Rehabilitation services should take place largely, although not exclusively, outside of the community mental health facility in order to symbolize the shift from a focus on illness to a focus on healthy behavior and the acquisition of regaining of skills. Most patients will participate simultaneously in maintenance/supportive therapy and rehabilitative therapy, but a greater emphasis should be placed on one or the other at any given point in time. I have found that in highly dependent patients with poor ego strength and an inability to tolerate groups and/or intimacy, supportive therapy must precede active rehabilitation.

Patients at risk for relapse may benefit from more protective rehabilitation experiences such as social groups located in the mental health center, occupational therapy activities, and sheltered workshops. Patients at low risk for relapse can be more actively engaged in community-based social groups, vocational/rehabilitation testing and training, problem-solving groups, and educational programs. Those who already have achieved a satisfactory level of social adjustment but still require some support can be used as volunteers or as paid workers to assist others less adjusted in the rehabilitative process.

Coordination

The final element necessary to the success of a community service network is a formal system of coordination. Coordination is required on an individual level each time a new patient enters the network and on a systems level as network components interact on program planning, implementation, and evaluation issues. Without it, the patient can become entangled in a web of services or, worse, disengaged entirely.

The psychiatric nurse is uniquely suited for the liaison/consultation role needed to coordinate the activities of both the professional and the natural helping networks. The nurse is equally accepted in professional and neighborhood circles and has long moved freely in both. Familiar to the lay public by virtue of her community health, occupational, and school nurse role, she is allowed access to slices of daily life not usually available to other health practitioners. In inpatient and outpatient settings, the nurse is a staple of daily care.

Nurses are grounded in psychological, physiological, and psychosocial theories of health and are recognized as skilled observers of behavior. All this fosters broad interpretation of patient data and makes it easy for them to interact with a wide variety of health professionals. Of course, a full range of caregivers—psychiatrists, neurologists, social workers, occupational therapists, transitional living counselors, and social/vocational rehabilitation counselors—is necessary to implement the professional helping network. But none of these professional workers share the nurse's wide base of theoretical preparation, medical and psychosocial orientation, and ready access to and acceptance in the natural helping network.

Nursing acquired its supportive, nurturing, low-threat image long ago, and has long been involved in the care of the chronically ill. Perhaps it is time to take advantage of its strategic location in both helping networks and use nurses to close the gaps in community-based care for chronically ill psychiatric patients.

References

1. Slavinsky, A., Tierney, J., and Krauss, J. Back to the community: a dubious blessing. *Nurs.Outlook* 24:370–373, June 1976.

2. Wing, J. K. The social context of schizophrenia. *Am.J.Psychiatry* 135:1333–1339, Nov. 1978.

3. U.S. President's Commission on Mental Health, Report to the President: Volume 2, Task Panel Reports. Washington, D.C., U.S. Government Printing Office, 1978, pp. 1–138.

4. Bassuk, E. L., and Gerson, S. Deinstitutionalization and mental health services. *Sci. Am.* 238:46–53, Feb. 1978.

5. California Mental Hygiene Department. *Worlds that Fail, Part I*, by D. Miller. Sacramento, The Department, 1965.

6. Rosenblatt, A., and Mayer, J. E. The recidivism of mental patients: a review of past studies. *Am.J.Orthopsychiatry* 44:697–706, Oct. 1974.

7. Solomon, Phyllis, and Doll, William. The varieties of readmission: the case against use of recidivism rates as a measure of program effectiveness. *Am.J.Orthopsychiatry* 49:230–239, Apr. 1979.

8. Greenblatt, M., and Glazier, E. The phasing out of mental hospitals in the United States. *Am.J.Psychiatry* 132:1135–1140, Nov. 1975.

9. Slavinsky, A. T., and others. *op.cit.*, p. 373.

10. Reich, R., and Seigal, L. The emergence of the Bowery as a psychiatric dumping ground. *Psychiatric Q.* 50:191–201, Fall 1978.

12. Reider, R. O. Hospitals, patients and politics. *Schizophr.Bull.* Issue 11:9–15, Winter 1974.

13. Evans, J. R., and others. Premorbid adjustment, paranoid diagnosis, and remission. Acute schizophrenics treated in a community mental health center. *Arch.Gen.Psychiatry* 28:666–672, May 1973.

14. Klerman, G. L. Better but not well: social and ethical issues in the deinstitutionalization of the mentally ill. *Schizophr.Bull.* 3(4):617–631, 1977.

15. Ozarin, L., and Sharfstein, S. The aftermaths of deinstitutionalization: problems and solutions. *Psychiatric Q.* 50:128-132, Summer 1978.

16. Grad, J., and Sainsbury, P. The effects that patients have on their families in a community care and control psychiatric service—a two-year followup. *Br.J.Psychiatry* 114:265–278, Mar. 1968.

17. Stevens, B. Dependence of schizophrenic patients on elderly relatives. *Psychol.Med.* 2:17–32, Jan. 1972.

18. Greer, C., and Wing, J. Living with schizophrenic patients. *Br.J.Hosp.Med.* July 1975, pp. 73–82.

19. Brown, G. W., and others. Influence of family life on the course of schizophrenic disorders: a replication. *Br.J.Psychiatry* 121:241–258, Sept. 1972.

20. Vaughn, C. E., and Leff, J. P. The influence of family and social factors on the course of psychiatric illness: a comparison of schizophrenic and depressed neurotic patients. *Br.J.Psychiatry* 129:125–137, Aug. 1976.

21. Naparstek, A. J., and Haskell, C. D. Neighborhood approaches to mental health services. In *Neighborhood Psychiatry*, ed. by L. B. Macht and others. Lexington, Mass., Lexington Books, Division of D. C. Heath and Co., 1977, pp. 31–42.

22. Hogarty, G. E., and others. Drug and sociotherapy in the aftercare of schizophrenic patients: Part 2. Two-year relapse rates. *Arch.Gen.Psychiatry* 31:603–608, Nov. 1974.

23. Goldberg, S. C. and others. Prediction of relapse in schizophrenic outpatients treated by drug and sociotherapy. *Arch.Gen.Psychiatry* 34:171–184, Feb. 1977.

24. Burgoyne, R. W. Effect of drug ritual changes on schizophrenics. In *Scientific Proceedings 128th Annual Meeting of the American Psychiatric Association, held at Anaheim, California May 1975.* Washington, D.C., American Psychiatric Association, 1976, pp. 254–255.

25. Manthey, Marie, and Kramer, Marlene. A dialogue on primary nursing. *Nurs.Forum* 9(4):366–379, 1970.

Chapter Thirty-Four

BURNED OUT

Christina Maslach

JUST BEFORE CHRISTMAS, A woman went to a poverty lawyer to get
help. While discussing her problems, she complained about the fact that
she was so poor that she was not going to be able to get any Christmas
presents for her children. The lawyer, who was a young mother herself,
might have been expected to be sympathetic to the woman's plight.
Instead, she found herself yelling at the woman, telling her, "So go rob
Macy's if you want presents for your kids! And don't come back to see
me unless you get caught and need to be defended in court!" Afterward,
in thinking about the incident, the lawyer realized that she had "burned
out."

Hour after hour, day after day, health and social service
professionals are intimately involved with troubled human beings. What
happens to people who work intensely with others, learning about their
psychological, social or physical problems? Ideally, the helpers retain
objectivity and distance from the situation without losing their concern for
the person they are working with. Instead, our research indicates, they are
often unable to cope with this continual emotional stress and burnout
occurs. They lose all concern, all emotional feeling, for the persons they
work with and come to treat them in detached or even dehumanized ways.

For the past few years, I have been studying the dynamics of
burnout in collaboration with co-workers at the University of California
in Berkeley. We have observed 200 professionals at work, conducted
personal interviews and collected extensive questionnaire data. Our sample
includes poverty lawyers, physicians, prison personnel, social welfare
workers, clinical psychologists and psychiatrists in a mental hospital, child-
care workers and psychiatric nurses. Our findings to date show that all of
these professional groups (and perhaps others that you can think of in

your own experience) tend to cope with stress by a form of distancing that not only hurts themselves but is damaging to all of us as their human clients.

For one thing, the worker's feelings about people often show a shift toward the cynical or negative. According to one social worker, "I began to despise everyone and could not conceal my contempt," while another reports, "I find myself caring less and possessing an extremely negative attitude." In many cases, professionals who have burned out from stress and can no longer cope begin to defend themselves not only by thinking of clients in more derogatory terms but even by believing that the clients somehow deserve any problems they have. As one psychiatric nurse reported to us, "Sometimes you can't help but feel, 'Damn it, they want to be there, and they're fuckers, so let them stay there.' You really put them down."

There is little doubt that burnout plays a major role in the poor delivery of health and welfare services to people in need of them. They wait longer to receive less attention and less care. It is also a key factor in low worker morale, absenteeism, and high job turnover (for a common response to burnout is to quit and get out).

Further, we found that burnout correlates with other damaging indexes of human stress, such as alcoholism, mental illness, marital conflict and suicide. The suicide rate of police officers, for example, is 6½ times higher than that of people in non-law enforcement occupations, and psychiatrists contribute more than their share of numbers to the suicide toll.

If stress cannot be resolved while on the job, then it is often resurrected at home. Sometimes the professional is unaware of the causes and wrongly attributes the increased fighting to something that has gone wrong in the family relationship. As one correctional officer put it, when talking about the pressures of working in prison, "None of my three wives understood."

Burnout varies in severity among different professions and is called by different names (some law enforcement groups refer to this suppression as the "John Wayne syndrome"), but the same basic phenomenon seems to be occurring across a wide variety of work settings.

In our project, we are uncovering the interpersonal stresses that plague these workers, learning what (if any) preparation they receive to cope and isolating the techniques that they use to "detach" themselves from clients or patients. Also, we seek to identify the human consequences for American society that result from use of such distancing techniques, and we are addressing ourselves to solutions. What can be done to prevent the destructive process of burnout?

The verbal and nonverbal techniques used to achieve detachment were remarkably similar among all the many professional groups we studied. By reducing the worker's emotional involvement, these techniques make a client seem less human, more like an object or a number.

We found that a change in the terms used to describe people was one way of making them appear more objectlike and less human. Some of these terms are derogatory labels ("They're all just animals" or "They come out from under the rocks"). Others are more abstract terms referring to large, undifferentiated units, such as "the poor," "my caseload" or "my docket."

Another way of divorcing one's feelings from some stressful event is to describe things as precisely and scientifically as possible. In several professions, the use of jargon (e.g., "a positive GI series," "reaction formation") typically serves the purpose of distancing the person from a client who is emotionally upsetting in some way.

Patients are often labeled by their immediate medical problem, such as "He's a coronary." While this aspect of the patient is the most important one that a physician should be attending to, the fact that it is often the only one means that the patient's complex humanness—his or her accomplishments, hopes and feelings and beliefs—is disregarded or ignored.

A related technique that we discovered involves recasting a volatile situation in more intellectual and less personal terms. For example, in dealing with a mental patient who is being verbally or physically abusive, a psychiatric nurse may try to stand back and look at the patient analytically so as not to get personally upset. "I think that if someone on the outside were to hit me, I would get really angry and hit them back," a nurse told us. "But I don't get angry if a patient hits me, because it's a different situation. The patients who strike out are not really angry at you—they're striking out in fear, or they're so out of it that they don't even know what they're doing. Sometimes a patient is striking out at the devil. So, at the moment, you happen to look like the devil, but it's not you personally that he's striking out at—so I don't get angry at that."

Another way of distancing is to make a sharp distinction between job and personal life. Many professionals whom we studied do not discuss their family or personal affairs with their co-workers, and they often refrain from discussing their experiences on the job with their spouses and friends. "My husband and I have an explicit agreement that neither of us will 'talk shop' at home. I'm in social work, and he's in clinical practice. Neither of us wants to burden the other with more emotion-arousing anecdotes from the day, as we each have had enough of our own to cope with," explained one of our subjects.

Some of the prison personnel even refused to tell people what their job was. In response to questions, they would only say, "I'm a civil servant" or "I work for the state." By leaving their work at the office and not reliving it once again at home, the emotional stress is confined to a smaller part of the professional's life.

One social worker in child welfare stated that if he did not leave his work at the office, he could hardly stand to face his own children. Likewise, when he was at work, he could not think of his family because he would then overempathize with his clients, leading to unbearable emotional stress. As one might expect, he doesn't have the usual family photos on the office desk. Rules forbidding staff to socialize with their patients or clients outside the job setting can help to bring about this clear distinction.

For many psychiatrists, a drawback of going into private practice is that job and private life can merge in disturbing ways. As one of our respondents put it, "Everytime you hear your telephone ring at night, you think, 'Oh, no—I hope it's not a patient.' At times it seems as if you can't ever get away from your patients' problems for some peace and quiet for yourself. When I worked at the hospital, there wasn't the same problem because when I went home for the day, another shift came on—and so I could relax in the evenings because I knew that if any of the patients needed help, there was someone else there to provide it."

Another technique for cooling emotion is to minimize physical involvement in a tense encounter. How does it happen? We observed a number of ways. Some people physically distanced themselves from others (by standing farther away, avoiding eye contact or keeping their hand on the doorknob) even while continuing a minimal conversation. Withdrawal was also achieved by communicating with the patient or client in impersonal ways—superficial generalities, stereotyped responses and form letters.

In some cases, professionals simply spend less time with their patient or client, either by deliberately cutting down the length of the formal interview or therapy sessions, or by spending more of their time talking and socializing with other staff members. Many of the psychiatric staff were able to point to specific patients with whom they limited their interaction. "There was one woman who was very suicidal. She had injured herself in some bizarre ways and had set herself on fire several times on the ward. She was extremely depressed, and I did a lot of work with her. One day I had to spend my entire eight-hour shift with her, and I was so down by the time I left that I knew that I had to limit my time with her. I wouldn't spend more than two hours with her because she really got to me after a while," a psychiatric nurse told us. Or, in another case: "There is a 13-year-old schizophrenic boy that I'm working with now who thinks he's a machine, or a 'mutant.' I like him, but he frustrates me tremendously. Sometimes all I can handle is a 30-minute conversation with him because he's very nongiving. Sometimes I deal with the frustration by separating myself from the patient. I won't spend as much time with him; instead, I'll spend more time with other patients whom we're achieving a little more with."

Related to withdrawal is the technique of "going by the book" rather than unique factors of a situation. It's another way of short-circuiting any personal involvement with a client or patient. By applying a formula, the professional can avoid having to think about the nature of the problems. Also, the emotional stress triggered by taking responsibility for unpopular or painful decisions can be eluded if a worker says, "I'm sorry, but it's not my fault those are the rules around here, and I have to follow them."

For the social welfare workers, one of the major signs of burnout was the transformation of a person with original thought and creativity on the job into a mechanical, petty bureaucrat.

For many of the people whom we observed, social outlets proved to be a more gratifying, if ironic, route to detachment. They solicited advice and comfort from other staff members after withdrawal from a difficult situation. Such social support eased the stress and pain, fostered a sense of distance from the situation and tended to neutralize the emotions. Reported one of the profession, "When we get together, we bitch a lot to each other. We hash things out. We laugh at it sometimes. We talk about it a lot and try new ways. It helps to talk about it, and if you can't see it another way, then somebody else might be able to."

Social support also led to a perception of diffused responsibility among staff members, which helped the individual worker to feel even more remote from troublesome clients. Another social technique was the use of humor. Joking and laughing about a stressful event reduced personal anxiety by making the situation seem less serious, less frightening and less overwhelming. The battlefield surgeons in M*A*S*H*, who made "sick" jokes and flirted with the nurses while they performed grave operations, are a particularly apt example of this technique at work. As one of our respondents put it, "Sometimes things are so awful and so frustrating that in order to keep from crying, you laugh at a situation that may not even be funny. You laugh but you know in your heart what's really happening. Nevertheless, you do it because your own needs are important—we're all human beings, and we have to be ourselves."

Many of these detachment techniques can be used by professionals either to reduce the amount of personal stress or to cope with it successfully while still maintaining concern for the people they must work with. However, because some forms of these techniques preclude any continued caring, we found that they often degenerated into the total detachment and dehumanization of burnout. In these cases, the worker's attempts at emotional self-protection came at the expense of the client, patient, child, prisoner, etc. The professionals donned such thick armor that nobody could get through.

At the moment, we cannot present a total solution to the problem of burnout. However, our work thus far has pointed to a number of factors that could reduce the harm done by burnout or prevent its occurrence altogether.

Burnout often leads to a deterioration of physical well-being. The professional becomes exhausted, is frequently sick and may be beset by insomnia, ulcers and migraine headaches, as well as more serious illnesses. Some of the prison guards reported physical problems with their back and neck, although only a few seemed to realize the psychosomatic nature of these ailments. "On the way home from my first day on the job," says one guard, "I realized that my neck hurt. The muscles were tight, and that caused me to have a headache. Perspiration was heavier than normal. Later on, I realized that my neck and back would begin to get stiff and sore and painful just before I went to the prison—and it would last until I got home again."

In order to cope with these physical problems, the worker may turn to tranquilizers, drugs or alcohol—"solutions" that have the potential for being abused. Better measures include regular vacations (where one can rest completely and "recharge one's batteries") and physical exercise. In a booklet on burnout, put out by the Drug Abuse Council, Dr. Herbert Freudenberger suggests, "Encourage your staff and yourself to exercise physically. If you want to run, do it. Play tennis, dance, swim, bicycle, exhaust yourself on the drums. Engage in any activity that will make you physically tired. Many times the exhaustion of burnout is an emotional and mental one that will not let you sleep."

Burnout often becomes inevitable when the professional is forced to provide care for too many people. As the ratio increases, the result is higher and higher emotional overload until, like a wire that has too much electricity flowing through it, the worker just burns out and emotionally disconnects. The importance of this ratio for understanding burnout is vividly demonstrated in the research on child-care workers that I recently conducted with Ayala Pines. We studied the staff members of eight child-care centers where staff-to-children ratios ranged from 1 to 4 to as high as 1 to 12.

The staff from the high-ratio centers worked a greater number of hours on the floor in direct contact with the children and had fewer opportunities to take a break from work. They were more approving of supplementary techniques to make children quiet, such as compulsory naps and the use of tranquilizers for hyperactive children. They did not feel that they had much control over what they did on the job, and overall they liked their job much less than did the staff from low-ratio centers.

Social welfare workers said that a high ratio of clients to staff was one of the major factors forcing a dehumanized view of clients. "There are just so many, you cannot afford to sympathize with them all," explained a social worker. "If I only had 50 clients, I might be able to help them individually. But with 300 clients in my caseload, I'm lucky if I can see that they all get their checks."

When staff ratios are low, then the individual staff member has fewer people to worry about and can give more attention to each of them. Also, there is more time to focus on the positive, nonproblem aspects of the person's life, rather than concentrating just on his or her problems. For example, in psychiatric wards with low staff-patient ratios, the nurses were more likely to see their patients in both good times and bad. Even though there were upsetting days, there were also times when the nurses could laugh and joke with the patients, play Ping-Pong or cards with them, talk with their families and so on. In a sense, these nurses had a more complete, more human, view of each patient.

Opportunities for withdrawing from a stressful situation are critically important for these professionals. However, the type of withdrawal that is available may spell the difference between burnout and successful coping. The most positive form of withdrawal that we observed is what we have called a "time-out." Time-outs are not merely short breaks from work such as rest periods or coffee breaks. Rather, they are opportunities for the professional to voluntarily choose to do some other, less stressful, work while other staff take over client/patient responsibilities. For example, in one of the psychiatric wards we studied, the nurses knew that if they were having a rough day, they could arrange to do something else besides work directly with patients. "There are times on the ward when I know that I'm not as capable of giving that much of myself, so I'll sit in the office and do a lot of paperwork. The way our schedule is, it gives you the opportunity to do that. You can withdraw and choose to attend meetings for a while. Or you can ask to get assigned to medications, so that you spend the entire day in the medicine room. Then, the only time you see patients is when you're calling on them for medicines." In this system, when one nurse took a time-out, the other nurses would cover for her and continue to provide adequate patient care.

In contrast to sanctioned time-outs were the negative withdrawals of "escapes." Here, the professional's decision to take a break from work always came at the expense of clients or patients, since there were no other staff people to take over. If the professional was not there to provide treatment or service, then people in need simply had to wait, come back another day or give up. The professionals were more likely to feel trapped by their total responsibility for these people; so they couldn't temporarily withdraw without feeling some guilt. When guilt was heaped upon the already heavy emotional burden they tenuously carried, the load often became too much to bear.

The use of sanctioned time-outs versus guilt-arousing escapes seemed to be primarily determined by the structure of the work setting. Time-outs were possible in well-staffed agencies that had shared work responsibilities, flexible work policies and, most importantly, a variety of job tasks for each professional, rather than just a single one. When institutional policies prevented the use of voluntary time-outs, we found lower staff morale, greater emotional stress and the inevitable consequence of more dissatisfied citizens, frustrated at not getting the care they needed.

The number of hours that a person works at a job is very likely to be related to that person's sense of fatigue, boredom, stress, etc. So one might suspect that longer working hours would lead to a higher burnout rate. However, our data reveal a somewhat different pattern of behavior. Longer hours are correlated with more stress and negative staff attitudes only when they involve continuous direct contact with patients or clients. Our study of child-care centers provides a good illustration of this point. Longer working hours were related to signs of burnout when the longer hours involved more work on the floor with children. They were more approving of institutional restraints on the children's behavior, and when they were not at work, they wanted to get as far away as possible from children and child-related activities. Staffers who worked just as many hours but spent a smaller proportion of time in direct contact with children did not develop such negative attitudes toward young people. Instead, they felt positively about them and about the child-care center in general. Perhaps the quality of caring, if not mercy, may have to be time-shared.

In many of the institutions we studied, there was a clear split in job responsibilities—either the professionals worked directly with clients or patients, or they worked in administration. As an example, most of the child-care workers spent all their time on the floor with the children, while the directors only had a few (if any) hours with the children and spent the rest of their time in administrative work and meetings. Burnout was more likely to occur for the workers. Often, they would then escape into administrative work.

We were initially surprised to discover how many social workers were returning to school to get advanced training for this kind of higher level, "nonclient" work (and we found it bitterly ironic that clients should be such outcasts in a profession that would not exist without them). As one social worker said, "We can all point to people who have burned out—who are cold, unsympathetic, callous and detached. And each of us knows that we have the potential to fit that role as well, if we haven't already. And that's why we're going back to school to become administrators or teachers or whatever—so that our client contact will be limited and we won't be forced to become callous in order to stay sane."

Our findings on the effect of prolonged direct contact suggest some job changes that would modify the amount of such direct contact. Possible work alternatives include shorter work shifts, greater opportunities for time-outs, or jobs that involve varied work responsibilities so that an individual staff person is not constantly required to be working directly with other people.

The availability of formal or informal programs in which professionals can get together to discuss problems and get advice and support is another way of helping them to cope with job stress more successfully. Contrary to the beliefs of some skeptics (one physician stated that such a system would only provide the nurses with another opportunity to chitchat rather than work), such support groups serve a very valuable function for their professional members. Burnout rates seem to be lower for those professionals who have access to such a system, especially if they are well-developed and supported by the larger agency.

Some of the psychiatrists reported being part of a social-professional support group when they were doing their residency. They would meet regularly to discuss problems that they were having in treating their patients, to vent frustrations or to report their successes. After leaving the hospital and entering private practice, some of these psychiatrists found that the lack of such a group was a serious, unanticipated loss to them. "I felt cut off, isolated—I didn't feel I had people whom I could turn to when problems arose, and whose opinions I could trust," one therapist told us. Some psychiatrists even made efforts to rejoin the hospital meetings of the residents, although not always successfully.

Since health and social service workers often experience strong emotional reactions, efforts must be made to constructively deal with these feelings and prevent them from being extinguished, as in burnout. We were surprised to find that many of our subjects did not know that other people were experiencing the same feelings they were; each of them thought their personal reaction was unique. And it was easy to keep this illusion, because they rarely shared feelings with colleagues. In many cases, workers felt that something was wrong with them—they were "bad persons" to have such feelings—and several had sought psychiatric help to deal with what they thought was personal failing.

Even though many of these professionals keep their feelings to themselves, it is painfully clear that they have a strong need to talk to someone about them. Throughout our work, we have been struck by the outpouring of emotional responses to our research from health and social service professionals. They are extremely eager to talk with us about the problems of detached concern and burnout. In fact, we often receive calls from other professional people who have heard about our research. For example, while we were collecting information from the staff of the psychiatric ward at a county hospital, several of the nurses from the alcoholism treatment ward contacted us and asked to be interviewed as well. All too often, their reason for volunteering for the research was "I know that I have burned out—but I want to understand why."

Our findings show that burnout rates are lower for those professionals who actively express, analyze and share their personal feelings with their colleagues. Not only do they consciously get things off their chest, but they have an opportunity to receive constructive feedback from other people and to develop new perspectives and understanding of their relationship with their patients/clients. This process is greatly enhanced if the institution sets up some social outlets such as support groups, special staff meetings or workshops. In general, we found that those professionals who are trained to treat psychological problems were better able to recognize and deal with their own feelings.

In contrast, prison guards who experienced great fear were constrained from expressing, or even acknowledging, it by an institutional macho code, one consequence of which was the channeling of this emotion into psychosomatic illnesses. According to one former prison guard, "Male identity is a killing factor within the all-male prison society. Concern of any kind is all too often translated as weakness. All new correctional officers must learn to control their emotions, especially the incredible fear. Each of us reacted to the fear in his own way, but we had no way to release tensions."

It seems clear from the research findings to date that health and social service professionals need to have special training and preparation for working closely with other people. While they are well trained in certain healing and service skills, they are often not well equipped to handle repeated, intense, emotional interactions with people. As one poverty lawyer put it, "I was trained in law, but not in how to work with the people who would be my clients. And it was that difficulty in dealing with people and their personal problems, hour after hour, that became the problem for me, not the legal matters per se."

In recommending that these professionals receive training in interpersonal skills, I do not mean to suggest that somehow these people are antisocial types who are personally unable to relate to other people. Rather, I believe that their occupations require them to operate in situations of unique stress, for which their previous life experiences have not adequately prepared them. Any of us, facing such a stressful set of circumstances, would probably burn out fairly quickly, but we expect these professionals not to do so. Such an expectation, however, is unwarranted unless they have careful training.

Such training should focus on the personal stress involved in the work—what its sources are, what the constructive and ineffective techniques for dealing with it are, what the possible changes in attitude and emotions are (and why they occur). In other words, professionals need to be made aware of the importance and relevance of their psychological state to their work with other people.

In addition, it is important that they understand their own motivations for entering their particular career and recognize the expectations they have for their work. As Freudenberger points out in his booklet, staff members can be on a variety of "trips": a self-fulfilling ego trip; a self-aggrandizement ego trip; a self-sacrificing, dedication-to-others ego trip; or a trip to deny their own personal problems.

Although many of our subjects stated that they wished they had had prior preparation in interpersonal skills, some reported that there was no time for it in their already packed curriculum. Others felt that such preparation was just "icing on the cake" and not an essential part of professional training. The view of several physicians was that the competent practice of medicine was all that they need to know to be successful in their career, and that any psychological training simply amounted to knowing how to make "small talk" with their patients. Such a skill was viewed as pleasant but unimportant. In my opinion, this viewpoint is sadly in error, for it trivializes an essential aspect of the doctor-patient relationship and fails to recognize that both the doctor and the patient are human beings whose personal attitudes and emotions can affect not only the delivery of health care, but also how and even whether it is accepted.

Is burnout inevitable? Some professionals seem to think so and assume that it is only a matter of time before they will burn out and have to change their job. The period of time most often cited in one psychiatric ward was 1½ years, in free clinics it was usually one year and some poverty lawyers spoke of a reduction of the former four-year-stint down to two. I would like to think that burnout is not inevitable and that steps can be taken to reduce and modify its occurrence. My feeling is that many of the causes of burnout are located not in permanent traits of the people involved, but in certain specific social and situational factors that can be influenced in ways suggested by our research.